D1300184

TO HEAL HUMANKIND

The "human right to healthcare" has had a remarkable rise. It is found in numerous international treaties and national constitutions, it is litigated in courtrooms across the globe, it is increasingly the subject of study by scholars across a range of disciplines, and—perhaps most importantly—it serves as an inspiring rallying cry for health justice activists throughout the world. However, though increasingly accepted as a principle, the historical roots of this right remain largely unexplored. *To Heal Humankind: The Right to Health in History* fills that gap, combining a sweeping historical scope and interdisciplinary synthesis. Beginning with the Age of Antiquity and extending to the Age of Trump, it analyzes how healthcare has been conceived and provided as both a right and a commodity over time and space, examining the key historical and political junctures when the right to healthcare was widened or diminished in nations around the globe.

To Heal Humankind will prove indispensable for all those interested in human rights, the history of public health, and the future of healthcare.

Adam Gaffney is a physician, writer, public health researcher, and healthcare advocate. An Instructor in Medicine at Harvard Medical School, he practices pulmonary and critical care medicine at the Cambridge Health Alliance. He is active in the single-payer advocacy organization, *Physicians for a National Health Program*, and lives in Cambridge, Massachusetts.

To Heal Humankind

The Right to
Health in History

Adam Gaffney

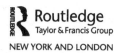

Routledge
Taylor & Francis Group

NEW YORK AND LONDON

First published 2018
by Routledge
711 Third Avenue, New York, NY 10017

and by Routledge
2 Park Square, Milton Park, Abingdon, Oxon, OX14 4RN

Routledge is an imprint of the Taylor & Francis Group, an informa business

© 2018 Taylor & Francis

Library of Congress Cataloging in Publication Data
A catalog record for this book has been requested

ISBN: 978-1-138-06720-2 (hbk)
ISBN: 978-1-138-06722-6 (pbk)
ISBN: 978-1-315-15843-3 (ebk)

Typeset in Minion
by Florence Production Ltd, Stoodleigh, Devon, UK

This book is dedicated to my mother and father,
who taught me how to think, and who encouraged me to act.

Contents

Acknowledgments

This book would have been little more than a pipe dream were it not for the tremendous encouragement and assistance I received from friends, family, colleagues, and mentors. My parents Frederick and Aileen remain steadfast in their support of my life and my work; my mother also helpfully read an early draft. My brother Nicholas has provided crucial support and encouragement, which I especially needed during the sometimes difficult years when this book was written. This book has no doubt been shaped intellectually by countless hours of discussion with my lifelong friend Michael Leonard, who read much of an intermediate-stage draft and provided very useful feedback. Ever since I approached him out of the blue at a conference, Howard Waitzkin has given his time and support selflessly and generously, including reviewing the entire nearly-final manuscript. Without Howard, the book would never have seen the light of day, and the example of his life and work provided much inspiration. Dean Birkenkamp has been thoughtful, encouraging, and unfailingly patient throughout the process of writing, and I owe him a debt of gratitude. My heroes, professors David Himmelstein and Steffie Woolhandler, provided crucial encouragement and opportunities for me in recent years; they also critically reviewed much of an advance draft. My interest in healthcare rights was very much propelled by my work in healthcare advocacy, and for this I am indebted to the example and comradeship of many *Physicians for a National Health Program* (PNHP) activists, including Oli Fein, Gordy Schiff, Mardge Cohen, Martha Livingston, Joanne Landy, and many others. I took two classes with Greg Grandin as an undergraduate, and have been learning from him ever since; Greg continues to support and encourage me, and also kindly read portions of the manuscript. My good friend, the admirable Jon Cohn, took on the task of editing a late version of this manuscript, and I remain in his debt. Even though I contacted both of them essentially out of the blue, historians Caroline Wazer and Calloway Scott generously reviewed parts of Chapter 1, providing very helpful comments. My uncle and scholar Grahame Shane provided insight at a very early stage in this book's conception, and he critically reviewed portions of an early draft. David Pomerico, Jeffrey Shyu, and Joe Duignan also read portions of drafts and provided useful feedback. Barron Lerner provided important guidance. Many others who cannot all be listed here provided inspiration, encouragement, and support over the years during which this book was written.

I should note that this is a work of synthesis and analysis, with a broad scope over both time and space, and as such it mainly relies on secondary sources. I therefore owe an enormous debt to the scholars and writers whose original work I rely on, discuss, and cite throughout. I apologize in advance if I have misconstrued any of the ideas or arguments of others, and more broadly for any errors that may have found their way into this book. Any such errors are mine alone.

Finally, all proceeds from this book will go to *Physicians for a National Health Program*, an organization that I am proud to be a part of, and which is doing much to keep the light of universal healthcare alive in the United States.

Introduction

The "human right to healthcare" has had an astonishing rise. Its history, as it is typically told, begins with the end of the Second World War. In 1946, it received one of its earliest articulations in the constitution of the newly formed World Health Organization: "The enjoyment of the highest attainable standard of health," its oft-quoted preamble boldly proclaims, "is one of the fundamental rights of every human being . . ."[1] Two years later, the United Nations adopted the Universal Declaration of Human Rights, which somewhat less grandly included a right to "medical care" among the socioeconomic goods now considered the natural birthright of all humankind. In the decades since, in some form or another, the right to health (and to healthcare) has found a place in a wide range of international treaties and national constitutions.[2] It has served as a compelling rallying cry for activists struggling for healthcare justice around the world, and in recent days as a more formulaic talking point for politicians seeking health system reform.

But where did this right come from, and what does it mean? Whereas the historical roots of the "human right" have been the subject of much scholarship, the "right to health" (and, more specifically, to healthcare, the predominant concern of this book) has been largely under-historicized.[3] This work is intended as a corrective, providing an early examination and analysis of the historical roots of the right to healthcare. It begins not—as is typical—with the post-Second World War rights declarations, but instead with antiquity, although it extends to the present day. (Its geographical scope is much more confined, with a regrettable emphasis on Europe and the United States, for several reasons.)[4] It aims to trace how ideas about socioeconomic rights—together with ideas and practices around the provision of "universal" healthcare—evolved from this early era to the present day. It seeks not to provide a comprehensive history of the right to healthcare, but instead—through an analysis of critical historical junctures—to begin an exploration of the origins, the meaning, and the relevance of this powerful and egalitarian aspiration for us today. An aspiration, it warrants mentioning, of great and growing potential benefit for billions around the globe.

But first, is there any merit in turning back earlier than the postwar era, when the first major "human rights" documents began to appear, and when the history of the right to healthcare usually begins? In his pathbreaking book *The Last Utopia: Human Rights in History*, scholar Samuel Moyn counters reams of scholarship that pinpoint the roots of human rights in this or that philosophical school or historical period—ranging from antiquity to the Enlightenment—and argues in contrarian fashion that the "human right" did not really emerge in an impactful sense until as recently as the 1970s. An essential feature of modern "human rights," in his line of argument, is that they trump the laws of the nation-state; in contrast, earlier rights (such as the "rights of man" of the Enlightenment) were citizen rights, to be realized through the power of the state, not over or above it. Thus, he contends, while these earlier rights were a form of "rights," they were not "human rights" in the manner understood today, that is, as constraints on governments. The human right was thus a fundamentally new concept, serving a distinct political purpose in a postcolonial age when the promise of an older utopian paradigm— that of democratic socialism—had begun to fade on both sides of the Iron Curtain.[5]

Yet though this argument may be persuasive from the perspective of the modern human rights discourse, it is rather problematic when turning to the specific case of the right to healthcare. The right to healthcare is—inherently—a social right that must be realized at the state level.[6] It is one of the social rights—together with housing and education—that T.H. Marshall, in his post-Second World War classic treatise *Citizenship and Social Class*, argued was remaking the meaning of citizenship in the twentieth century, in a day and age when "human rights" talk was still in its infancy.[7] And indeed, whereas international instruments can be wielded to protect human rights on the supranational level—international tribunals can punish human rights transgressors, international troops can enforce treaties, and so forth—states ultimately create rights to healthcare *through the establishment of health systems*. Health systems that universally provide access to healthcare as a public good—particularly if this access is (largely or entirely) *free* and (to the extent possible) *equitable*—produce universal social rights to healthcare, regardless of whether this is conceived or achieved within a human rights paradigm. The history of the right to healthcare, in other words, is inextricably bound up with the history of healthcare universalism.[8] The "right to healthcare" thus has a history of its own, connected to but also independent from the "human right" considered more broadly.

This book thus traces the story of the "right" (and, later, the socioeconomic right) from its beginnings in the natural law and natural rights tradition of the ancient world, the Middle Ages, and (later) the Enlightenment, through the ages of revolution and of industry, and ultimately to the contemporary era. It interweaves into this history the story of the "universalist-medical ethos," which is to say, instances and movements wherein individuals, groups, or states proposed or endeavored to make medical care universal. This is the story of early medical charity and the advent of the hospital, of the ethics of healthcare and the social duties of the healthcare provider, and of proposals and programs for the implementation of universal healthcare systems. The relationship between these developments and the concept of the socioeconomic right is admittedly complex and contradictory. Ultimately, however, the development of health systems should be seen as central to the idea and practice of treating healthcare as a right, even when ideas about "rights" or "human rights" are far from the ideological or rhetorical core of such systems.

In fact, the temporal link between the *discourse* and the *praxis* of healthcare rights is rather weak. As this book will explore, the creation of some novel universal health systems in the postwar era—like that of the National Health Service (NHS) in Britain—was accomplished without much talk about the "right" to healthcare. Yet the NHS nonetheless created, in a very concrete and meaningful sense, a legal right to healthcare. And ironically, even as the human right to health movement got underway in the 1980s and 1990s, rights to healthcare were, in a practical sense, under assault in many places, a topic that will be explored in the final chapter. For instance, in the developing world, international financial organizations like the World Bank were wielding their considerable political and economic muscle to pressure low-income countries—particularly in Africa—to impose charges ("user fees") on the poor for the use of health services, to the great detriment of the health of these populations—indeed, at the cost of countless lives lost.[9] Meanwhile, nations in both the developing and developed world were taking steps towards health system privatization in ways that sometimes threatened the right to healthcare for their citizens.

Thus, whereas the human right to healthcare is indeed a recent rhetorical convention and ethical notion, ideas and practices around the right to healthcare— that is, around healthcare universalism—stretch back considerably further. Yet a conceptualization of a "right to healthcare" developed over time in tension with the far more typical practice of providing healthcare as a commodity or consumer good. In some moments and places, healthcare was conceived of and provided by right on the basis of needs; more typically, it has been a service sold on the basis of means, like other commodities.

The first aim of this book then is to trace what might be termed a healthcare "rights-commodity dialectic" through history, an approach colored by the idea of welfare "decommodification" of sociologist Gøsta Esping-Andersen. Esping-Andersen proposed a landmark (though highly criticized[10]) typology of the "three worlds" of welfare under capitalism. The emergence of capitalism, he noted, led to an almost complete individual dependence on the "cash nexus" for survival. This was met by qualitatively different welfare responses among various advanced capitalist nations, which he clustered into liberal, conservative, and social-democratic regimes. Under the social-democratic response, welfare benefits undergo what he called "de-commodification," which "occurs when a service is rendered as a matter of right, and when a person can maintain a livelihood without reliance on the market."[11] Healthcare "decommodification" is contextualized in this book in a similar light: it occurs with the creation of a social right to access to healthcare that is *independent of one's market position*,[12] and through which individuals can obtain equitable health care *without being forced to enter the cash nexus*. Thus, to the extent that these two configurations of healthcare—as social right and as commodity—are oppositional and exclusive, it is reasonable to speak of a healthcare right-commodity dialectic.

The second aim of the book is to examine *how* healthcare rights are realized. Where and why rights to healthcare goods were fought for—and achieved—relates little to changing interpretations of rights and more to political struggle and economic change. Though ideas about equality have existed since antiquity, constituencies strong enough to challenge social, economic, and, indeed, healthcare inequalities have usually been too scattered over time and space to challenge the status quo in a meaningful way. Potent proposals for social welfare, including healthcare, most often arose when such constituencies became sufficiently mobilized to at least be perceived as a credible threat: examples in Europe include (among others) the eras of the English Civil War, the French Revolution, the Revolutions of 1848, and the years following the Second World War; in the United States, such periods include the New Deal Era and the Civil Rights era; and in the developing world, as we will see, revolutionary moments during the post-colonial period were most critical (to generalize broadly). The emergence of such political challenges, in turn, can only be understood in the setting of the innovations, disruptions, and profound strains imposed by an economic system that evolved not gradually, but in great fits and starts, whether that be the advent of industrial capitalism in the nineteenth century or of economic crises like the Great Depression in the twentieth.

Similarly, the successes and the failures in the achievement of the human right to healthcare in the twenty-first century—the healthcare right-commodity dialectic today—have to be understood in the context of the latest stage of global economic history, what is often called "neoliberalism." The mobilization of corporate power in the past few decades has often served to substantially favor the commodification of healthcare services throughout the globe, to constrain the vision of universal healthcare in both the developing and developed world, and to restrict the potential of healthcare reform in the United States. Still, the story is by no means all negative: during these very same decades, there have been activist movements and even major political achievements that have helped enhance the right to healthcare, in ways small and large, in countries throughout the world.

The fate of the "right to healthcare"—whether it will rise to a universal reality, remain a privilege for some classes or some nations, or shrink to little more than pleasant but irrelevant rhetoric—will, in the final analysis, depend on the outcome of such struggles.

Notes

1   World Health Organization, *Constitution of the World Health Organization*, 1948, accessed March 8, 2015, www.Who.Int/Governance/Eb/Who_Constitution_En.Pdf.

2   Two key works on the history of the right to health in international law are: John Tobin, *The Right to Health in International Law* (Oxford: Oxford University Press, 2012) and Brigit C.A. Toebes, *The Right to Health as a Human Right in International Law* (Antwerpen: Intersentia/Hart, 1999).

3   An early chapter in Tobin's volume is an exception to this. Tobin's chapter is notable in beginning before the Second World War era, and in drawing connections between ideas of public health and of human rights. Tarantola, in contrast, provides a cursory look at the right

to health which begins in the post-Second World War era. Tobin, *The Right to Health in International Law*, 14–43; Daniel Tarantola, "A Perspective on the History of Health and Human Rights: From the Cold War to the Gold War," *Journal of Public Health Policy* 29, no. 1 (2008): 42–53.

4   Although the first chapter and the last two chapters have a global scope, the other chapters concern events only in Europe and the US. This regrettable Western-centrism reflects the necessity of making choices as well as the limitations of the author. In particular, the complete exclusion of indigenous healing traditions, whether in America or Africa, is a significant deficiency. Additionally, it is worth mentioning that this is a short book about a large issue, and is by no means intended to be complete or authoritative. It is instead a synthesis and an analysis of selected moments in selected places, with the aim of beginning a discussion about the rise and emergence of the human right to healthcare in history. Although I turn to some of the most important documents, I mainly rely on a large number of scholars and writers, whose work I discuss and cite throughout. Finally, the overall approach of this book can reasonably be critiqued as idiosyncratic, and others might reasonably trace the right to health in very different ways, with either a narrower scope (e.g. focusing on the modern *human* right to health movement) or a broader one (e.g. looking at the practice of healthcare in cultures throughout the globe).

5   Samuel Moyn, *The Last Utopia: Human Rights in History* (Cambridge, MA: Belknap Press of Harvard University Press, 2010).

6   Farmer notes that NGOs working in low-income nations must "learn how to strengthen the public sector, since only governments can guarantee their citizens' rights." Paul Farmer, "Challenging Orthodoxies: The Road Ahead for Health and Human Rights," *Health and Human Rights* 10, no. 1 (2008): 10.

7   T. H. Marshall, "Citizenship and Social Class," in *Citizenship and Social Class* (London: Pluto Press, 1992).

8   Hoffman's outstanding book, which I cite many times in this book, similarly deals with the evolution of healthcare "rights" outside of the narrow spectrum of the human rights discourse/paradigm. Beatrix Rebecca Hoffman, *Health Care for Some: Rights and Rationing in the United States since 1930* (Chicago: University of Chicago Press, 2012).

9   Rick Rowden, "The Ghosts of User Fees Past: Exploring Accountability for Victims of a 30-Year Economic Policy Mistake," *Health and Human Rights* 15, no. 1 (2013): 175–85.

10   Bambra puts the criticisms of Esping-Andersen's work in three categories: theoretical, methodological, and empirical. Clare Bambra, "Going Beyond the Three Worlds of Welfare Capitalism: Regime Theory and Public Health Research," *Journal of Epidemiology and Community Health* 61, no. 12: 1098–102.

11   Gøsta Esping-Andersen, *The Three Worlds of Welfare Capitalism* (Princeton, N.J.: Princeton University Press, 1990), 21–2.

12   Bambra employs a very similar definition. Clare Bambra, "Cash Versus Services: 'Worlds of Welfare' and the Decommodification of Cash Benefits and Health Care Services," *Journal of Social Policy* 34, no. 02 (2005): 201.

1
Health, Rights, and Welfare
Antiquity to the Early Modern Era

"If we believe," Aristotle is quoted as saying, "men have any personal rights at all as human beings, they have an absolute right to such a measure of good health as society, and society alone is able to give them."[1] Such a statement implies that not only human rights—but also the *human right to health*—can be traced back to the fourth century BCE. It suggests an impressive continuity of the human right to health throughout history, and might be thought of as providing an ancient philosophical grounding for the work of health rights activists today.

Alas—perhaps not surprisingly—these are not Aristotle's words. A scholar who investigated this oft-cited quotation's origins was unable to find any semblance of it in Aristotle's corpus.[2] Its first known use was apparently in a speech given by Robert F. Kennedy (and from where he got it is unclear), and it subsequently appeared in print in a 1979 book dealing with the right to health.[3] It then made its way forward to the present, periodically appearing in articles and books. Its continued life speaks to an understandable desire to legitimize an idea by imbuing it with the authority and prestige of the past. But it also shows that the temptation to perceive a chain of historical continuity for an idea—especially an idea one believes in or struggles for—is strong.

Although recognizing the real perils of this temptation, this chapter nonetheless begins in antiquity. The point in turning to the distant past is not to "find" some predecessor to modern ideas about socioeconomic rights to goods like healthcare, but instead to trace the twists and turns of how healthcare was produced, provided, and perceived along a rights-commodity divide. This is not so much the history of the right to health, as its prehistory. But it is a rich and complex prehistory. Although an explicit conceptualization of a "right to health" did not emerge until the twentieth century, ideas about "natural rights" evolved over the centuries, and (arguably) came to include one *socioeconomic* right of the poor by the High Middle Ages. Additionally, a discourse and a practice around the notion of providing healthcare to the excluded and marginalized—a "universalist-medical ethos"— emerged in parallel to these philosophical developments. Indeed, by the early modern period, some writers even explicitly called for the state provision of healthcare to the poor. Though no doubt quite removed from the explicit declaration of social and economic rights of the post-Second World War era, these developments are crucial early moments in the larger story of the right to healthcare. They are the ambiguous and contradictory beginnings of a long story of what seems to be a diffusely identifiable human impulse: the delivery of healthcare to every individual regardless of economic means.

Rights and Welfare in the Ancient World

When do human rights begin? The debate, no doubt, is a thorny one, and depends upon whether we are thinking of human rights as a philosophical idea, a basic moral concept, or a particular pair of words in the English language. Some, for instance, assert that in the Western tradition, a common thread connects modern ideas of human rights to earlier concepts stretching back to the ancient world. Before the era of "human rights," there was the "rights of man" discourse of the Enlightenment. And before that, there was a discourse around "natural rights" and "natural law" during the Middle Ages and antiquity. Legal scholar Hersch Lauterpacht argued that this long intellectual heritage provided crucial stimulation for the struggle for international human rights of the mid-twentieth century,[4] and the philosopher Ernest Cassirer argued that the "rights of man" of the Enlightenment had its intellectual roots in the natural law theory that emerged in early modern Europe.[5]

Yet the "natural law" of antiquity (or, for that matter, of the early modern period) was starkly different from modern-day "human rights."[6] As the classicist Moses Finley has noted with some justification, the ancient Greeks and Romans not only lacked, but "would have been appalled by," our notion of rights.[7] In Plato's *Gorgias*, for instance, the sophist Callicles uses "natural law" (possibly the earliest known use of the term) to mean that, in nature, the mighty deservedly dominate the meek.[8] Moreover, Plato and Aristotle do not seem to be particularly concerned with "rights," whether political or socioeconomic or otherwise. The meaning of the Greek words doesn't quite match up, it has been noted, while an emphasis on individual human liberty, often regarded as a necessary precursor to moral rights, was not recognized.[9] For example, although Plato's Socrates disagrees with Thrasymachus's "might makes right" argument in the *Republic*, he does so by finding true justice in a rigidly stratified, dystopic republic.[10]

Some scholars have contended, however, that Aristotle's idea of justice in his *Politics* "entails a theory of rights" (though lacking a single equivalent word or phrase to describe them), and that these "nascent rights"—mainly political rights owed *only* to the citizens of the city-state—amounted to the "historical seed" from which natural rights would later emerge.[11] Others, in contrast, have seen no substantial role for rights in the overall political theory of Aristotle.[12] And while they note that Aristotle did discuss the idea of "natural law" in such works as the *Rhetoric* and *Nicomachean Ethics*,[13] what he meant by this concept seems to have little to nothing in common with modern human rights. For instance, not only did he not articulate a right to health, but he also strenuously emphasized the essential and *natural inequality* of the human race.[14] And while Plato proposed common property for some as part of his utopic political vision, neither he nor

Aristotle argued that human beings inherently deserved—or had a right to—any particular social or economic goods, much less healthcare.[15]

Yet before dismissing the legacy of antiquity entirely, it is important to briefly note that others did propose universalist ethical ideas and—to some extent—an *equality* (of sorts) among human beings under the Law of Nature. This more egalitarian conceptualization of natural law emerged from the works of some of the sophists, Greek philosophers of the fifth and fourth centuries BCE.[16] The sophists counterpoised *physis* (nature) with *nomos* (norms or conventions), seeing various merits in each.[17] While, for some sophists (like Callicles) an emphasis on the superiority of *physis* over *nomos* might simply mean a doctrine of "might makes right," for others it was used to emphasize natural human equality over unjust human conventions.[18] Remarkably, it also seems that sophists were among the earliest in history to argue that slavery itself was inherently unnatural—or against *physis*—and therefore unjust.[19] Some sophists also stressed that Greeks and foreigners were fundamentally the same;[20] that "everyone shares a sense of justice and civic virtue";[21] that nobility of birth was "something altogether empty";[22] and that there should be "equality of education as well as equality of property."[23]

It was during the Hellenistic Era that the doctrine of natural law (the *ius naturale* in Latin) was articulated and analyzed by philosophers of the Stoic school. The "immutable law" proposed by the Stoics, Lauterpacht wrote, knew of "no distinction between rich and poor, of Greek and barbarians."[24] Against Aristotle, for example, Cicero contended that there is "no essential difference within mankind," and that "we are all constrained by one and the same law of nature."[25] However, Cicero's (and other Stoics') ideal of natural law still overall had little in common with modern human rights ideas: in the humanitarian realm, Cicero was fairly accepting of gladiatorial slaughter or atrocities in war, while from a social and economic perspective, he condemned economic redistribution and land reform.[26] Nonetheless, the ambiguous, conflicted Stoic formulation of the natural law—which declared men free in theory even while it condoned slavery in practice—was built into the foundation of Roman law during Justinian's reign in the Byzantine Empire, through which it had an enormous impact on the Western intellectual tradition to the present day.[27]

But putting aside for the moment the question of the impact of the *ius naturale* on human rights theory, one might also ask whether these philosophical ideas played any role in efforts to make for a more just or fair society, to deliver socioeconomic goods—if not healthcare *per se*—to the poor. Seneca—whose Stoicism was of a more egalitarian bent than that of Cicero[28]—argued that men should show mercy to others, such as by providing aid to the unfortunate, "as one human being to another"—not out of pity, but in order to extend "assistance and benefit," especially to disadvantaged groups like the elderly, the poor, and the disabled.[29] From a political perspective, there is also some limited and controversial evidence that some of the egalitarian ideas of philosophies like Stoicism may have contributed to efforts for social and economic change. The Stoic-taught tribune Tiberius Gracchus, for instance, famously moved to redistribute land downward in the era of the Roman Republic; this could be interpreted as a "measure of public philanthropy," one historian has noted, but at the same time was also meant to "eliminate the need for private charity or public aid . . ."[30] Some (but not others) have asserted that a Stoic influence might have underlain the Spartan Revolution of the third century BCE in Greece, in which two Spartan kings, during a period of rising economic inequality, sought to eliminate debts and redistribute some land.[31] And (possibly) amidst the regional unrest unleashed by this revolution, some have also seen an egalitarian thrust in the words of the Cynic poet and politician Cercidas, who denounced inequality and called for the redistribution of wealth, and possibly for efforts to help the sick.[32] Still, it seems to be a stretch to construct from such fragments some sort of Stoic social welfare ethos. Indeed, many Stoics—Cicero and Seneca included—moved into (and out of) circles of great power and wealth, perhaps because—as one historian notes—their "natural law concepts easily justified the established order."[33]

What can we say about the idea of welfare for the poor or sick in antiquity more broadly? According to some scholars, the idea of a social imperative to help the poor, sick, and unfortunate was largely nonexistent in this era.[34] Finley, for instance, argued that the concept behind the phrase "[b]lessed are the poor" was not to be found in Greco-Roman values: "The very poor," he wrote, "aroused little sympathy and no pity throughout antiquity."[35] Indeed, assisting the poor might simply reinforce their innate slothfulness (an idea that would have a long shelf-life): as the Roman dramatist Plautus put it, "To give to a beggar is to do him an ill service."[36] At the same time, the Greeks did have a complex and evolving notion of *philanthropia* (the origin of the English word "philanthropy"); the word means "love of mankind," though it had something of a paternalistic or hierarchical connotation for the Greeks.[37] It was first used to describe Prometheus's gift of fire to humankind, and more generally could mean the gods' love for humanity.[38] By the fourth century, the word was employed as a "curb on brutality," possibly under the strain of prolonged and vicious war.[39] But it seems its meaning slowly transformed over the years. With the emergence of Stoicism, for instance, it gained a more egalitarian connotation, suggesting a general benevolence towards all.[40] For Diogenes Laertius, it meant a number of things, including hospitality or charity to those in need.[41] It was also invoked in texts on medical practice that were drawn on by physician-writers like Galen. However, as one historian notes, the hospitality implied by *philanthropia* was essentially a privatized endeavor, and within such "ideological boundaries, there was initially no public duty toward the sick in ancient Greece. Illness remained a private concern."[42]

Public welfare under the Greeks, was thus, in other words, limited—albeit perhaps with some exceptions, such as payments to the disabled poor in Athens.[43] With respect to healthcare, if one needed the services of a physician, generally speaking, she had to pay for it. In later centuries—whether in Western Europe, the Byzantine Empire, or the Islamic world—the sick poor could have recourse to the charitable hospital. However, despite the existence of Roman *valetudinaria*, or specialized hospitals for slaves and soldiers, there was no real equivalent of the charitable hospital in antiquity, no explicit centers of medical care for the poor.[44]

Medical care was, by and large, treated as a commodity like other goods and services.

Yet if there was no right—legal or moral or otherwise—for the poor to healthcare in antiquity, the reality was in fact more complex. In the ancient world, two "health services" are sometimes cited by scholars as potential sources of care for the poor: the temples of Asclepius, the god of medicine, and a diffuse and heterogeneous group of "public physicians" who, some have posited, treated the poor for free as a public service. Additionally, some Greek and Roman physicians advocated, at times, the provision of medical treatment outside the cash nexus. To some extent, in other words, there may have been some limited tension within the healthcare rights-commodity dialectic, even in this early era.

Ancient Healthcare: From the Temples of Asclepius to a Greek "State Health Service"

For those unable to afford the fees of physicians (or maybe for those turned away by them), the Temples of Asclepius may have functioned as a source of healthcare for centuries. Asclepius is best known as the Greco-Roman god of medicine, and he first appears in Homer's *Iliad* as a great and mortal physician. Hesiod describes him as the son of Apollo, sent to Hades for having committed the sin of resurrecting a patient from the dead. He was later deified, becoming the god of medicine and the father of a line of physicians, and a (confused) version of his snake-wrapped staff much later became a modern symbol of the medical profession in the United States. The god-physician Asclepius rapidly achieved enormous fame in antiquity: his cult and his temples spread throughout the Mediterranean world, from Greece to Asia Minor to Rome. For about a thousand years, people would come to these temples—sometimes traveling from afar—in the hope of finding a cure for their ailments. Once they arrived, they would pass the night inside the temple. Asclepius would then (it was said) visit them in their dreams and perform some medical feat—whether performing surgery or just providing instructions—that would hopefully leave them cured.[45]

No doubt visitors came to the temples of Asclepius for a variety of reasons. However, one major reason for Asclepius's popularity—offered by Emma Edelstein and Ludwig Edelstein in their influential book on the cult—was that he served as a provider of healthcare for that large swath of the ancient world who could not afford the fees of physicians. The temple of Asclepius provided care, they argued, to both rich and poor sufferers alike. "[I]t was one of his claims to fame and admiration that he took care of the poor . . ." they describe, noting that he was thought of as the "god of the destitute."[46] Medical historian Henry Sigerist concurred with their judgment, noting that whereas physicians were in the *business* of providing healthcare and thus not required to treat the poor, the "indigent sick man could always seeks the god's [Asclepius's] help."[47] Some scholars have also pointed to the hostels adjacent to the temples, where sufferers could go while waiting to be cured. These buildings were open to both the rich and the poor, and so in some sense prefigured the Christian charitable hospital.[48] Was Asclepius's medicine, then, a sort of pre-commodified form of healthcare for the ancient world? Can we construe tension along a rights-commodity dialectic even at this early stage—between the Greek physician on the one hand, and the temples of Asclepius on the other?

Perhaps not. Before concluding that this cult represented some sort of incipient system of universal healthcare, it is important to note that the temples may not have been purely egalitarian ventures. For instance, what exactly did the temple priests want from the patients who sought Asclepius's help? While some scholars emphasize that the temple required only small gifts, thanks, or sacrifices, it may be the case that such "gifts" (or even cold cash) were not only appreciated, but required.[49] New scholarship has cast doubt on the theory that Asclepius represented a form of charitable or even less costly healthcare: those hoping to be cured, it has been argued, first had to pay the priests a negotiated sum.[50] Moreover, Greeks of the fifth century BCE may not have gone to the temples for inexpensive or free care, but for another reason altogether: to be treated for conditions that physicians would typically refuse to treat, namely chronic or incurable diseases.[51] This was no doubt an important service, and in any event it is easy to imagine that patients sought cures from Asclepius for a variety of reasons, sometimes economic. Additionally, it is worth noting that these shrines may also have functioned as a stage for the display of wealth and prestige by elites, who would sometimes pay for elaborate dedications at them[52] (perhaps roughly analogous to elite donations to large medical centers in the present day, in exchange for their names plastered on the hospital or medical schools). Still, Asclepius remained greatly popular as a source of care for a broad swath of the population into late antiquity—indeed into the sixth century CE—when paganism was finally suppressed, and the god of medicine brought to heel.[53]

If Asclepius did not then primarily serve as a source of healthcare for the poor, what can be said of the established healers of the Hippocratic tradition? Hippocrates himself is an obscure figure, purported to have descended from Asclepius, and it is unknown if any of the works typically credited to him were indeed authored by him.[54] That said, it is worth asking what the Hippocratic corpus had to say about the delivery of healthcare to the poor. The famous Hippocratic oath contains various ethical commandments, yet it says nothing about distributive healthcare justice. However, the profit-oriented approach of established healers was sometimes criticized *even in antiquity*. In a long rant against the (predominantly Greek) medical profession, for instance, Pliny the Elder wrote of physicians' "avarice, their greedy bargains made with those whose fate lies in the balance, the prices charged for anodynes, the earnest-money paid for death, or their mysterious instructions . . ." The profession was condemned by his forefathers, he wrote, "chiefly because they refused to pay fees to profiteers in order to save their lives."[55]

In fairness, however, in one Hippocratic work—the *Precepts*—the problem of physician fees—and of providing healthcare to those of limited means—received a far more nuanced discussion.[56] The Hippocratic *Precepts* offers a somewhat more egalitarian approach, especially as compared with that of the contemporaneous Empiricists, who spoke more frankly about moneymaking as the main pursuit of a physician.[57] For example, the *Precepts* warns that a physician "must not be anxious about fixing a fee," as "such a worry" might "be harmful to a troubled patient . . ." Here, however, the writer is not so much urging the reader to humanitarian feats as he is suggesting that an emphasis on payment will not be good for the psychological health, and therefore medical outcome, of the patient. However, the text continues, "the quickness of the disease, offering no opportunity for turning back, spurs on the good physician not to seek his profit but rather to lay hold on reputation . . . it is better to reproach a patient you have saved than to extort money from those who are at death's door." The emphasis here is still more on the importance of the physician's honor over his or her wallet, than it is on any incipient conceptualization of the patient's "right" to be treated. Still, the treatise goes a bit further, perhaps even suggesting that there is an *imperative* to treat those who are unable to afford care: the author asks the reader "not to be too unkind, but to consider carefully your patient's superabundance or means." Indeed, it exhorts, "Sometimes *give your services for nothing*, calling to mind a previous benefaction or present satisfaction" (emphasis added), and "if there be an opportunity of serving one who is a stranger in financial straits, give full assistance to all such."[58]

Moreover, in the Roman era, maybe under the influence of Stoicism, some medical writers exhibited a perhaps even greater egalitarian concern, with *philanthropia* placed closer to the center of a doctor's duties. Galen of Pergamum, for example, the most prominent physician not only of Rome but of the entire pre-Renaissance Western medical tradition, emphasized the importance of *philanthropia* in medicine: he claimed that he cared for the poor and that indeed, he did not even take payment from his patients. He also recounted a story about Hippocrates—whom he held in the highest regard—in which the father of medicine allegedly turned down a position from a Persian ruler so that he could continue to care for the Greek poor.[59] It has also been said that Galen "prided himself on treating senators and slaves with the same scrupulousness."[60]

The Roman physician Scribonius Largus, who lived in the first century CE and was also influenced by Roman Stoicism, likewise articulated a more egalitarian mission for medicine.[61] In one text, he emphasizes the ideas of *humanitas* (or "humane feeling and kindness") and *misericordia* ("compassion").[62] Although in part he was simply advocating the use of drug therapy (then a matter of controversy), he conceptualizes the practice of medicine as "an enterprise of compassion" that is "based in an evolution of Greek *philanthropia*," in which "the physician will serve beyond self-interest."[63] Notably, Largus contends in this text that medicine "does not measure a man's worth according to his wealth or character, but *freely offers its help to all who seek it*, and never threatens to harm anyone" (emphasis added).[64] For Largus, one scholar argues, *philanthropia* was "an essential feature of the true physician."[65]

Care for the poor of antiquity was also provided by the system of "public physicians," which some historians have described as a precursor to universal healthcare. These municipal physicians became a topic of historical conversation in the eighteenth century, and by the nineteenth century, French historians were positing the existence of a network of Greek and/or Roman public physicians that together constituted something of a system of free public medical care.[66] The earliest mention of a public physician comes from a Greek historian who describes some "former lawgivers who had required that private citizens when ill should enjoy the services of physicians at state expense."[67] A public physician was later alluded to in a passage in Aristophanes in which a peasant requests medical care, and is instructed to instead seek out the public physician.[68] Centuries later, a scholiast annotated the text, and defined the word used for public physician as "the physicians appointed by the state being public officers . . . accustomed to attend upon the sick without fee."[69] More evidence emerges during the Hellenistic era, when a large number of inscriptions were made praising public physicians for various "distinguished services."[70] Some interesting bits of evidence come from these inscriptions, which date back to the fourth century BCE.[71] One doctor, for example, was rather remarkably praised for having "treated all equally, poor and rich alike, slave and free."[72] Similarly, another doctor was honored for having ". . . saved many of the townsfolk . . . when they were in a critical condition, accepting no fee . . ."[73] Drawing on this sort of evidence, the classicist A.G. Woodhead somewhat breathlessly concluded in 1952 that a "state health service is not as new an institution as is generally supposed," that it "existed in the ancient world in Greek lands" and in fact constituted the "most comprehensive and widespread State Health Service that the world has yet seen," providing care regardless of the means or the liberty of the patient.[74]

But did, as the historian Louis Cohn-Haft later asked, the ancient Greeks really have a system of socialized medicine?[75] His answer is a clear *no*.[76] There is little question that municipal physicians existed; what is unclear, however, is whether they actually were *required* to provide free care to the poor, and also what this role meant in different periods and regions.[77] Cohn-Haft argued that the inscriptions which form most of the evidence about this supposed national health service demonstrate that *not* accepting fees was considered exceptional—something deserving of praise. Why, he asks, would public physicians be celebrated for merely doing their job?[78] Cities may have simply hired such a doctor in order to ensure that they had at least one resident physician.[79] Perhaps all that can be concluded, therefore, was that there *was* a system of public physicians, and that these physicians took on a variety of roles (which differed over time and by location), some of whom were praised for caring for all—including poor or slaves—for free.[80] In sum, just as Aristotle cannot be said to have proclaimed a right to healthcare, the ancient Greeks cannot be said to have created socialized medicine.

Considered together, the ideas and practices cited in this section thus amount to mere fragments of a more egalitarian healthcare ethos: by and large, there seems to have been only some weak strain in the health rights-commodity dialectic of this era, with medical care still mainly a good to be purchased by those who could afford it, who were generally people of means.

India and China: Hospitals and the Ethics of Egalitarianism

Similar fragments can be found outside the West. In South Asia, a number of scholars have identified charitable medical facilities, sometimes described as hospitals, as far back as ancient times. Such institutions, which might be described as instances of an early "universalist-medical ethos," seem to have been inspired in part by Buddhism, perhaps not surprising given the religion's founding tenets and myths. As one scholar puts it, "Buddha's interest in medicine formed part of his compassion for living beings and for the sick."[81] Buddha himself was said to have proclaimed, "Whoever, O monks, would nurse me, he should nurse the sick."[82] Buddhism may have also influenced the creation of some of the earliest known "hospitals," perhaps as far back as the fourth century BCE.[83]

Scholars have also noted a public role in the provision of medical welfare in ancient India. Though treatment at home was more typical, the state would provide for the lodging and care of those who didn't have access to assistance from others, in particular during the reign of King Asoka.[84] In the aftermath of a horrific war, Asoka purportedly felt great repentance, relinquishing militarism and turning to non-violence and "Dharma."[85] According to the messages he had written on rocks throughout the empire, he also appears to have embraced religious tolerance and to have taken on some interesting social welfare projects.[86] For instance, he set up an office of "Dharma officials," according to one edict, who were to provide help to (among others) "the poor and the aged, to secure the welfare and happiness and release from imprisonment of those devoted to Dharma."[87] With respect to healthcare, he claimed in one of his edicts that in many territories, "everywhere provision has been made for two kinds of medical treatment, treatment for men and for animals."[88] Additionally, "[m]edicinal herbs, suitable for men and animals, have been imported and planted wherever they were not previously available."[89] The institutions set up during this period and later have been described as "either regular hospitals for the poor and the needy or poorhouses equipped with medicines," as well as dispensaries having a "charitable character."[90] Their charitable purpose can be gleaned from a contemporary description by a traveling Chinese Buddhist by the name of Fa-Hien (CE 405–411).[91] Fa-Hien wrote how the town's nobility established:

> [H]ouses for dispensing charity and medicines. All the poor and destitute in the country, orphans, widowers, and childless men, maimed people and cripples, and all who are diseased, go to those houses, and are provided with every kind of help, and doctors examine their diseases. They get the food and medicines which their cases require, and are made to feel at ease . . .[92]

Ancient China saw some similar developments, including the construction of hospital-like institutions with what seems to have been an explicitly charitable function. During the same century in which Fa-Hien traveled to India, the first permanent hospital-like institutions in his home country were established. Although the first institution was built by a Buddhist prince in the fifth century

CE, a state hospital that focused on the care of those who were indigent and suffering from debilitating diseases was constructed some two decades later. As Joseph Needham puts it, this hospital "had a distinctly charitable purpose, being intended primarily for poor or destitute people suffering disabling diseases . . ." Subsequent centuries saw a contest of sorts for control over these institutions between Buddhists and the government, with hospitals previously under the control of monasteries progressively taken over by the state. By the Sung dynasty, Needham describes "a wide variety of State institutions at work," including hospitals for the elderly and the poor and also for foreigners, together with orphanages, government pharmacies, and ambulatory clinics.[93]

In addition, egalitarian ideas about what we might call "healthcare equality" can be found in Chinese texts dealing with medical ethics, and the historian Paul Unschuld's translation and compilation of unabridged, annotated excerpts of these texts makes for fascinating reading in this regard.[94] The earliest Chinese author he discusses is Sun Szu-miao (c. 581?–682 CE), a physician whose work reflects both Taoist and Buddhist ideas.[95] (The influence of Buddism on medicine in China might potentially be thought of as analogous to the role played by Christianity in the West, discussed in the next section.) His text emphasizes that "Great Physicians" must develop a sensibility of sympathy and compassion (a point made in several other texts).[96] He further articulates the doctrine that the Great Physician must treat all patients—regardless of wealth or status—equally:

> If someone should seek help because of illness or on the ground of another difficulty, [a Great Physician] should not pay attention to status, wealth or age, neither should he question whether the particular person is attractive or unattractive, whether he is an enemy or a friend, whether he is Chinese or a foreigner, or finally, whether he is uneducated or educated. He should meet everyone on equal ground; he should always act as if he were thinking of himself.[97]

Other writers cited by Unshculd explicitly emphasized Buddhist medical notions, the importance of compassion, the idea that physicians should not be motivated by pecuniary gain, and the principle that rich and poor patients deserve equal healthcare. Some of these writers lived beyond the chronological confines of this chapter, but are worth citing insofar as they speak to this intellectual tradition. For instance, the Confucian Chu Hui-ming (c. CE 1590) noted that "there is no difference between the poor and the rich, once they have reached the crossroads between life and death"; physicians should not seek enrichment, he argued, but rather aim to "direct their full attention to those who remain dependent [on others] and should render their greatest compassion to those who have no one else to whom they could turn."[98] Similarly, Kung Hsin, a Confucian physician alive in the early seventeenth century, wrote that "[a] patient's wealth or poverty is of no concern" to the enlightened physician, who "prescribe[s] drugs according to a formula which is valid for everyone."[99] Hsü Yen-tso (fl. CE 1895) harkened back to the Buddhist tradition by noting that "In the Buddhist classics we read:

'The whole world is equal.' Physicians should be guided by this opinion." He went further by recognizing the double damage that disease inflicted on the indigent: not only must they suffer from the disease itself, but their already tenuous livelihood would be threatened by their incapacity.[100] Doctors who only helped those who were wealthy were, he argued, of no real help to humankind.[101]

In sum, drawing on a variety of traditions—including Buddhism, Taoism, and Confucianism—Chinese medical writers in some instances seem to have put forth an egalitarian and decommodified philosophy of healthcare in which all patients, regardless of economic or social status, deserved *equal* medical treatment. "In antiquity," noted Chu Hui-ming, "it was said: 'there are no two kinds of drugs for the lofty and the common; the poor and the rich receive the same medicine.'"[102] These words well summarize this notion that medical needs are universal, and should not depend on means.[103] Such a sentiment contrasts with the typical reality of healthcare today, with two-tiered or multi-tiered health systems entrenched in most nations throughout the globe, including the United States.

However, what emerges from the various institutions and ideas explored in this section—from Chinese and Indian "hospitals" to the egalitarian ideas found in Chinese medical texts—is something of a universalist-medical ethos: premodern attempts or endorsements of a public obligation to provide—if not a right to receive—healthcare to all. A somewhat similar ethos was also beginning to emerge, around the same time, in the West.

Christianity, the Hospital, and the "Charitable Imperative" to Healthcare

The medieval era represented a major break from a classical tradition in which sickness and poverty were viewed as a mark of shame. As one historian describes, as opposed to the ancient world, ". . . Christianity displayed a marked philanthropic imperative that manifested itself in both personal and corporate concern for those in physical need."[104] Now, on the one hand, the advent of new forms of charitable medical care should clearly not be seen as tantamount to any sort of right to healthcare. Christian medical charity represented a private initiative to provide some care to some of the sick poor, delivered in a hierarchical framework. On the other hand, the advent of charitable healthcare for the poor represents an important shift within the health rights-commodity dialectic: if not creating a right to healthcare for the poor, it nonetheless provided a decommodified form of healthcare, together with something of a moral and societal obligation to provide it.

What were the origins of this novel orientation towards poverty and charity? Some scholars stress the legacy of antiquity, arguing that the early Christians inherited the classical notion of *philanthropia* but expanded it into a more egalitarian and universalistic ethos.[105] Others underscore the humanitarian strain within Judaism, noting the humanizing influence of the Judaic notion of the *imago Dei*, the concept that God made humanity in his own image.[106] An interest in the welfare of the poor and an emphasis on charity is part of the Hebrew tradition, and in conjunction with the Christian concept of universal *agape*, or love, may have contributed to the Christian charitable impulse.[107] Some also stress the specifically *medical* overtones of the new religion. The parable of the Good Samaritan, for instance, emphasizes the importance of providing care for the unfortunate, not only for those within one's faith or group but also for those outside it.[108] Some early Christian theologians also articulate the image of Jesus as doctor. Early in the second century CE, Bishop Ignatius opined that "[t]here is only one physician, first subject to suffering and then beyond it, Jesus Chris our Lord."[109] Origen promoted the concept of Jesus as "the Great Physician" in the third century CE.[110] He wrote that Jesus had followed the "method of a philanthropic physician who seeks the sick so that he may bring relief to them and strengthen them," connecting (as did Galen and the Hippocratic writer of the *Precepts*) medicine and *philanthropia*.[111] Jesus was also a healer in a more literal sense: there are forty-one separate instances in the New Testament gospels of Jesus's performing an exorcism or an act of healing.[112]

Finally, the Christian era saw a new—and more positive—conceptualization of poverty and sickness, and a shift away from the classical disgust of both. "The poor will always be with you," Jesus famously said to his followers.[113] A new concept, not reflected in ancient notions of *philanthropia*, emerged: *philoptôchos*, or "lover of the poor."[114] Similarly, there was a transformation in the social meaning of sickness: infirmity was now not necessarily considered—as it sometimes was in classical times—something shameful or sinful.[115] In contrast, for Christians, sickness was imbued with a spiritual significance, and the sufferer was thought to deserve compassionate care.[116]

This theological emphasis was accompanied by the early emergence of institutional medical charity. In his *Apologeticus*, Tertullian notes that bishops were to provide "to the invalid commiseration; to the strangers a shelter, to the hungry food; to the thirsty drink; to the naked clothing, to the sick visitation, to the prisoners assistance."[117] Early local church parishes had some social welfare duties, with church deacons entrusted with the task of providing alms to the needy.[118] The organization created by the early Church was, historians have pointed out, the first in classical antiquity that "effectively and systematically cared for its sick."[119] The Church also played an important and novel role in the provision of charitable care—to both pagans and Christians—during the horrific Plague of Cyprian in 250 CE.[120] Some have contended that Christianity's emphasis on healing and charitable care may have contributed to the growth of the religion.[121]

However, while poor relief and charity were delivered on several levels, it is the hospital that best typifies medieval medical charity. In an age of greatly limited therapeutics, the sick could nonetheless benefit through the provision of *care*, in the form of shelter, food, and nursing. This was something early societies could deliver, however lacking their knowledge of human biology and therapeutics, and it was a type of care that was largely not available to the poor in pre-Christian Europe. Today, anyone who has so much as received—much less been bankrupted by—a hospital bill might find the concept of a hospital as a purely charitable endeavor rather quaint. Certainly, over the course of the twentieth century, hospital care increasingly became a commodified good. Yet hospital care initially arose as a non-commodified charitable service. "Charitable care" is even sometimes included as one of the features that *defines* the hospital.[122] As historian Michael Mollat points out, "Until quite recently the poor were almost the only clients of hospitals, places in which they felt truly at home."[123]

Hospitals first arose in the Byzantine world. This is perhaps not surprising, given the strong Byzantine emphasis on social welfare that drew on an egalitarian conceptualization of *philanthropia*.[124] Institutions called "poorhouses"—places for the sick and the poor to reside—appeared early in the fourth century CE in the Eastern Empire. At some point in the century, hostels called *xenones* (affixed to churches) that housed the sick poor, appeared. The hospital proper emerged later in the century: these institutions, which went by different names (such as *xenodocheia* and *nosokomeia*), were more explicitly geared towards the *care* of the sick poor, particularly those near the end of their lives.[125] St. Basil of Caesarea is sometimes commended for building the "first hospital" in the second half of the fourth century in modern-day Turkey: his hospital was notable for the fact that it included a staff of physicians who lived in the building.[126] Again, this hospital served an explicitly charitable purpose: the early Church historian Sozomenos called it "the most celebrated hospice for the poor."[127] The Byzantine emphasis on charitable hospital care is perhaps best exemplified by the hospital of Pantocrator, built later in the Middle Ages: the hospital seems to be of the highest quality of its era, with one bed for each patient, generous physician staffing, a pharmacy, specialist wards, and a nutritious diet with a special allocation of funds given to patients to buy additional food.[128]

Hospitals spread widely throughout the Byzantine Empire in the coming centuries. In Western Europe, however, they diffused at a far slower pace. Hospitals initially arose within monasteries, and only by the High Middle Ages did numerous and sometimes quite large institutions appear, usually endowed by monarchs, nobles, guilds, and towns.[129] Medical practitioners were largely absent from these institutions until the sixteenth century.[130] Hospitals also spread to (and were transformed by) the Arab-Islamic world, where they seem to have reached a more advanced form. These facilities, called the "crowning achievement" of Islamic medicine, indeed sound rather impressive, with inpatient and outpatient areas, specialized wards, rounds by physicians, and pharmacies.[131] But again, the crucial point is that these were fundamentally charitable institutions: admission (including food, shelter, and medical treatment) was free, and patients were sometimes even given a sum of money at the time of their discharge to assist them as they looked for work.[132] To varying extents, these hospitals were also notable in that they provided healthcare regardless of the religion or racial background of the patients.[133]

Thus, to summarize, during the Middle Ages—whether in the Byzantine Empire, Western Europe, or the Arab-Islamic Caliphate—a novel tradition of medical charity emerged. This tradition arose, to some extent, on the backbone of a conceptualization of the dignity of the poor and the sick.[134] Of course, simply tracing the rise of these institutions says little about the actual experience of those who used them. Though we might find descriptions of the more refined Islamic and Byzantine models impressive, it is easy to imagine that most of these hospitals were likely grungier, skimpier, and terribly unpleasant places to be sick. Many people went to hospitals simply because they were poor, and had no other choice, and no doubt—in some instances—conditions could be grim. More broadly, it seems easy to conclude that hospitals did not meet the healthcare needs of the population.[135] They existed in part to serve the healthcare needs of the poor, but also to serve the spiritual needs of those who donated to them, to whom they offered the hope of salvation.[136] This mechanism of funding no doubt impacted their design, function, accessibility, and hierarchical structure.

But although the provision of charitable healthcare to some of the poor in this era did not amount to a "right" to healthcare, it is not fair to characterize medieval medical charity as nothing more than a paternalistic institution only meant to save the souls of rich donating elites. The historian Colin Jones has argued that there was a moral *expectation* to provide for the poor—even in the age before the welfare state—that amounted to what he calls a "charitable imperative" that goes beyond our traditional conceptions of charity. "The concept and the practices of charity," he writes, "were enmeshed within a matrix of moral obligation, religious dutifulness, and social exigency and expectation. Although the phrase sounds oxymoronic to twentieth-century ears, the idea of a 'charitable imperative' lay at the heart of medieval and early modern poor relief."[137] Jones contends that a framework which draws a well-defined line between voluntary charity and modern medical state welfare is reductionist and, indeed, inaccurate.[138] Private medical charity cannot be so clearly separated from the provision of healthcare by the state: such charities, for instance, have been supported by government for centuries.[139] At the same time, however, it is clear that the medieval "charitable obligation" does not equate with a "right to healthcare." As Jones and Jonathan Barry note of the pre-welfare state period more generally, an indirect, charity-based approach to welfare has advantages for a state, insofar as it allows it to escape "public admission that care was the *right* of the poor, rather than the gift of the rich . . ."[140] Thus, however compelling the "matrix of moral obligation" might have been, and however many of Europe's poor received care as a result of the "charitable imperative," such care by no means amounted to a "right" to medical care.

Still, though the poor had no right to medical care in the Middle Ages, some have suggested that they possibly had one socioeconomic right. The aforementioned "charitable imperative" or "philanthropic imperative," as the next section examines, was grounded—to some extent—in ideas about how property was conceived under the *ius natural*, or the natural law.

The Natural Rights of the Poor

Around the same time that "natural law"—with its contradictory orientation towards slavery and liberty—was incorporated into the Justinian code in the sixth century CE, *property* also came to acquire something of a conflicted meaning within natural law. Did natural law protect the right to property, or was property common to all under natural law? Some millennia later (as the final chapter of this book explores), a somewhat similar question was asked with a rather different twist: Does international law protect the right to intellectual property to goods like medications, or should such essential medications be common to all under the human right to healthcare, as it is enshrined in international law? In the Middle Ages, the discourse around property rights informed the medieval concept of charity—indeed, it led to the emergence of what one might call the first socioeconomic natural right.[141]

The problematic place of property in natural law emerged as the days of classical antiquity closed and those of the Christian era dawned. Archbishop of Seville Saint Isidore (c. 560–636)—sometimes dubbed the "last scholar of the ancient world"—dealt with the issue in *Etymologies,* in which he delineated specific rights (like liberty) that fell under the umbrella of natural law, in what one scholar refers to as "the most important definition of *ius naturale* in the European legal tradition."[142] Notably, among the "examples of natural law" in his list he includes "the common possessions of all persons."[143] Property was—in some sense—conceived as common to all in this highly influential passage. "Under the *ius naturale*," as Richard Tuck puts it more generally, "everything had been held and used in common."[144]

However, the Western world was, at that moment, in the process of descending into what is (perhaps unfairly) called the "Dark Ages," and there was no further major elaboration of natural law theory for centuries.[145] It was not until the eleventh or perhaps late twelfth century, when Europe entered into something of a medieval renaissance, that natural law again came under scholarly evaluation.[146] Scholars turned with renewed interest to the analysis and organization both of the recently discovered Justinian code and of the large, disorganized mass of church law (or "canon law").[147] In the twelfth century, Gratian—a monk and scholar based in Bologna—systematized the unruly corpus of canon law into a greatly influential compilation known as the *Decretum,* while the glossator Joannes Teutonicus wrote an important interpretation of Gratian's work called the *Glossa Ordinaria.*[148] As the historian Brian Tierney explains, these and other canonists found themselves in something of a predicament in their considerations of the place of property in natural law. On the one hand, they sought to defend the right to property, but on the other, they had to contend with various church writings (like that of Isidore) that proposed that property was common under natural law.[149] They also had to reckon with the "primitive communism" of early Christian communities.[150]

This very old Christian communism was, according to Tierney, less problematic than the texts of the early Church fathers. In addition to the passage of Isidore, Gratian quoted some passages of St. Clement of Rome, who had (allegedly) written that the "use of all things that are in the world ought to be common to all men."[151] Gratian also referenced a similar passage from another Christian theologian, who contended that "[n]o one may call his own what is common, of which if he takes more than he needs, it is taken with violence."[152] His work left unresolved a serious incongruity: property could be legally owned under human law but seemed to be "common" under natural law—and, problematically, natural law superseded human law.[153]

Tierney describes two ways that this theoretical gap was closed. One response was that of Aquinas, who some have controversially argued initiated the modern human rights tradition.[154] Aquinas followed the ancient line that slavery and private property were, in some sense, inconsistent with natural law, but added that they were joined to natural law for societal benefit: "In this sense, *the possession of all things in common and universal freedom* are said to be of the natural law," he wrote, "because, namely, the distinction of possessions and slavery were not brought in by nature, but devised by human reason for the benefit of human life."[155] Aquinas essentially resolved the dilemma of common property by interpreting natural law as the way things had been under a "primitive state of things, without permanent validity."[156] It is true that he did acknowledge that the poor had a claim to the property of the rich when in "imminent danger," but for Aquinas, this claim was greatly limited: even hunger might not be sufficient grounds for such redistribution.[157]

The more radical response was that of canonists Huguccio and Teutonicus. As Tierney notes, these two created a new meaning of "common" adopted by their successors. In his *Glossa Ordinaria*, Teutonicus notes that by at least one definition, "according to this law of nature all things are called common, *that is they are to be shared in time of necessity. . . .*"[158] In other words, natural law did not demand the elimination of property *per se*, but it did, in theory, establish an *imperative* to share with those in need. The work of Teutonicus thereby tied together "natural law theory and the obligation of charity," and indeed this notion would thereafter become "a fundamental tenet of medieval sociology . . ."[159] Medieval charity, in Tierney's perspective, was therefore not merely a gift: it was an obligation, to some extent *grounded in natural law*. As he puts it, these canonists were essentially arguing that "the poor had a *right* to be supported from the superfluous wealth of the community."[160] Charity "formed part of the moral economy," another historian has argued along similar lines, "something to be expected *as of right* by the poor, in times of difficulty or phases of the life cycle . . ." (emphasis added).[161]

The poor thereby came to have one theoretical socioeconomic right in the Middle Ages: the right to assistance in time of need. Such assistance might be considered a right in that, if it was not given freely, it might justifiably be taken.[162] "One who suffers the need of hunger seems to use his right," argued thirteenth-century jurist Hostiensis, "rather than to plan a theft."[163] The English bishop William Lyndwood later even argued that the poor need not delay until hunger had set in to take what they needed—at that point, they would be too weak to help themselves.[164] And critically, by the thirteenth century, some canonists even went so far as to assert that the imperative of the rich to give to the poor might even be *legally enforceable*.[165] This more radical theoretical grounding of medieval charity—including medieval *medical charity*—is very important. Not only was the hospital care of this period a form of decommodified healthcare for the poor, but it was also—to some extent—enmeshed into this theoretical framework of natural rights.[166] "The jurists' analysis of the rights of the poor," notes Kenneth Pennington, "represented another strand in rights thinking . . .",[167] and it is a strand that is frequently neglected in historical discussions of human rights.[168] An undercurrent of such "rights thinking" informed ideas about charity—including the medical charity—of this era.

However, as time passed, things begin to change, particularly in the wake of the "Black Death" in the fourteenth century (and the wars and famine that accompanied it). In the Late Middle Ages—after the plague and the popular revolts that it may have prompted—the poor were viewed with increased distaste and fear, resulting in a new and often more severe orientation towards charity with a greater state role.[169] Associated changes in social and economic conditions no doubt played a role as well, with the growth of the landless poor in some parts of Europe, the rise of a more mobile workforce, the expansion of the commercial agrarian economy, and the increasing dispossession of peasants by the "enclosure" of land for sheep-rearing.[170] By the years of the Renaissance, the general perception was that bands of vagabonds were threatening Europe.[171] With time, the poor were divided into the "deserving" and the "undeserving"; whereas the former should receive aid, the latter should be carefully watched and punished.[172] Imposing a work obligation on the able-bodied poor and eliminating unauthorized charity were increasingly emphasized.[173] At the same time, charity—including church poor relief and hospitals—became inadequate in light of the needs of a growing population of the poor.[174] In addition to the traditional patient of the hospital—the disabled and the socially marginalized—were the growing numbers of other groups in need: As Mollat puts it, ". . . these institutions failed to recognize the existence of the working poor and were overwhelmed by the growing numbers of vagabonds and other social outcasts."[175]

English Poor Law—which some have conceptualized as a precursor to the modern welfare state[176]—was one example of an evolving response to the challenges of this era. The roots of the "Poor Law" extend back into the early Middle Ages, when poor relief was predominantly a Church affair (the centuries after the Black Death, however, saw increasing government involvement in its operation).[177] This canonical form of poor relief formed the basis for the Elizabethan Poor Law, which was also made possible by the fusion of Church and State in England by Henry VIII.[178] The Elizabethan Poor Laws of 1597 and 1601 remained fundamentally intact until the early nineteenth century.[179] But the essential features of this poor law, Tierney argues, should be seen as (in part) arising from the long tradition of canonical poor relief—and the theory of charity underlying it—of the Middle Ages:

> From the reception of Gratian's *Decretum* in the mid-twelfth century to the final codification of the Elizabethan poor law in 1601, a single developing tradition without any sudden break or reversal of policy can be traced. . . . The acknowledgement that society had to provide for the impotent poor through established public authority, the rule that each parish should support its own poor, the principle of compulsory poor relief contributions—all these things were old and canonical.[180]

In other words, to some highly limited extent, the English Poor Law provided something of a "right to relief," funded by taxes on the community.[181] Indeed, T. H. Marshall went so far as to call a later iteration of the Poor Law—the so-called Speenhamland system that supplemented the wages of the working poor—as a "substantial body of social rights . . ." Indeed, at least in that era, he contended that the Poor Law functioned "as the aggressive champion of the social rights of citizenship."[182]

Notably, there was also a medical component to the Poor Law. Although it did not explicitly provide for healthcare, it did seek to aid the "lame, impotent, old, blind, and such other among them being poor and not able to work."[183] "[I]n time," notes historian George Rosen, "the scope of this provision came to include medical care."[184] Parishes, for instance, sometimes provided healthcare to their poor by contracting with a private physician.[185] "The parish had an obligation to the parishioner," notes historian Christopher Hamlin, "whether the need was food or physick [medicine]."[186] As Hamlin adds, this duty may not often have been achieved in practice, though it remained important as a political conception. But if the English Poor Law guaranteed some concrete benefits to the poor and sick, it also had vindictive, controlling aspects. The relief of the poor went hand-in-hand with repressive labor laws and efforts to punish vagrants.[187] As social reformers Sidney and Beatrice Webb would later put it in a frequently cited phrase, the English Poor Law was an instance of "[r]elief of the poor within a Framework of Repression."[188] It was thus a Janus-faced institution: in part arising from a tradition in which relief was conceived of as a theoretical *right* of the poor, it was also an attempt to control its beneficiaries.

Both the emergence of a discourse and practice of medical charity and the articulation of a notion of a limited socioeconomic right speak to the complexity of the dialectic around the rights of the poor of this era. But under the strains of economic and political change, more direct calls for the redistribution of socioeconomic goods emerged in the early modern period. In particular, explicit proposals for the public provision of healthcare appeared by the seventeenth century, shortly after the English Civil War, including from a lawyer by the name of John Cooke.

The English Civil War and Universal Healthcare

The years of the English Civil War were eventful for Cooke, a barrister who started life as the son of a destitute farmer, and who ended it hung, drawn, and quartered for the crime of regicide. Cooke was not, it seems fair to say, one to shrink from controversial causes. In 1646, for instance, he represented radical activist "Freeborn" John Lilburne, a "Leveller" who took seriously the idea of natural rights and equality.[189] A few years later, Cooke prosecuted Charles I in what one biographer and human rights lawyer has enthusiastically termed "the first war crimes trial of a Head of State."[190] Cooke did something else remarkable: he proposed that healthcare—inclusive of the services of physicians, surgeons, and apothecaries—be provided for free to the nation's poor.

More broadly, this era saw the evolution of ideas both about natural rights and about the state provision of healthcare to the poor. In 1642, the English Civil War broke out between King Charles I on one side and Parliament on the other, culminating in the monarch's defeat and later decapitation. What began largely as a power struggle between political elites came in some instances to have a potent popular component. Indeed, in the revolutionary milieu of these years, ideas about political equality, socioeconomic justice, and even "universal" healthcare were articulated. At the same time, the abstract and ethereal meaning of "natural rights" evolved into a far more concrete construct.

Two notable radical political groups in this regard were the "Levellers," a pejorative label given by supporters of the King to a group of writer-activists that emerged late in the Civil War,[191] and the Diggers. The Levellers were radical democrats, demanding much more equal representation in Parliament—that is to say, for semi-universal suffrage (excluding women and servants, however).[192] Notably, they drew on the ancient language of natural rights and natural law, which they imbued with fresh and provocative political importance.[193] According to Justinian's *Institutes*, under the law of nature, "all men are originally born free."[194] The Leveller Lilburne, the aforementioned client of Cooke's, went further in writing that "all men were born to equal natural rights."[195] Yet while "natural law" for the Levellers led to individual *political rights*, for the Diggers it led to *socioeconomic rights*, namely common ownership and use of the land.[196] Gerrard Winstanley, the most prominent of the Diggers, also promoted the advancement and application of science in his pamphlet *Law of Freedom*.[197] His communitarianism extended to free healthcare. In one section of the book entitled "Laws to restore slaves to freedom," he proposed that if "[i]f any persons be sick or wounded, the surgeons . . . shall go when they are sent for to any who need their help, but require no reward, because the common stock is the public pay for every man's labour."[198]

Others less radical than Winstanley also proposed systems in which healthcare would be provided to the poor. Before the outbreak of the war, for instance, Samuel Hartlib, in his 1641 *A Description of the Famous Kingdome of Macaria*, described a utopian society in which a "College of Experience" would "deliver out, yearly, such medicines as they find out by experience," and years later, he proposed a mechanism of providing free physician care to the poor.[199] More notably, John Cooke put forward the "Poor Man's Case" in his 1648 pamphlet *Unum Necessarium*.[200] Cooke again adopted the essential argument we have already traced, namely that under natural law, the poor deserved some of the wealth of the rich: "[T]he rule of charity is, that one man's superfluity should give place to another man's conveniency, his conveniency to another's necessity, his lesser necessities to another's extremer necessities, and to the mechanical poor to relieve the mendicant poor in their extremer need, and this is but the Dictate of the Law of Nature. . . ."[201] He proposed a number of methods to realize this redistribution. Mines (which he called "Nature's presents"), for instance, might appropriately contribute to the "poor man's box."[202] He also dealt more specifically with the great problems that the poor faced when they became sick. "[H]ow many people in this Kingdom die yearly," he mused, "that can never get any physician to visit them in their sickness; and how many poor people are there about London that had rather die then fee an apothecary's bill . . . "[203] This was particularly a problem, Cooke explained, because sickness—specifically the Plague—most usually struck the poor.[204] He encouraged physicians to "deal kindly" with the sick poor, as their fees might be more damaging than the disease itself (in light of the typical treatments of the time, that was sadly true).[205] But he went further, arguing that physicians, apothecaries, and surgeons (like lawyers) should actually be "assigne[d]" to the poor, *in forma pauperis.*[206] Some have argued that together, Cooke's healthcare propositions made him "the visionary who first proposed a national health service" for Britain.[207]

Others made other sorts of proposals for an expanded public role in health-care. The physician and scientist William Petty, for instance, called for the establishment of hospitals and the planning of healthcare personnel so as to meet society's needs.[208] We could also "pursue the means of acquiring the public good and comfort of mankind a little further," he wrote, by constructing teaching hospitals.[209] Samuel Herring went even further, making the case for a publicly-funded system of healthcare provided *free at time of use.* In a letter to Oliver Cromwell he wrote that "the poor throughout this Commonwealth, should be provided for, so that none should be found begging . . . that houses should be built and bought in city, town and country, for old people to be cherished in . . ."[210] He argued that, like the lawyer, the physician "should be maintained out of the public treasury, and *should be made incapable of receiving any monies from the people*; and every county should be supplied with a competent number of them . . ." (emphasis added).[211]

This reformist, egalitarian spirit extended beyond the years of the Civil War and Commonwealth to that of the Restoration. Perhaps the most interesting example here is the Quaker merchant and philanthropist, John Bellers (1654–1725).[212] Bellers, whose work possibly reflects the influence of the Diggers, proposed a variety of welfare institutions, inclusive of a system of universal healthcare.[213] In his *An Essay Towards the Improvement of Physick . . .* , Bellers explicitly proposed not only that the poor should receive free healthcare, but that it was the *state's responsibility* to provide it. As medical historian George Rosen put it, such a proposal was all but tantamount to "an eighteenth century plan for a national health service."[214]

Bellers begins by estimating the collective toll of inadequate healthcare for the poor (he was no doubt misguided in his evaluation of the therapeutic utility of the medical care of his day, but this is beside the point). "[I]t may be reasonably supposed," he wrote, "that a hundred thousand . . . die yearly of *curable* diseases; for want of *timely advice,* and *suitable medicines.*"[215] He therefore contended that if "*the safety of the people be the supreme Law,*" then Parliamentary legislation "for the improvement of MEDICINE" was necessary.[216] The magnitude of the problem meant that private charity was insufficient, and state support necessary: "It is too great a burden to be left upon the shoulders," as he put it, "or to the care of the physicians alone, no private purse being able to bear the needful charges of it:

especially considering the necessity of many .... [T]here is the more Reason to expect the STATE should bear a good part of the expense of it."[217]

He offered a multitude of proposals to accomplish these goals. First, "there should be built ... HOSPITALS for the POOR. ... And to have *physicians* and *surgeons* suitable, to take care of the SICK."[218] He also proposed that "in every hundred of a county, and parish of a city, there be appointed one *doctor* and *surgeon* (and more, if needful) to take care of the sick *poor* in them...."[219] He additionally envisioned a general improvement in medical science, which would include a prize for medical achievements, public regulation of medicine, and publicly funded laboratory research efforts.[220] But importantly, Bellers understood the fundamental problem with requiring payment for medical care at the time of service for those with few resources. As he argues, when workers become ill and therefore unable to work, "they have little or nothing to give for physick [medicine] ... therefore without some provision be made, multitudes of them must fall by untimely deaths."[221]

There is something extraordinary about these proposals. This chapter has chronicled various early instances and exhortations towards charitable medical care, but Bellers went beyond these in arguing that the government had a systematic *responsibility* to ensure that all had access to healthcare. Though he did not use the language of rights, he was describing a public system that would provide medical care to the poor *as of right*.

But what was to be the fate of these varied radical ideas, whether of the Levellers or Diggers, of Cooke or Hartlib, or (later) of Bellers? For the earlier figures, a turn of events in the political sphere constrained their proposals to the realm of theory. The monarchy was crushed, but Cromwell soon assumed dictatorial powers of his own. The Levellers were crushed.[222] Cooke was tortured and killed by the regime. And the Poor Law policy of Cromwell's Commonwealth reflected an even more severe attitude towards poverty, with little of the egalitarian and innovative spirit of the thinkers discussed.[223] The benefits of the Civil War, whatever its popular support, seem to have accrued largely to economic elites,[224] and no expanded access to healthcare—much less a "right" to it—was to emerge in these years—or indeed, for centuries.

Conclusions

Healthcare has never functioned as a pure market commodity.[225] The *idea* of an ethical obligation to provide healthcare to the sick poor outside the confines of the "cash nexus"—as demonstrated in different ways and to varying degrees in a variety of Greek, Roman, Chinese, Indian, and medieval contexts—clearly has deep roots in a number of different world cultures. In classical antiquity, for instance, physicians were sometimes praised for providing free care for all, whether free or enslaved. In the Chinese ethical texts, one can find an emphasis on an obligation to treat the poor and rich equally. The Edicts of Asoka, meanwhile, perhaps demonstrate some sort of commitment to healthcare on the public level. And in the medieval era, novel forms of institutionalized charitable medical care—in the form of the charity hospital—emerged and evolved in the Byzantine East, Western Europe, and the Arab-Islamic world. Such systems, of course, operated in parallel to a more commodified healthcare arena, available only to those who had the money to pay for it. Indeed, it is difficult to have a sense of the adequacy of any of these provisions, and to some extent, this chapter has said very little about the actual medical lives of the poor. Though there very well may be a healthcare rights-commodity dialectic snaking through history, so far this has been a tension mostly in the realm of *ideas*.

Ideas, however, can have an influence that outlasts the era of their genesis. The Middle Ages saw the rise of a "charitable imperative" to provide healthcare to the sick poor, an obligation grounded in egalitarian religious values about poverty and sickness. And the period also arguably "produced" one socioeconomic right: the limited and largely theoretical natural right of the poor, under natural law, to the property of the rich in times of desperation. During and after the English Civil War, some went further in arguing that the poor deserved *more* than charity and that the government had some sort of *duty* to provide healthcare to the poor, which it could achieve by appointing physicians to the poor or building hospitals for them. In such proposals one perceives the seeds of a social "right to health," one that emerged simultaneously with and to some extent in parallel to evolving ideas about political "natural rights."

These developments, however, also show how feeble ideas can be. Without a powerful political movement to carry it forward, universal healthcare—like universal suffrage—remained in the realm of ideas: of historical interest, no doubt, but of little use to those actually living, and dying, without it.

Notes

1 An internet search reveals some variations on this quote. This version is that offered by Edmund D. Pellegrino, *Aristotle and the Right to Health Care: A Cautionary Tale: Appendix to Scope Note 20* (Washington, DC: Kennedy Institute of Ethics, National Reference Center for Bioethics Literature, 2008), accessed November 21, 2015, https://repository.library.georgetown.edu/bitstream/handle/10822/556875/sn20.pdf?sequence=1&isAllowed=y.

2 Ibid.

3 James Taranto, "Fake but Aristotelian?," *The Wall Street Journal*, October 16, 2009, accessed November 21, 2015, http://www.wsj.com/articles/SB1000142405274870432200457447734286 4992048; Pellegrino, *Aristotle and the Right to Health Care: A Cautionary Tale*.

4 Hersch Lauterpacht, *An International Bill of the Rights of Man* (New York: Columbia University Press, 1945), 3–4.

5 For Cassirer it is Grotius who "bridges the gap" between antiquity and modernity. Ernst Cassirer, *The Philosophy of the Enlightenment* (Princeton, NJ: Princeton University Press, 2009), 236, 248–9.

6 Again, Moyn emphasizes these differences. Samuel Moyn, *The Last Utopia: Human Rights in History* (Cambridge, MA: Belknap Press of Harvard University Press, 2010).

7 Essentially, he argues, there was no limit to state power. M. I. Finley, *The Ancient Economy*, updated ed. (Berkeley: University of California Press, 1999), 154.

8 Watson and Guthrie both note that he likely used the term with a sense of paradox. Gerard Watson, "The Early History of 'Natural Law'," *Irish Theological Quarterly* 33, no. 1 (1966): 66; W. K. C. Guthrie, *The Sophists* (Cambridge: Cambridge University Press, 1971), 103–6, 118; Plato, *Gorgias*, trans. Robin Waterfield (Oxford: Oxford University Press, 1994), 66.

9   Indeed, as Tuck notes, the Romans actually used *ius* (a word which would later come to mean right) to mean a liberty. H. L. A. Hart, "Are There Any Natural Rights," *The Philosophical Review* 64, no. 2 (1955): 166–7 n4; Richard Tuck, *Natural Rights Theories: Their Origin and Development* (Cambridge: Cambridge University Press, 1979), 26.

10 Plato, *The Republic*, trans. A. D. Lindsay (New York: Knopf, 1992), I. 338.

11 Fred D. Miller, "Aristotle and the Origins of Natural Rights," *The Review of Metaphysics* 49, no. 4 (1996): quotes on page 878, 880 and 907.

12 Richard Kraut, "Are There Natural Rights in Aristotle?," *The Review of Metaphysics* 49, no. 4 (1996): 757.

13 For instance, in *Nicomachean Ethics*, he made a famous argument contending that "by nature" there is one best constitution "everywhere," while in the *Rhetoric*, he notes that "Universal law is the law of nature." Max Solomon Shellens, "Aristotle on Natural Law," *Natural Law Forum* 4, no. 1 (1959): 72–100; Aristotle and F. H. Peters, *Nicomachean Ethics* (New York: Barnes & Noble Books, 2005), 1134b–35a; Aristotle and W. Rhys Roberts, *Rhetoric*, Dover thrift ed. (Mineola, NY: Dover Publications, 2004), 1373b.

14 He proposed, for instance, the perverse notion of the "slave by nature," who was little more than a "living piece of property . . . a tool in charge of other tools." Aristotle, *The Politics*, trans. T. A. Sinclair (Harmondsworth: Penguin Books, 1984), 1254a9; David Brion Davis, *The Problem of Slavery in Western Culture* (New York: Oxford University Press, 1988), 70–1.

15 A point made by Samuel Fleischacker, *A Short History of Distributive Justice* (Cambridge, MA: Harvard University Press, 2004), 20.

16 Tony Burns makes the case that the Sophists elaborated an egalitarian natural law (which for some made slavery unjust). Tony Burns, "The Tragedy of Slavery: Aristotle's Rhetoric and the History of the Concept of Natural Law," *History of Political Thought* 24, no. 1 (2003): 16–36.

17 Hippias of Elis, for instance, championed *physis* over *nomos*. *The First Philosophers: The Pre-Socratics and Sophists*, trans. Robin Waterfield (Oxford: Oxford University Press, 2009), 250–1; Guthrie, *The Sophists*, 21–2, 48.

18 Guthrie, *The Sophists*, 102, 117–18.

19 David George Ritchie, *Natural Rights* (London: George Allen & Unwin Ltd, 1924), 25; Davis, *The Problem of Slavery in Western Culture*, 69, 72–3; Aristotle, *The Politics*, 1253b14; Burns, "The Tragedy of Slavery"; Guthrie, *The Sophists*, 118.

20 Antiphon, *The First Philosophers: The Pre-Socratics and Sophists*, trans. Robin Waterfield (Oxford: Oxford University Press, 2009), 264.

21 Protagoras' words per Plato; his argument is made by way of allegory through a story about Hermes and Zeus. Plato, *Protagoras and Meno*, trans. W. K. C. Guthrie (Harmondsworth: Penguin, 1956), 323A; Ellen Meiksins Wood, *Citizens to Lords: A Social History of Western Political Thought from Antiquity to the Middle Ages* (London: Verso, 2008), 59–62.

22 Lycophron the Sophist per Aristotle, quoted in Guthrie, *The Sophists*, 154.

23 Phaleas' opinion according to Aristotle. Ibid., 152; Aristotle, *The Politics*, 1266b24 .

24 Lauterpacht, *An International Bill of the Rights of Man*, 19.

25 Marcus Tullius Cicero, *On Obligations*, trans. P. G. Walsh (Oxford: Oxford University Press; repr., 2008), III. 27; Marcus Tullius Cicero, "The Laws," in *The Republic and the Laws* (Oxford; New York: Oxford University Press, 1998), I. 30.

26 Richard A. Bauman, *Human Rights in Ancient Rome* (London: Routledge, 2000), 23–4, 122–4; Fleischacker, *A Short History of Distributive Justice*, 21.

27 Slavery, according to Justinians' *Institutes* (echoing the Stoic-influenced Ulpian), ". . . is contrary to the law of nature . . . by that law all men are originally born free." George Holland Sabine, *A History of Political Theory*, 3d ed. (New York: Holt, 1961), 160, 167–9; Ritchie, *Natural Rights*, 38; Tony Honoré, "The Cosmopolis and Human Rights," 2nd ed., *Ulpian: Pioneer of Human Rights* (Oxford: Oxford University Press, 2002; repr., Oxford Scholarship Online, 2010), doi: 10.1093/acprof:oso/9780199244249.003.0003, 79–80; Davis, *The Problem of Slavery in Western Culture*, 83; "The Institutes 535 CE," *The Medieval Sourcebook*, Fordham University, accessed

March 7, 2014, http://www.fordham.edu/halsall/basis/535institutes.asp; Anthony Pagden, "Human Rights, Natural Rights, and Europe's Imperial Legacy," *Political Theory* 31, no. 2 (2003): 174.

28   Seneca was responsible for the "humanization" of Stoicism, according to Campbell. He indeed would later criticize Roman cruelty in war, gladiatorial combat, its treatment of slaves, and in one instance its racism. Lucius Annaeus Seneca, *Letters from a Stoic*, trans. Robin Campbell (London: Penguin; repr., 2004), 41, 90–6; Bauman, *Human Rights in Ancient Rome*, 69–70, 85, 121; Sabine, *A History of Political Theory*, 153; Robin Campbell, Introduction to *Letters from a Stoic, by Seneca* (London: Penguin, 2004; repr., 2004), 17.

29   Lucius Annaeus Seneca, *Dialogues and Essays*, trans. John N. Davie (Oxford: Oxford University Press, 2008), 216–17.

30   Arthur Robinson Hands, *Charities and Social Aid in Greece and Rome* (London: Thames & Hudson, 1968), 16.

31   The Spartan King Cleomenes, who attempted this program, was tutored, as several historians point out, by the prominent Stoic Sphaerus of Bosporus. Thomas Africa, on the other hand, calls the Spartan Revolution–Stoicism connection "extremely tenuous." Tarn nonetheless deems it a "social revolution." W. W. Tarn, "The Social Question in the Third Century," in *The Hellenistic Age: Aspects of Hellenistic Civilization*, ed. J. B. Bury, et al. (Cambridge: The University Press, 1923), 108–40; Paul Cartledge, *Ancient Greek Political Thought in Practice* (Cambridge: Cambridge University Press, 2009), 113–19; Christos P. Baloglou, "Cleomenes III's Politico-Economic Reforms in Sparta (235–222 BC) and Cercidas' Economic Thought," in *Political Events and Economic Ideas*, ed. Ingo Barens, Volker Caspari, and Bertram Schefold (Cheltenham: Edward Elgar, 2004), 193–5; Thomas W. Africa, "Stoics, Cynics, and the Spartan Revolution," *International Review of Social History* 4, no. 3 (1959): 469.

32   Cercidas asks that the city ". . . have a care for Paean [a Greek god of healing, or physician to the gods], and for Sharing – she is indeed a goddess – and Retribution that walketh the earth." Tarn (similar to Baloglou) interprets Cercidas here to mean that his city "must heal the sick and give to the poor while they have the chance . . ." While dismissing the role of genteel Stoicism in such unrest, Africa concedes that if any philosophy played a role, it was indeed the "leveling austerity of the genuinely radical Cynical school." Tarn, "The Social Question in the Third Century," 136–7; Africa, "Stoics, Cynics, and the Spartan Revolution," quote on page 465; Donald Reynolds Dudley, *A History of Cynicism from Diogenes to the 6th Century A.D* (New York: Gordon Press, 1974), 79–81, Cercidas quote on 79; Baloglou, "Cleomenes III's Politico-Economic Reforms in Sparta (235–222 BC) and Cercidas' Economic Thought," 196–9.

33   Africa, "Stoics, Cynics, and the Spartan Revolution," 463.

34   Gary B. Ferngren, *Medicine & Health Care in Early Christianity* (Baltimore: Johns Hopkins University Press, 2009), 87.

35   Finley, *The Ancient Economy*, 38–9.

36   Quoted in Hands, *Charities and Social Aid in Greece and Rome*, 65.

37   Ferngren, *Medicine & Health Care in Early Christianity*, 87.

38   John Ferguson, *Moral Values in the Ancient World* (London: Methuen, 1958), 103; Ferngren, *Medicine & Health Care in Early Christianity*, 87; Demetrios J. Constantelos, *Byzantine Philanthropy and Social Welfare*, 2nd (rev.) ed. (New Rochelle, NY: A.D. Caratzas, 1991), 3.

39   Bauman, *Human Rights in Ancient Rome*, 10–19, quote on page 11.

40   Ferngren, *Medicine & Health Care in Early Christianity*, 92.

41   Bauman, *Human Rights in Ancient Rome*, 10; Ferguson, *Moral Values in the Ancient World*, 102.

42   Guenter B. Risse, *Mending Bodies, Saving Souls: A History of Hospitals* (New York: Oxford University Press, 1999), 44.

43   Hands, *Charities and Social Aid in Greece and Rome*, 137–8; Constantelos, *Byzantine Philanthropy and Social Welfare*, 6.

44   Gary B. Ferngren, *Medicine and Religion: A Historical Introduction* (Baltimore: Johns Hopkins University Press, 2014), 89–90.

45 The paragraph's discussion of the facts about Asclepius and his temples synthesizes facts found in the following sources: Henry E. Sigerist, *A History of Medicine*, vol. 2, *Early Greek, Hindu, and Persian Medicine* (New York: Oxford University Press, 1961), 51–67; Risse, *Mending Bodies, Saving Souls*, 20–33; Ferngren, *Medicine and Religion*, 50–2, 68; Bronwen Lara Wickkiser, *Asklepios, Medicine, and the Politics of Healing in Fifth-Century Greece: Between Craft and Cult* (Baltimore: The Johns Hopkins University Press, 2008), 1–2.

46 Emma J. Edelstein and Ludwig Edelstein, *Asclepius: A Collection and Interpretation of the Testimonies* (Baltimore: The Johns Hopkins Press, 1945), 2: 175–6.

47 Sigerist, *A History of Medicine*, 2: 72.

48 Ibid., 72–3; Edelstein and Edelstein, *Asclepius*, 2:176; Hands, *Charities and Social Aid in Greece and Rome*, 132.

49 Hector Avalos, *Health Care and the Rise of Christianity* (Peabody, MA: Hendrickson, 1999), 92–3; Risse, *Mending Bodies, Saving Souls*, 32; Sigerist, *A History of Medicine* 2: 44; Edelstein and Edelstein, *Asclepius*, 2: 175–7.

50 Wickkiser, *Asklepios, Medicine, and the Politics of Healing in Fifth-Century Greece*, 4–5.

51 Ibid., for instance, 8, 26–9, 58–9.

52 This is a point made in a personal communication by historian Calloway Scott, e-mail communication to the author, September 13, 2016.

53 Edelstein and Edelstein, *Asclepius*, 2: 257.

54 Ferngren, *Medicine and Religion*, 41.

55 Pliny the Elder, *Natural Histories*, Book XXIX, accessed October 16, 2016, http://www.masseiana.org/pliny.htm#BOOK%20XXIX. I was directed to this work and section by historian Caroline Wazer, personal e-mail communication, August 16, 2016.

56 Several scholars have discussed the *Precepts* along these lines; I've followed them to this text and have benefited from their analysis. For instance, Ferngren, *Medicine & Health Care in Early Christianity*, 88; Louis Cohn-Haft, *The Public Physicians of Ancient Greece* (Northampton, MA: Dept. of History of Smith College, 1956), 20; Hands, *Charities and Social Aid in Greece and Rome*, 131.

57 Hands, *Charities and Social Aid in Greece and Rome*, 132.

58 The quotes from this paragraph are all from Hippocrates, "Precepts," in *Hippocrates*, ed. Jeffrey Hendersen (Cambridge, MA: Harvard University Press), 317–19.

59 This paragraph thus far relies on Ferngren, *Medicine & Health Care in Early Christianity*, 92–5. See also Edmund D. Pellegrino and Alice A. Pellegrino, "Humanism and Ethics in Roman Medicine: Translation and Commentary on a Text of Scribonius Largus," *Literature and Medicine* 7, no. 1 (1988): 22–38.

60 Edelstein and Edelstein, *Asclepius*, 2: 175.

61 Pellegrino and Pellegrino, "Humanism and Ethics in Roman Medicine: Translation and Commentary on a Text of Scribonius Largus."

62 Ibid., 29.

63 Ibid., 32, 35.

64 Ibid., 26. A different translation of this passage appears in Ferngren, *Medicine & Health Care in Early Christianity*, 94.

65 Ferngren, *Medicine & Health Care in Early Christianity*, 95.

66 Vivian Nutton, "Archiatri and the Medical Profession in Antiquity," *Papers of the British School at Rome* 45 (1977): 191n1; Louis Cohn-Haft, *The Public Physicians of Ancient Greece*, 1.

67 This point and the quote are from Cohn-Haft, *The Public Physicians of Ancient Greece*, 8–9.

68 Ibid., 10–11.

69 Quoted by ibid., 33.

70 Ibid., 11.

71 Vivian Nutton, "Medicine in the Greek World, 800–50 BC," in *The Western Medical Tradition: 800 BC–1800 AD* (Cambridge: Cambridge University Press, 2009), 38.

72 Quoted in Cohn-Haft, *The Public Physicians of Ancient Greece*, 37.

73 Quoted in Hands, *Charities and Social Aid in Greece and Rome*, 132.

74 A. G. Woodhead, "The State Health Service in Ancient Greece," *Cambridge Historical Journal* 10, no. 03 (1952), quotes on page 235 and 250. Constantelos asserts this as well. Constantelos, *Byzantine Philanthropy and Social Welfare,* 8.

75 Cohn-Haft, *The Public Physicians of Ancient Greece,* 32.

76 Ibid.

77 For a comparative look, see Nutton, "Archiatri and the Medical Profession in Antiquity."

78 Cohn-Haft, *The Public Physicians of Ancient Greece,* 35–7.

79 Ibid., 44–67.

80 Hands suggests that Cohn-Haft is primarily arguing from an *absence* of evidence, but seems to agree with his overall skepticism. He also notes that there is no good reason to believe that the situation changed much under the Romans (Cohn-Haft dealt only with the Greeks). Hands, *Charities and Social Aid in Greece and Rome,* 132–40.

81 Poonam Bala, *Medicine and Medical Policies in India: Social and Historical Perspectives* (Lanham: Lexington Books, 2007), 34.

82 Quoted in ibid.; Paul U. Unschuld, *Medical Ethics in Imperial China: A Study in Historical Anthropology* (Berkeley: University of California Press, 1979), 62.

83 C. G. Uragoda, *A History of Medicine in Sri Lanka from the Earliest Times to 1948* (Colombo: Sri Lanka Medical Association, 1987), 23–4, 35.

84 O. P. Jaggi, *Medicine in India: Modern Period* (New Delhi: Oxford University Press, 2000), 70.

85 Stanley A. Wolpert, *India,* 3rd ed. (Berkeley, CA: University of California Press, 2005), 36; Richard McKeon, Foreword to the *Edicts of Asoka,* trans. N. A. Nikam and Richard McKeon (Chicago: University of Chicago Press, 1978), xi–xii.

86 Several writers make note of the health-related significance of Asoka, and/or quote from these inscriptions. For instance, Jaggi, *Medicine in India,* 70; Bala, *Medicine and Medical Policies in India,* 35; Henry Ernest Sigerist, "An Outline of the Development of the Hospital," *Bulletin of the Institute of the History of Medicine* (1936), 576–7.

87 *The Edicts of Asoka,* trans. N. A. Nikam and Richard McKeon (Chicago: University of Chicago Press, 1978), 59.

88 Ibid., 64. Joppi's translation of this inscription refers to "hospitals for men and hospitals for animals." The point about Asoka's Buddhist ethic extending to animals is made by Bala. Jaggi, *Medicine in India,* 70; Bala, *Medicine and Medical Policies in India,* 35.

89 *The Edicts of Asoka,* 64.

90 Jaggi, *Medicine in India,* 70; Bala, *Medicine and Medical Policies in India,* 35.

91 Jaggi, *Medicine in India,* 70.

92 This version of the quote is from Fa-Hien, "The Travels of Fa-Hien," *The Literature of China: with critical and biographical sketches* (New York: Colonial Press, 1900), accessed December 19, 2015, http://hdl.handle.net/2027/pst.000002381930, 252. It is cited or alluded to in several other works which directed me to it, for instance: Jaggi, *Medicine in India,* 71; Sailendra Nath Sen, *Ancient Indian History and Civilization,* 2nd ed. (New Delhi: New Age International Publishers, 1998), 216.

93 This paragraph relies throughout on Joseph Needham and Lu Gwei-Djen, "Medicine and Chinese Culture," in *Clerks and Craftsmen in China and the West: Lectures and Addresses on the History of Science and Technology* (Cambridge: Cambridge University Press, 1970), 277–9.

94 Unschuld, *Medical Ethics in Imperial China.*

95 Ibid., 25.

96 Ibid., 30.

97 Ibid.

98 Unschuld, however, notes that Chu-ming completely ignores the patient's perspective, and also advocated physicians not taking on cases bound to be unsuccessful ("prognosis"). Ibid., 60–2, quote on 62.

99 Ibid., 68–9, quote on 69.

100 Ibid., 108, quote on 112.

101 Ibid., 112.

102   Ibid., 63.
103   However, it's important to also not make too much of this: although a number of writers
       emphasized such egalitarian ideas here and there, this was not by any means the primary thrust
       of these texts. Indeed, Unschuld mainly conceptualizes the development of Chinese medical
       ethics as part of a process of professionalization, and indeed as a "protective mechanism" for
       physicians who might be liable for the poor outcomes of their patients. Ibid., 12–13, 120.
104   Ferngren, *Medicine and Religion*, 84.
105   Ibid., 114; Constantelos, *Byzantine Philanthropy and Social Welfare*, 3–13.
106   Ferngren, *Medicine & Health Care in Early Christianity*, 97–8.
107   Ibid., 98; Vivian Nutton, "Medicine in Late Antiquity and the Early Middle Ages," in *The Western
       Medical Tradition: 800 B.C.–1800 A.D* (Cambridge: Cambridge University Press, 1995), 73.
108   Ferngren, *Medicine and Religion*, 76–7.
109   Quoted in Amanda Porterfield, *Healing in the History of Christianity* (Oxford: Oxford University
       Press, 2005), 44.
110   Ibid., 53.
111   Quoted by Ferngren, *Medicine & Health Care in Early Christianity*, 107.
112   Porterfield, *Healing in the History of Christianity*, 21.
113   Quoted in Michel Mollat, *The Poor in the Middle Ages: An Essay in Social History* (New Haven:
       Yale University Press, 1986), 1.
114   Ferngren, *Medicine & Health Care in Early Christianity*, 121–2.
115   Ferngren, *Medicine and Religion*, 78–9; Henry E. Sigerist, *Medicine and Human Welfare* (New
       Haven: Yale University Press, 1941), 17.
116   Ferngren, *Medicine and Religion*, 79.
117   Quoted in Constantelos, *Byzantine Philanthropy and Social Welfare*, 12.
118   Nutton, "Medicine in Late Antiquity and the Early Middle Ages," 77.
119   Ferngren, *Medicine and Religion*, 84.
120   Ferngren, *Medicine & Health Care in Early Christianity*, 118–21.
121   Avalos, *Health Care and the Rise of Christianity*, 3, 15; Porterfield, *Healing in the History of
       Christianity*, 44; Ferngren, *Medicine & Health Care in Early Christianity*, 139.
122   Ferngren, *Medicine & Health Care in Early Christianity*, 124.
123   Mollat, *The Poor in the Middle Ages*, 146.
124   Constantelos, *Byzantine Philanthropy and Social Welfare*, 202–3.
125   These facts on poorhouses, *xenones*, *xenodocheia* and *nosokomeia* are all drawn from Ferngren,
       Medicine and Religion, 90–2.
126   These facts about Basileias are found in Ferngren, *Medicine & Health Care in Early Christianity*,
       124–7, quote on 126. Also, George Rosen, "The Hospital: Historical Sociology of a Community
       Institution," in *From Medical Police to Social Medicine: Essays on the History of Health Care*
       (New York: Science History Publications, 1974), 275–6.
127   Quoted in Constantelos, *Byzantine Philanthropy and Social Welfare*, 119.
128   Ibid., 135–6; Timothy S. Miller, *The Birth of the Hospital in the Byzantine Empire*, Johns
       Hopkins pbk. ed. (Baltimore: Johns Hopkins University Press, 1997), 13–21.
129   Rosen, "The Hospital: Historical Sociology of a Community Institution."
130   Colin Jones, *The Charitable Imperative: Hospitals and Nursing in Ancien Régime and
       Revolutionary France* (London: Routledge, 1989), 12.
131   Lawrence I. Conrad, "The Arab-Islamic Medical Tradition," in *The Western Medical Tradition:
       800 B.C.–1800 A.D* (Cambridge: Cambridge University Press, 2009), 135–6.
132   Ibid.
133   Ferngren, *Medicine and Religion*, 128–9.
134   Mollat, *The Poor in the Middle Ages*, 11.
135   Mollat states that it's difficult to have an accurate sense of the ratio of an area's population to
       the number of hospitals. He notes that in Iberia and in the south of France, the fact that there
       were many hospitals doesn't mean that many patients were actually treated. Ibid., 146–8.
136   A point by made by Rosen, "The Hospital: Historical Sociology of a Community Institution,"
       284. As Jones notes, this critique was made by a number of Enlightenment writers, including

Montesquieu and Condorcet. Colin Jones, "Picking up the Pieces: The Politics and Personnel of Social Welfare From the Convention to the Consulate," in *Beyond the Terror: Essays in French Regional and Social History, 1794–1815* (Cambridge: Cambridge University Press, 1983), 55.

137 Jones, *The Charitable Imperative*, 1.

138 Jones also sees a false dichotomy in the frequent contrast drawn between Christian charity and non-Christian apathy. Jonathan Barry and Colin Jones, "Introduction" in *Medicine and Charity before the Welfare State* (London; New York: Routledge, 1991), 2–3, 11; Colin Jones, "Charity before c. 1850," in *Companion Encyclopedia of the History of Medicine*, ed. W. F. Bynum and Roy Porter (London: Routledge, 1997), 1469–70.

139 Barry and Jones, "Introduction," in *Medicine and Charity before the Welfare State*, 2.

140 Ibid., 2–3.

141 The first point in this sentence—that the discourse around natural law and property contributed to conceptualizations of charity—derives from Tierney, whose book I am indebted to throughout this section. Brian Tierney, *Medieval Poor Law: A Sketch of Canonical Theory and Its Application in England* (Berkeley: University of California Press, 1959).

142 Kenneth Pennington, "Rights," in *The Oxford Handbook of the History of Political Philosophy*, ed. George Klosko (Oxford: Oxford University Press, 2013), 534–5. This title ("last scholar of the ancient world") is frequently used, for instance by Rens Bod, *A New History of the Humanities: The Search for Principles and Patterns from Antiquity to the Present* (Oxford: Oxford University Press, 2013), 103.

143 Quoted in Pennington, "Rights," 534.

144 Tuck, *Natural Rights Theories*, 18.

145 According to Pennington, nothing much happened in this regard between Isidore and Gratian. Pennington, "Rights," 535.

146 Tuck contends that the "first modern rights theory" arose from the efforts of jurists who began re-examining Roman law in the twelfth century. Jean Porter, "From Natural Law to Human Rights: Or, Why Rights Talk Matters," *Journal of Law and Religion* 14, no. 1 (1999–2000): 80; Tuck, *Natural Rights Theories*, 13.

147 Tierney, *Medieval Poor Law*, 7–8.

148 Ibid., 7–8, 16.

149 Ibid., 26–8.

150 Ibid., 26–7; Alan Ryan, *On Politics: A History of Political Thought from Herodotus to the Present* (New York: Liveright Pub. Corp., 2012), 2: 207–8.

151 Quoted in Tierney, *Medieval Poor Law*, 27.

152 Quoted in Pennington, "Rights," 537.

153 Tierney, *Medieval Poor Law*, 29–30.

154 Whereas previous writers had spoken of *ius* in an "objective" way (i.e. not belonging to a person, but instead meaning "the just thing"), Aquinas, according to John Finnis, used them also in a "subjective sense" (meaning something that a "subject" held). John M. Finnis, "Aquinas on Ius and Hart on Rights: A Response to Tierney," *The Review of Politics* 64, no. 03 (2002): 407–10.

155 Thomas Aquinas, "Summa Theologica," in *Basic Writings of Saint Thomas Aquinas* (New York: Random House, 1945), 780.

156 Tierney, *Medieval Poor Law*, 31–2.

157 This point is made by Hont and Ignatieff, which are also the source of the Aquinas quote. Istvan Hont and Michael Ignatieff, "Needs and Justice in the *Wealth of Nations*: An Introductory Essay," in *Wealth and Virtue: The Shaping of Political Economy in the Scottish Enlightenment* (Cambridge: Cambridge University Press, 1983), 26–7, Aquinas quoted on 27; Fleischacker, *A Short History of Distributive Justice*, 29.

158 Quoted in Tierney, *Medieval Poor Law*, 32.

159 Ibid., 33 and 35.

160 Ibid., 38.

161 S. J. Woolf, *The Poor in Western Europe in the Eighteenth and Nineteenth Centuries* (London; New York: Methuen, 1986), 39.

162 Pennington, "Rights," 537–8; Tierney, *Medieval Poor Law*, 37–8.

163 Quoted in Pennington, "Rights," 537–8.

164 Tierney, *Medieval Poor Law*, 36.

165 Ibid., 38, 125–7; Porter, "From Natural Law to Human Rights: Or, Why Rights Talk Matters," 87–8.

166 Again, the point about the connection between overall medieval charity and natural rights is that of Tierney.

167 Pennington, "Rights," 537.

168 A point Moyn makes about the absence of discussion of economic rights in Lynn Hunt's work on rights during the Enlightenment. Moyn, *The Last Utopia*, 247 n50.

169 "One of the most important effects of the Black Death," argues Robert Gottfried, "was its role in the provocation of popular rebellion . . ." Mollat, *The Poor in the Middle Ages*, 290–3; Jones, *The Charitable Imperative*, 3; Robert Steven Gottfried, *The Black Death: Natural and Human Disaster in Medieval Europe* (New York: Free Press; Collier Macmillan, 1983), 97–103, quote on 97; Derek Fraser, *The Evolution of the British Welfare State: A History of Social Policy since the Industrial Revolution*, 4th ed. (Basingstoke: Palgrave Macmillan, 2009), 38.

170 Wood notes that though it is true that some historians have cast doubt on the quantity of evictions that actually occurred in the sixteenth century, observers at the time (including the monarchy itself) certainly connected the Enclosure Acts with a growing class of dispossessed peasants. Ellen Meiksins Wood, *Liberty and Property: A Social History of Western Political Thought from Renaissance to Enlightenment* (London: Verso, 2012), 213; Tierney, *Medieval Poor Law*, 112–13.

171 Gaston V. Rimlinger, *Welfare Policy and Industrialization in Europe, America, and Russia* (New York: John Wiley and Sons, 1971), 13; Mollat, *The Poor in the Middle Ages*, 290–3; Tierney, *Medieval Poor Law*, 113.

172 Jones, "Charity before c. 1850," 1473; Mollat, *The Poor in the Middle Ages*, 290–3; Woolf, *The Poor in Western Europe in the Eighteenth and Nineteenth Centuries*, 18; Gilbert, Bentley B. Gilbert, *The Evolution of National Insurance in Great Britain: The Origins of the Welfare State* (London: Michael Joseph Ltd., 1966), 52.

173 Jones, *The Charitable Imperative*, 3; Mollat, *The Poor in the Middle Ages*, 291.

174 Mollat, *The Poor in the Middle Ages*, 266–71, 286.

175 Ibid., 266–71, quote on 271; Rosen, "The Hospital: Historical Sociology of a Community Institution," 284–5.

176 Fraser, *The Evolution of the British Welfare State*, 45.

177 E. M. Leonard, *The Early History of English Poor Relief* (New York: Barnes & Noble, 1965), 3–10.

178 Tierney, *Medieval Poor Law*, 131.

179 Leonard, *The Early History of English Poor Relief*, 294.

180 Tierney, *Medieval Poor Law*, 132.

181 Leonard, *The Early History of English Poor Relief*, 1.

182 T. H. Marshall, "Citizenship and Social Class," in *Citizenship and Social Class* (London: Pluto Press, 1992), 14–15

183 Quoted in George Rosen, "Medical Care and Social Policy in Seventeenth Century England," *Bulletin of the New York Academy of Medicine* 29, no. 5 (1953):159.

184 Ibid., 179.

185 Ibid., 170.

186 Christopher Hamlin, *Public Health and Social Justice in the Age of Chadwick: Britain, 1800–1854* (Cambridge: Cambridge University Press, 1998), 20.

187 Leonard, *The Early History of English Poor Relief*, 9; Fraser, *The Evolution of the British Welfare State*, 38–40.

188 Quoted in Rimlinger, *Welfare Policy and Industrialization in Europe, America, and Russia*, 18.

189 The facts about Cooke in this paragraph are from Geoffrey Robertson, "England's Bravest Barrister," *Counsel*, September 2005; Geoffrey Robertson, Introduction to *The Levellers: The Putney Debates* (London: Verso Books, 2007), xxviii.

190 Robertson, "England's Bravest Barrister," 25.

191   Robertson, "Introduction" in *The Putney Debates: The Levellers*, xv.

192   Sabine, *A History of Political Theory*, 487–8.

193   An overall point discussed by Richard A. Gleissner, "The Levellers and Natural Law: The Putney Debates of 1647," *Journal of British Studies* 20, no. 1 (1980): 74–89. See also Sabine, *A History of Political Theory*, 484.

194   "The Institutes 535 CE," *The Medieval Sourcebook.*

195   Quoted in Gleissner, "The Levellers and Natural Law: The Putney Debates of 1647," 75.

196   Sabine, *A History of Political Theory*, 491.

197   George Rosen, "Left-Wing Puritanism and Science," *Bulletin of the Institute of the History of Medicine* 15 (1944): 375–80.

198   His spelling has been modernized. Gerrard Winstanley, "The Law of Freedom in a Platform," in *The Law of Freedom and Other Writings*, ed. Christopher Hill (Harmondsworth: Penguin, 1973), 387. Rosen discusses Winstanley's ideas about the promotion of science in this book. Rosen, "Left-Wing Puritanism and Science," 375–80.

199   Both the facts here and the quote from Hartlib are drawn from George Rosen, *From Medical Police to Social Medicine: Essays on the History of Health Care*, 1st ed. (New York: Science History Publications, 1974), 160–1.

200   Other writers have pointed to Cooke's proposal of a system of free healthcare for the poor, and I have followed their lead to him and his work, including ibid., 161; Robertson, "England's Bravest Barrister," 25. I have modernized Cooke's spelling.

201   His spelling has been modernized. John Cook, *Unum Necessarium* (London: Printed for Matthew Walbancke at Grayes Inne Gate, 1648), accessed December 17, 2015, http://gateway.proquest.com.ezp-prod1.hul.harvard.edu/openurl?ctx_ver=Z39.88-2003&res_id=xri:eebo&rft_id=xri:eebo:citation:99864028, 13.

202   His spelling, punctuation, and capitalization has been modernized. Ibid., 3.

203   His spelling, punctuation, and capitalization have been modernized. Ibid., 61.

204   Ibid., 64.

205   His spelling has been modernized. Ibid., 61.

206   Ibid.

207   Robertson, "England's Bravest Barrister," 25.

208   George Rosen, "Economic and Social Policy in the Development of Public Health," *Journal of the History of Medicine and Allied Sciences* 8, no. 4 (1953): 178–9.

209   His spelling and capitalization have been modernized. William Sir Petty, "The Advice of W.P. To Mr. Samuel Hartlib for the Advancement of Some Particular Parts of Learning" (London: [s.n.], 1648), accessed 2015, http://gateway.proquest.com.ezp-prod1.hul.harvard.edu/openurl?ctx_ver=Z39.88-2003&res_id=xri:eebo&rft_id=xri:eebo:citation:13292085, 9. I owe this citation to Rosen. Rosen, "Economic and Social Policy in the Development of Public Health," 180–1.

210   His spelling has been modernized. Samuel Herring, "Original Letters and Papers of State, Addressed to Oliver Cromwell" (London: Printed by William Bowyer, and sold by John Whiston bookseller, at Boyle's Head in Fleet-Street, 1743), http://hollis.harvard.edu/primo_library/libweb/action/dlDisplay.do?vid=HVD&search_scope=default_scope&docId=HVD_ALEPH012273696&fn=permalink, 100–1. I followed Christopher Hill's lead to Herring and these specific passages; Hill wrote that Herring "demanded a free national health service." Christopher Hill, *The World Turned Upside Down: Radical Ideas During the English Revolution* (Harmondsworth: Penguin, 1991), 298.

211   His spelling has been modernized. Ibid., 101.

212   George Rosen, "An Eighteenth Century Plan for a National Health Service," *Bulletin of the History of Medicine* 16, no. 5 (1944), 430.

213   Margaret James, *Social Problems and Policy During the Puritan Revolution, 1640–1660* (New York: Barnes & Noble, 1966), 340.

214   This is the title of an article by George Rosen, in which he discusses and quotes extensively from John Bellers' *ESSAY Towards the IMPROVEMENT of PHYSICK . . .* In this section, I turn towards Bellers' *Essay*, which was reprinted in 1935. However, I am indebted to Rosen, whose article

directed me to Bellers' work. Rosen, "An Eighteenth Century Plan for a National Health Service"; John Bellers, "An Essay Towards the Improvement of Physick . . ." in *John Bellers, 1654–1725: Quaker, Economist and Social Reformer* (London: Cassell and company, 1935), 109–43.

215   His spelling and capitalization have been modernized. Bellers, "An Essay Towards the Improvement of Physick . . .", 110.

216   His spelling and capitalization have been modernized. Ibid., 111

217   Modernization as above. Ibid., 112.

218   As above. Ibid., 114.

219   As above. Ibid., 116.

220   Rosen, "An Eighteenth Century Plan for a National Health Service," 436; Bellers, "An Essay Towards the Improvement of Physick . . .", 114–18.

221   His capitalization has been modernized. Bellers, "An Essay Towards the Improvement of Physick . . .", 134.

222   Robertson, "Introduction" in *The Putney Debates: The Levellers*, xxix–xxxii.

223   James, *Social Problems and Policy During the Puritan Revolution, 1640–1660*, 301–2.

224   Christopher Hill, *The Century of Revolution, 1603–1714* (New York: Norton, 1982), 128; Christopher Hill, *The World Turned Upside Down*, 13.

225   Health economist Gavin Mooney sees at least two problems with treating healthcare as just another market commodity: it ignores the impact or benefit of healthcare for communities, and it ignores benefits of healthcare outside its impact on health alone. Gavin H. Mooney, *The Health of Nations: Towards a New Political Economy* (London; New York: Zed Books, 2012), 41–2.

2
Enlightenment and Revolution
The Rights—and the Health—of Man

In 1793, the political tides turned against the Marquis de Condorcet, a French mathematician, philosopher, and politician who ran afoul of the insurgent Jacobins during the heady, radicalized days of the French Revolution. Fearing for his life, Condorcet fled to avoid arrest, and managed to remain safe in hiding for some months. Though he was sick, desperate, and betrayed—the ominous rise and fall of the guillotine was spreading throughout the nation—Condorcet nonetheless chose (at the urging of his wife) to pursue a book of fantastic optimism, his famous *Sketch for a Historical Picture of the Progress of the Human Mind*, with his few remaining days.[1] Condorcet's reflections on equality, human welfare, and the endless possibilities of medicine in the final section of this book say a great deal about how far ideas about human rights and health had come during the course of the Enlightenment.

For though the philosophers of the French Enlightenment may not have invented the concept of "inalienable rights," they were—by and large—the "first to make a real moral gospel of this idea and to embrace it passionately," as the philosopher Ernst Cassirer puts it.[2] The "natural rights" thought of in earlier centuries did not necessarily reject slavery, much less economic injustices or the repression of women. Condorcet, in contrast, minced no words in condemning with appropriate acidity the injustices of racial inequality, religious intolerance, and the "inequality of rights between the sexes."[3] In his *Sketch*, he called for the elimination of inequality among nations and the attenuation of inequality within nations.[4] To accomplish the latter, he proposed "greater equality of education" together with a system of social security (including provisions for the elderly, widows, and children) to attenuate inequalities of wealth.[5] Rights and equality, for Condorcet, were not confined to the narrow civil realm: they had unambiguous social and economic consequences. But with respect to medical care and health, his optimism about the future became even more heroic.

Condorcet argued that with some combination of preventative healthcare, better nutrition, healthier housing, the elimination of both "misery and excessive wealth," and the progress of medical science, disease could ultimately be eliminated, the "human species might be capable of indefinite progress," and the human lifespan would trend towards infinity.[6] One might question whether that would be a positive, possible, or sustainable goal, but the optimism of his vision is nonetheless striking. And though Condorcet was a unique individual, for many others during the Enlightenment (and especially during this age of revolution), "natural rights" would come to have increasingly egalitarian implications.

In his article on "Natural Liberty" in the *Encyclopédie*, for instance, Louis de Jaucourt restated the age-old notion (traceable back to Roman law) that "naturally all men are born free." Yet unlike the natural law theorists of earlier periods, he saw this as necessitating a genuine anti-slavery ethos; indeed, he criticized the Christian nations that, "independent of natural law," had enslaved Africans for use in their fields and mines.[7] In 1770, the French writer Abbé Raynal published a history of European colonialism that tore apart Europe's despicable regime of slavery; indeed it even forecast a slave revolution (which prompted the author's exile).[8] Jacques-Pierre Brissot de Warville, who later founded France's first abolitionist society (and who, like Condorcet, was persecuted by the Jacobins), argued that the nation's judicial system brutally violated the "sacred rights" of humanity.[9] Furthermore, by the end of the eighteenth century, men and women spoke unambiguously not only of rights *from* oppression and injustice, but also of rights *to* social and economic goods, including healthcare. While the 1789 *Declaration of the Rights of Man*, for instance, did not include any such rights in its articles, some explicitly contended that it *should*.[10] Indeed, during the French Revolution, systems of social welfare and universal healthcare were not only advocated, but in some cases pursued.

Yet if the egalitarian ambition of the era remains impressive, and perhaps even inspiring, its ramifications were far more problematic, and its legacy more complex. Still, if we are to accept the notion that the Enlightenment in some sense bequeathed the human right to modern times (as some but not all contend), then so too must its legacy be said to envelop the notion of the socioeconomic right—inclusive, perhaps, of the right to healthcare.

The Reform of Man, Health, and Hospital

Now, overly ambitious proposals for the perfection of mankind were, to some extent, standard Enlightenment fare. However, more concrete, explicit ideas about social welfare were prominent in the literature of pre-Revolution France, including an explicit articulation of the state's responsibility for the *health* and *healthcare* of its citizens.[11] Montesquieu, for instance, in his *Spirit of the Laws* contended that "alms given to a naked man in the street do not fulfill the obligations of the state, which owes all its citizens an assured existence, food, proper clothing, and a mode of life not incompatible with health," and also that "the state is often obliged to provide for the needs of the aged, the sick and the orphans."[12] François de la Mothe-Fénelon (1651–1751), meanwhile, proposed a system of public welfare for the ill and unemployed.[13] Similarly, the Abbé de Saint-Pierre (1658–1743), famous for his proposal for an international peace organization, argued that the poor had a right to aid from the state.[14] Contributors to that epitome of Enlightenment intellectual production—the *Encyclopédie* of Denis Diderot and Jean le Rond d'Alembert—similarly proposed the expansion of social welfare. An article on

"Jurisprudence," for instance, concludes with an affirmation of the state's responsibility to hospitalize the poor and aid the "deserving poor."[15]

Another Frenchman concerned with healthcare was the philanthropist Claude Humbert Piarron de Chamousset (1717–1773), who was also known for his plans for Paris's postal system. In his *Plan d'une maison d'association*, Chamousset proposed a system of health *insurance*, as part of a more comprehensive welfare system, in which those who are well pay for the healthcare of those who are sick through regular insurance contributions. He suggested that such a system would be especially important for those not poor enough to receive free charitable care, but not sufficiently wealthy to be able to purchase medical care in their homes.[16] Chamousset's proposal was particularly novel in that it was the insurance *contribution* that created the *obligation* to receive care.[17]

Yet other thinkers, writing in a utopian genre influenced by such British works as Thomas More's *Utopia*, were even more ambitious, advocating approaches to expanding the poor's access to assistance and healthcare in an even more universal direction.[18] The utopias that these writers envisioned, in many instances, included provisions either for healthcare for the poor or for truly universal medical care for all. These societies ranged from social welfare states to communist republics. In *The Year 2440*, Louis Sebastian Mercier (1740–1814), a writer who—like Condorcet and Brissot—became a Girondin politician during the Revolution, envisaged a futuristic utopia in France in which a progressive system of education and medical care was available to all citizens.[19] Healthcare is described as a right: "Every man has a right to call in their [physicians'] aid; all their glory consists in recalling the bloom of health; and, if the unfortunate patient cannot produce an adequate salary, which is very rare, government takes the expense upon itself."[20] Hospitals, in this utopia, will have been greatly humanized, and "the poor sick have now no other calamities to endure but those imposed on them by nature," and they also "have the attendance of physicians, eminent for their charity as for their skill. . . . By this means health is restored under their humane services . . ."[21]

But perhaps the early French utopian thinker with the greatest impact on posterity was Morelly, an eighteenth-century figure about whom very little is known (e.g., either his birthplace or his first name).[22] In his 1755 *Code de la Nature*, Morelly set forth a utopian scheme for a socialistic society, including provisions for healthcare for all citizens.[23] In his proposed utopian cities, "a spacious and commodious building will be put up on the most healthful site," in which "any sick Citizen will find lodging and care."[24] Another building will serve as "a comfortable shelter for all infirm and decrepit Citizens" who will "be comfortably lodged, fed, and maintained . . ."[25] What is striking here is that Morelly is proposing not a system of healthcare for the *poor*, but instead a single system of public, universal, and—importantly—*equal* healthcare for all: "All sick Citizens," he describes, "without exception . . . will be cared for with the same meticulousness and cleanliness as in the bosom of their Families, and without distinction or preference."[26] As will be argued in Chapter 6, a notable feature of some post-Second World War universal health systems was exactly this configuration towards healthcare *equality*. But additionally, for Morelly, the government of each town would be "concerned with proper management and service in these houses, and will see to it that they are not wanting in anything necessary or agreeable, whether for the restoration of health, the progress of convalescence, or finally to while away the tedium of infirmity."[27]

The progressive healthcare spirit of the era, however, was manifest not only in the realm of ideas, but also in the more practical work of those who sought to improve the *quality* of healthcare for the poor. After all, some of the hospitals of this era were awful institutions, relied upon by the sick poor who often had no other recourse.[28] Many of these institutions were viewed as death traps—and particularly dirty, crowded, and miserable ones. In the *Encyclopédie*, for instance, Diderot describes the Hôtel-Dieu, the largest of Paris' hospitals, rather horrifically, with patients "packed three, four, five, or six into a bed, the living alongside the dead and dying, the air polluted by this mass of sick bodies, passing the pestilential germs of their afflictions from one to the other, and the spectacle of suffering and agony on every hand."[29] But in the decade before the French Revolution, reformers sought to raise the quality of these charitable institutions, culminating most notably in an ambitious proposal to reconstruct the Hôtel-Dieu, which was partly destroyed by a fire in 1772.[30] Louis XIV was eventually convinced—in part through the influence of Condorcet—to invite the Academy of Science to name a commission to study the reform of this ancient institution.[31] The commission relied greatly on the ophthalmologist Jacques Tenon—who both contributed to its official reports and published his own highly detailed observations in a book, *Memoirs on Paris Hospitals*—together with a number of other illustrious intellectuals.[32]

Tenon's writing not only detailed what hospital care in France looked like at the time, but also presented an Enlightenment picture of how, practically speaking, it *might* look.[33] His *Memoirs* proved highly influential, and became a source for the work of the Committee on Mendicity (which will be examined shortly), the body charged with public assistance and medical reform during the French Revolution.[34] Like Diderot, Tenon emphasized the contemptible crowding of the indigent, which in the preface to *Memoirs* he calls "a monstrous arrangement, more suitable for prolonging diseases" that would "destroy rather than restore and preserve health."[35] He found the hospital's maternity care to be particularly atrocious: according to his figures, while maternal mortality in childbirth approximated 1 percent in Dublin hospitals and 2 percent at a British hospital, it was around a startling 7 percent in the Hôtel-Dieu.[36] In one instance, he invoked the language of rights in his condemnation of this state of affairs: "The state to which women are condemned is even worse than that of the men," he wrote, adding that "women have a right to the same assistance as men, and we propose that this be provided in the new hospitals."[37]

It should be noted, however, that Tenon was in no way dismissive of the hospital's underlying mission. Indeed, in the first sentence of his *Memoirs*, he notes one praiseworthy and unique aspect of the Hôtel-Dieu: its provision of *universal* (in an almost literal sense) healthcare. The Hôtel-Dieu, in his words,

[A]dmits anyone at any time, regardless of age, sex, country, or religion; patients with fevers, injuries, contagious and noncontagious diseases, the insane susceptible to treatment, pregnant women and girls, are all admitted: it is, therefore, the hospital for the poor and sick, not only from Paris and France, but from the rest of the universe. Its doors, like the arms of Providence, are always open for those who seek refuge. . . . It is therefore a town rather than a hospital . . . a capital where all persons have right of asylum and are received as citizens of the same country, as children of the same family: it is the sanctuary of humanity.[38]

The commission (and Tenon) argued for the hospital to be replaced with four smaller hospitals, constructed to meet the needs of the individual patient, which could serve the nation's poor with dignity.[39] Large hospitals had a public mission, and thus were to be run by the government.[40] Tenon diverged from the commission by additionally proposing the construction of a health center in the middle of Paris that would include a hospital, an emergency room, and an ambulatory care facility to help the poor avoid unnecessary hospitalization.[41] He also argued that the number of hospitals should be proportional to the *per capita* number of sick and poor in a given municipality.[42] More broadly, Tenon and the commission sought to transform the hospital away from its religious and hierarchical medieval roots into a humane, secular, and modern institution: "As a public and secular house of healing, available to all men with health needs, the hospital's confessional, charitable, punitive quality was irrelevant. . . . Each was entitled equally to basic right of life, dignity, and the enjoyment of health . . ."[43] These reforms revolutionized how patients were viewed—from the hospitalized pauper to what historian Dora Weiner has called the dignified, empowered "citizen-patient" in her important examination on this era.[44]

Tenon was hopeful that reform was not a mere pipe dream: reason, he argued, had made governments "more attentive to the pressing needs of the sick and destitute" and philosophers more aware of the "incontestable rights of humanity."[45] However, while hospital trustees forestalled reform, world-historic events were unfolding on the national stage.[46] The year that the hospital commission filed its third and final report—1788—was a time of worsening economic and political crisis in France.[47] The French Revolution was about to change the course of history in a manner we grapple with still. And though Tenon's proposals fell by the wayside, his egalitarian hopes—in which the state took responsibility for the health of the poor—was revived in the wake of the Revolution.

Human Rights and Revolution

In the Enlightenment and over the course of the American, French, and Haitian Revolution, the meaning of natural rights—and, following its use in Rousseau's *Social Contract*, the so-called "rights of man"—underwent a historical transformation.[48] They were both (1) universalized/globalized (to an extent), and they

(2) came to explicitly include socioeconomic goods. With respect to the first phenomenon, in the early days of the American Revolution, a particular and local concept of "British freedom," or of the rights of the "freeborn Englishman," was the predominant concern; however, over the course of the war, "rights" were (at least in theory) increasingly contextualized as universal, and as pertaining to all *equally*.[49] The English-born Thomas Paine, for instance, most famously universalized rights in championing the cause of American independence.[50] The American cause, he noted, was "in a great measure the cause of all mankind," and it was waged against an enemy that was "declaring War against the *natural rights of all Mankind*. . ." (emphasis added).[51] (Of course, despite the grandiose language of universality, much of the population was excluded from enjoying even the most basic of human rights: the institution of slavery was not merely preserved, but in fact tragically *reinforced* by the Revolution.)[52] Revolutionaries in France also drew on the language of universal rights. "Men are born and remain free and equal in rights," the Declaration of the Rights of Man and Citizen stated, with the purpose of government amounting to nothing less than the "preservation of the natural and imprescriptible rights of man."[53] Later, the convergence of a powerful and historic Haitian slave revolt with radical ideas about the "rights of man" in France culminated in the revolutionary Jacobin decree of 1794 that abolished slavery in the French colonies.[54] But the revolutionary period also saw the development of the idea of the *socioeconomic right,* and is thus a moment of significant consequence in the history of the right to healthcare.

That was not the intention of the majority of the Revolution's makers, of course, for whom the rights of property were among the most sacred of rights (duly enshrined in the *Declaration of the Rights of Man*). However, changing political fortunes let loose dormant demands for social and economic change, as the already adverse situation of the French people had rapidly deteriorated in the years before the Revolution, and with traditional forms of charity recognized as inadequate.[55] Understandably, for the poor of France, livelihood—mere survival—was likely the greater concern than aspirations about theoretical natural rights. For instance, in advance of the meeting of the Estates-General in May 1789, electoral assemblies created delineations of specific grievances, or *cahier de doléances*, that gave voice to popular economic concerns, including demands for assistance and work for the poor.[56] One *cahier*, for instance, asked that the Estates-General set up a system of public assistance for the poor in the constitution.[57] Stephen P. Marks notes that a declaration of rights included in the *cahier de doléance* submitted by the commune of Nemours included a heavy emphasis on social and economic rights, ranging from assistance to the disabled to public education.[58] "[A]lthough the Declaration of 1789 limits its concern with equality to matters of taxation and property," he concludes, "the concerns of a more socially democratic approach to equality as social justice were voiced, and might have found expression in the text had more time been spent on it."[59]

An even more explicit (and enormously more influential) declaration of socioeconomic rights was famously made during these years by Thomas Paine, who had re-emerged on the world stage after returning to Great Britain following the victory of the American Revolution. In the second part of his *Rights of Man* (penned in response to Edmund Burke's condemnatory 1790 *Reflections on the Revolution in France*), Paine moved in a new (and very popular) direction. Paine essentially proposed a comprehensive system of social assistance, explicitly drawing on the language and concept of *rights*. Poor families, he argued, should receive government support for each young child.[60] Among the aged, the needy—who, he notes, were often forced to work until their death—also deserved a system of aid, and so should receive a pension beginning at age 50.[61] This aid, he importantly noted, "*is not of the nature of a charity, but of a right*" (emphasis added).[62] Additional aid should be made available for the education costs of children, insofar as "a nation under a well-regulated Government should permit none to remain uninstructed."[63] Sums should also be granted to women following the birth of a child as well as to couples following marriage.[64] The government also needed to create a system of employment for the urban poor, and a progressive system of estate taxation that could help fund such measures.[65]

Of course, many others had previously put forth proposals before for social welfare, governmental programs, and assistance for the poor: part of what made Paine's points original was that he grounded them in the theory of *natural rights* (or rather, the "rights of man"). As he later wrote in his pamphlet *Agrarian Justice*, "In advocating the case of the persons thus dispossessed, it is a right and not a charity that I am pleading for."[66] Paine's *Rights of Man* would have a tremendous influence in coming years. In Great Britain, over the year following its publication, some 200,000 copies of the second part of the *Rights of Man* were sold.[67] "[T]he success of the Second Part was phenomenal," notes historian E. P. Thompson. Indeed, "Paine, in this chapter, set a course towards the social legislation of the 20th century."[68] Unsurprisingly, Paine's radical arguments, particularly coming from a man who a decade earlier had helped provoke the American Revolution, displeased many. He was burned in effigy and summoned before the court; with authorities rapidly closing in, he fled to France, where he had been given honorary citizenship and indeed elected to the National Convention.[69]

Just as Paine's *Rights of Man* was inflaming readers throughout England, unfolding events in France seemed to make possible—if only fleetingly—some of his proposals. The era of possibilities, however, was to prove short-lived, with the aims of reformers soon subordinated to the demands of total war and the dictates of the Terror.

The French Revolution: Healthcare and the Rights of Man

In July 1789, the National Constituent Assembly assumed power in France. It was not long before it had to address the problem of poverty.[70] In late December 1789, a deputy from the Paris Commune made the case to the National Constituent Assembly that deputies must address the problem of the poor: "They are no longer serfs," stated Pierre-François Boncerf of the Society of Agriculture, "but what have they gained? If they are no longer bound to the soil; if they are no longer chattels of a master who, whatever else he might be, at least had an interest in their survival;

if they are free, and hence citizens, what use to them is that fine title, that apparent liberty?"[71] Along similar lines, Fretéau de Saint-Just and Jean-François Lambert asserted that the Assembly should draw on the principles of the Declaration of the Rights of Man and Citizen and create a committee that would provide assistance to those who lacked property.[72] The following month, the Assembly responded to the advice of the deputy François Alexandre Frédéric, duc de la Rochefoucauld-Liancourt, to appoint a "Committee on Mendicity" to address the issue of "beggary."[73] Many members appointed to this body, which was chaired by Liancourt, were involved in the charity debate of the preceding two decades.[74]

The work of the Committee on Mendicity, which extended throughout the period of the National Constituent Assembly, has been described as "the first . . . to recognize the reality of a social dimension in the French Revolution."[75] The Committee's proposals, scholars suggest, were radical, and seemed to rest on an implicit philosophical claim that the natural rights of humankind included socioeconomic rights. Charity would not suffice as a cure to poverty, for poverty was the result of the economic system itself; aid, therefore, should be given as a right.[76] Liancourt contended that everyone had one important socioeconomic right: *le droit à la subsistence*, or the "right to subsistence," which he contended deserved a spot in the Declaration of the Rights of Man.[77] He argued, some note, that it was the task of France to include the rights of the poor in its constitution—rights that no other state had yet recognized.[78] With respect to healthcare, the Committee seems to have been influenced by the ideas of pre-Revolutionary thinkers like Tenon; Liancourt, for instance, wrote to Tenon in June 1790 to request his *Memoirs on the Paris Hospital.*[79]

The proposals of Liancourt's Committee on Mendicity seem bold. Some argue that had the nation actually achieved them, France would have gained during these years a system of public assistance, including relief for the poor, disabled, and elderly together with a public healthcare system.[80] Medical care would have been made available for free to the sick poor (preferably in their home), and would have been delivered by a publicly-paid physician assigned to each rural district or town.[81] Municipalities with more than 4,000 people would be required to have general hospitals, while the largest cities would also have specialty hospitals.[82] All French people would have equitable access to hospital care, which would be publicly-financed.[83] Such proposals for public healthcare can be seen as a sharp turn within the healthcare rights-commodity dialectic—in the realm of ideas, if not practice. As the historian Lisa DiCaprio concludes, the Committee's proposals "were equivalent to a plan for a national health care service that presumed the right of the indigent to free medical treatment either at home or in a hospital."[84]

The Constituent Assembly also created a Health Committee, consisting of physician deputies.[85] The Health Committee accepted as the essential basis for its proposals the *New Plan for French Medicine* (drafted by the Royal Society) that dealt with various issues relating to medical education, practice, and research, but which also addressed the problem of providing healthcare for the whole nation.[86] To provide such care, the *New Plan* proposed a system of public doctors, who were to be educated and salaried at government expense, and who would provide free care for the poor and also have a number of public health duties.[87] The Health Committee's Draft Legislation stated that: "Each canton shall provide for a physician who shall care for poor patients in their homes free of charge . . . These doctors shall provide care to all those families. The doctors shall visit the sick in their homes as soon as asked or informed and treat their infirmities, illnesses or wounds."[88] Weiner calls the proposals of the Committee of Mendicity and the Health Committee "complementary," noting that together they constituted a "national health-care network."[89]

Yet, however sweeping such proposals may sound, the actual achievements of the Committee on Mendicity and the Health Committee were minimal, scholars suggest. The Committee of Mendicity was supposed to not only devise a new system of social assistance for the nation, but also manage the nation's existing charitable support system, including its hospitals, which had lost many of their traditional sources of funding.[90] The state, meanwhile, had many competing priorities for its funds—soon to include seemingly endless war.[91] While the Constituent Assembly did manage to implement a system of workshops for the unemployed, it largely ignored the Committee on Mendicity's other proposals.[92] By the time of its dissolution in September 1791, the Constituent Assembly had acted on essentially none of either committee's proposals due to inadequate funds.[93] The Constituent Assembly was replaced by the Legislative Assembly, which had a "Committee of Public Assistance" in place of both; however, it had to deal with the burden of responding to rising requests for poor aid that were coming in from around the country.[94] Additionally, by nationalizing church property, the Revolution had undercut an independent source of funding for the Church-supported hospitals, but failed to adequately replace it.[95]

In any event, time was running short: a new more radical stage of the French Revolution was about to begin.[96] This would have a complex impact on social welfare, and healthcare, in the young Republic.

Social Rights in the Jacobin Endgame

The National Convention, which came to power in September of 1792, soon declared the end of the monarchy and the beginning of the first French Republic. Yet although the subsequent Jacobin era is linked in the minds of many predominantly with the Reign of Terror, it also deserves credit for practical (if short-lived) efforts to expand social welfare, including healthcare: "[T]he egalitarian agenda of the Jacobin phase of revolution was not fatally locked within an inevitable spiral of violence or bound to generate a police state mentality," historian Jean-Pierre Gross has argued; instead, "some imaginative political initiatives . . . were bent on achieving social harmony by peaceful and lawful means and in some instances actually succeeded in doing so."[97]

While disentangling these strands of Jacobinism may seem morally fraught, a genuine egalitarian ethos does seem to have pervaded the ideas, proposals, and plans of many Jacobins, though this was an ethos (to a degree) shared by many Girondins as well, which Gross makes clear. The Declaration of the Rights of the

Man of 1793 is a case in point. Following the dissolution of the monarchy, a drafting committee—chaired by Condorcet and including Thomas Paine—convened to draft a new Constitution and Declaration of Rights.[98] The final version of that Declaration was heavily based on Condorcet's draft.[99] Though the 1793 Declaration retained strongly worded political rights, it is perhaps most notable for its bold proclamation of new socioeconomic rights, which had been absent in the 1789 Declaration.[100] According to the Declaration, "[p]ublic relief is a sacred debt" that requires the provision of either work or welfare to "unfortunate citizens." Additionally, "[e]ducation is needed by all," and so should be put "at the door of every citizen."[101] This explicit inclusion of socioeconomic rights was a historical milestone.

Moreover, the National Convention pursued a number of social welfare programs and policies from 1793 to 1794. In March and June of 1793 it passed laws funding poor relief, healthcare, and work (albeit while also making begging illegal).[102] A decree passed in June 1793 proposed to provide the services of physicians, nurses, midwives, and apothecaries to the sick poor.[103] The Jacobins pursued a variety of local and concrete social welfare projects, including a program that provided for free healthcare for armaments workers (along with pay for sick leave and disability and death benefits).[104] They also apparently made attempts to improve hospital quality.[105] The following year, they passed a law which created a system of pensions that would be provided to certain categories of the rural poor as well as to fund the salaries of three "health officers" per district who would deliver healthcare to these individuals.[106] Other Jacobin social welfare projects (of varied scale and success) included the division and distribution of the land of the émigrés, an "egalitarian food policy," and the founding of primary schools in some districts.[107]

No doubt there was a real egalitarian impulse behind such policies and laws, but their actual impact was much more limited. "Decree after decree proclaimed the eradication of mendacity and the end of chronic deprivation," notes Gross, "and ever larger appropriations were ear-marked with seemingly reckless abandon for poor relief . . . all to no lasting effect."[108] As the historian William Doyle notes, such reforms would have been extraordinarily difficult even in the "best of times."[109] In contrast, this was a moment when France was engaged in total war with most of its neighbors, while at the same time suppressing internal revolt. Perhaps not surprisingly, these underfunded social welfare measures played second fiddle to France's more bellicose priorities.[110] In some instances, the Jacobins did positive harm: for instance, when they nationalized hospitals in July 1794 without having the resources to maintain them.[111] More darkly, the onset of the Reign of Terror in September 1793 provoked divisions that took thousands of lives and spelled the end of this egalitarian agenda altogether. Despite his radicalism, Paine was himself arrested and imprisoned, narrowly escaping death only as the result of an errantly placed chalk mark.[112] Condorcet, meanwhile, was forced into hiding; caught and captured, the genius was soon found dead in his prison cell.[113]

The end of the Terror did not mean, however, a return to ambitious social welfare plans.[114] On the contrary, Revolutionary systems of public assistance—

however inadequate and unfunded—simply "sank without a trace," in the words of Jones, leaving essentially nothing in their wake.[115] Nor would they re-emerge. And while an effort was made to restore the charity of the old institutions, no real effort was undertaken to harmonize these efforts in a national, systematic manner.[116] Although some municipal programs persevered, the Thermidorian government instead "relied primarily on political repression rather than redistribution of wealth to address the desperate demands of the indigent."[117]

Conclusions

The idea of the socioeconomic right—including the right to healthcare—might be seen by some as an extrapolation, expansion, or perhaps distortion of the classic Enlightenment rights to life, liberty, and property. This view is false. As reviewed in this chapter, many thinkers argued that the Enlightenment principles of equality and the "rights of man" could, and should, be applied to problems of social policy. The civil-political right and the socioeconomic right share a common genetic origin; indeed, they might be seen as the paired strands of a single intellectual-historical double helix. This is nowhere better seen than in the single most influential human rights text of the era: Thomas Paine's *Rights of Man*, which dealt with both the political and socioeconomic rights of humankind.

But moving past Enlightenment thought, what overall verdict should be drawn of the French Revolution's actual impact on human welfare, and on the healthcare rights-commodity dialectic? Historians remain divided. Doyle's conclusion in his general history of the Revolution is damning. Nobody, he argued, "suffered more than the poor and the sick . . . from the blind destruction of established institutions before viable alternatives had been devised and funded. In no sphere was more human damage done by the French revolutionaries' failure to match rhetoric with reality."[118] Rosen, less bleakly, credits the Revolution with establishing the legal principle of assistance and for seeking to set up a nationwide system of relief that included healthcare.[119] Alan Forrest asserts that the Committee of Mendicity aimed to transform social provision from a charity to " a basic human right, a debt owed by the nation to its citizens," and more generally calls the Revolutionary efforts "a most imaginative experiment in public welfare provision . . ."[120] Colin Jones, while emphasizing the Revolution's disastrous impact on existing systems of charity and healthcare, acknowledges its importance in the field of ideas.[121] Gross faults fiscal disarray, the competing demands of war, and the Thermidorean reaction for cutting short the promise of "Jacobin egalitarianism."[122] DiCaprio draws an enthusiastic connection between this era and the success of the French post-Second World War welfare state, which she calls "a reassertion of revolutionary social welfare principles . . ."[123] Weiner takes an even longer, more optimistic view, crediting the reformers for creating a goal for future generations: "*the declaration of the citizen's right to healthcare* set a target toward which our societies have striven since the French Revolution" (emphasis added).[124] From this more positive perspective, the Revolution indeed constituted an important shift in the healthcare rights-commodity dialectic.

There is, to some extent, less difference than there might seem between these arguments. The proposals of the Revolutionaries were in some instances grandiose and impractical, but in other instances reasonable and achievable. Some individuals were likely aided, but the undercutting of existing charity no doubt harmed many more. A portion of the shortcomings were the fault of the reformers, though some were the consequence of larger events and foreign forces. But at the same time, is the gap between revolutionary reality and rhetoric really that much greater in the case of socioeconomic rights as it is in the case of the political rights that were declared during this era? On the other side of the Atlantic, for instance, it was proclaimed that all men were created equal, yet the profound barbarity of slavery not only endured, but was enshrined in the new nation's institutions.[125] This historical reality does not render the idea of equality meaningless. In the sphere of philosophy and example, the Revolution did achieve something great: it advanced the ideal that all humans had rights—not only of life itself, but also of a life happy, healthy, wise, and free—a dream which has surfaced time and time again, sometimes resurgent, sometimes in retreat, to the present day.[126]

Of course, such soaring aspirations had little meaning for most. "How consoling for the philosopher who laments the errors, the crimes, the injustices which still pollute the earth and of which he is often the victim is this view of the human race, emancipated from its shackles," noted Condorcet in his final work, soon before his own capture and death. "Such contemplation is for him an asylum . . . [T]here he lives in thought with man restored to his natural rights and dignity . . ."[127] Yet such contemplation was presumably less inspiring for the great mass of the sick and the poor, whose rights were still neglected by a society that nonetheless proclaimed them so powerfully.

Notes

1   These details on Condorcet are drawn from Keith Michael Baker, "Introduction" in *Condorcet: Selected Writings*, 1st ed. (Indianapolis: Bobbs-Merrill, 1976), xxxiii–xxxv. Of note, I use the phrase "The Rights—and the Health—of Man" in the title instead of a gender-neutral term because I am referencing the "rights of man."

2   Ernst Cassirer, *The Philosophy of the Enlightenment* (Princeton, NJ: Princeton University Press, 2009), 250.

3   Marie-Jean-Antoine Nicolas Caritat de Condorcet, "Sketch for a Historical Picture of the Progress of the Human Mind," in *Condorcet: Selected Writings* (Indianapolis: Bobbs-Merrill, 1976), 274.

4   Ibid., 258. His views, however, of the role that European nations would play in civilizing the rest of the world are retrograde.

5   Ibid., 254–66.

6   Ibid., 279–80.

7   Louis de Jaucourt, "Natural Liberty," trans. Thomas Zemanek, *The Encyclopedia of Diderot & d'Alembert Collaborative Translation Project* (Ann Arbor: Michigan Publishing, University of Michigan Library, 2009), accessed December 29, 2015, http://hdl.handle.net/2027/spo.did2222.0001.246. Originally published as "Liberté naturelle," Encyclopédie ou Dictionnaire raisonné des sciences, des arts et des métiers, 9: 471–2 (Paris, 1765).

8   Lynn Hunt, *The French Revolution and Human Rights: A Brief Documentary History* (Boston: Bedford Books of St. Martin's Press, 1996), 9–10, 51–5.

9   Lynn Hunt, *Inventing Human Rights: A History*, 1st ed. (New York: W.W. Norton & Co., 2007), 105–6, Brissot quoted on 105.

10   For instance, as we shall see, the La Rochefoucauld-Liancourt. Jean-Pierre Gross, *Fair Shares for All: Jacobin Egalitarianism in Practice* (Cambridge: Cambridge University Press, 1997), 5.

11   Though I directly quote from some of the available English versions of these texts (or sections of them), I am indebted to Rosen's direction to these texts, as well as to his analysis and direction of them, throughout this section. George Rosen, "Mercantilism and Health Policy in Eighteenth Century French Thought," *Medical History* 3, no. 04 (1959): 259–77.

12   Quoted in ibid., 263.

13   Ibid., 260–1.

14   Ibid., 262–3.

15   Dora B. Weiner, *The Citizen-Patient in Revolutionary and Imperial Paris* (Baltimore: Johns Hopkins University Press, 1993), 22–3.

16   These details on Chamousset thus far in the paragraph are from Rosen, "Mercantilism and Health Policy in Eighteenth Century French Thought," 269–70.

17   Pierre Rosanvallon, *The New Social Question: Rethinking the Welfare State* (Princeton: Princeton University Press, 2000), 12.

18   The connection between the English utopian tradition and the French is emphasized by Frank Edward Manuel and Fritzie Prigohzy Manuel, *French Utopias: An Anthology of Ideal Societies* (New York: Shocken Books, 1966), 1.

19   Rosen, "Mercantilism and Health Policy in Eighteenth Century French Thought," 266–7.

20   The quotes are from Louis-Sébastien Mercier, *Astræa's Return or, the Halcyon Days of France in the Year 2440: A Dream*, trans. Harriot Augusta Freeman (London, 1797), *Eighteenth Century Collections Online*, Gale, Harvard Library, accessed July 6, 2015, http://id.lib.harvard.edu/aleph/012408570/catalog, 43–4. I owe this citation to Rosen, and followed him to these passages: Rosen, "Mercantilism and Health Policy in Eighteenth Century French Thought," 267.

21   Mercier, *Astræa's Return*, 24.

22   Albert Fried and Ronald Sanders, *Socialist Thought: A Documentary History* (Garden City, N.Y.: Anchor Books, 1964), 17; Manuel and Manuel, *French Utopias: An Anthology of Ideal Societies*, 91.

23   Again, I followed Rosen's lead to these passages of Morelly, which are available in excerpt form (translated into English) in: Morelly, "Code de la Nature," in *French Utopias: An Anthology of Ideal Societies*, ed. Frank Edward Manuel and Fritzie Prigohzy Manuel (New York: Schocken Books, 1966), 102–17. See: Rosen, "Mercantilism and Health Policy in Eighteenth Century French Thought," 265–6.

24   Morelly, "Code de la Nature," 105.

25   Ibid., 105–6.

26   Ibid., 106.

27   Ibid.

28   As Weiner puts it, the poor considered the Hôtel-Dieu "a refuge they sought only to die." Dora B. Weiner, "Introduction" in *Memoirs on Paris Hospitals*, by Jacques Tenon (Canton, MA: Science History Publications, 1996), ix.

29   Quoted in Weiner, *The Citizen-Patient in Revolutionary and Imperial Paris*, 22.

30   Weiner, "Introduction" in *Memoirs on Paris Hospitals*, by Jacques Tenon, vii–viii.

31   Ibid., x.

32   Ibid., xi.

33   Ibid., vii.

34   Ibid., xvii.

35   Jacques Tenon, *Memoirs on Paris Hospitals* (Canton, MA: Science History Publications, 1996), 14.

36   Ibid., 18.

37   Ibid., 17.

38   Ibid., 7.

39   Weiner, *The Citizen-Patient in Revolutionary and Imperial Paris*, 32–3; L. S. Greenbaum, "'Measure of Civilization': The Hospital Thought of Jacques Tension on the Eve of the French Revolution," *Bulletin of the History of Medicine* 49, no. 1 (1975): 45.

40   Greenbaum, "'Measure of Civilization': The Hospital Thought of Jacques Tension on the Eve of the French Revolution," 45.

41   Weiner, "Introduction" in *Memoirs on Paris Hospitals*, by Jacques Tenon, xxi.

42   Tenon, *Memoirs on Paris Hospitals*, 43.

43   Greenbaum, "'Measure of Civilization': The Hospital Thought of Jacques Tension on the Eve of the French Revolution," 44–5.

44   Weiner, "Introduction" in *Memoirs on Paris Hospitals*, by Jacques Tenon, xiii; Weiner, *The Citizen-Patient in Revolutionary and Imperial Paris*.

45   Quoted in Greenbaum, "'Measure of Civilization': The Hospital Thought of Jacques Tension on the Eve of the French Revolution," 54.

46   Weiner, *The Citizen-Patient in Revolutionary and Imperial Paris*, 33.

47   Weiner, "Introduction" in *Memoirs on Paris Hospitals*, by Jacques Tenon, xiii.

48   Hunt, *Inventing Human Rights: A History*, 23–4. On the French Revolution, see Hunt, *The French Revolution and Human Rights: A Brief Documentary History*. On the importance of the Haitian Revolution, see Robin Blackburn, *The American Crucible: Slavery, Emancipation and Human Rights* (London; New York: Verso, 2011). Samuel Moyn, on the contrary, has more recently disputed the relevance of the Rights of Man tradition to modern human rights. *The Last Utopia: Human Rights in History* (Cambridge, MA: Belknap Press of Harvard University Press, 2010), 24–7.

49   Eric Foner, *The Story of American Freedom* (New York: W.W. Norton; repr., 1999), 13–15.

50   Ibid., 15.

51   Thomas Paine, "Common Sense," *Thomas Paine: Collected Writings* (New York: Library of America, 1995), 5–6.

52   Foner, *The Story of American Freedom*, 37; Blackburn, *The American Crucible: Slavery, Emancipation and Human Rights*, 168.

53   *Declaration of the Rights of Man*, 1789, http://avalon.law.yale.edu/18th_century/rightsof.asp.

54   Blackburn, *The American Crucible*, 188–97, 203, 322; Hunt, *Inventing Human Rights: A History*, 28.

55   Lisa DiCaprio, *The Origins of the Welfare State: Women, Work, and the French Revolution* (Urbana: University of Illinois Press, 2007), 16–21; Charles Coulston Gillispie, *Science and Polity in France: The Revolutionary and Napoleonic Years* (Princeton: Princeton University Press, 2004), 47; Alan I. Forrest, *The French Revolution and the Poor* (Oxford: Basil Blackwell, 1981), 16; Georges Lefebvre, *The French Revolution* (New York: Columbia University Press; repr., 1965), 116–17.

56   DiCaprio, *The Origins of the Welfare State*, 30–1.

57   Ibid., 31.

58   Stephen P. Marks, "From the 'Single Confused Page' to the 'Decalogue for Six Billion Persons': The Roots of the Universal Declaration of Human Rights in the French Revolution," *Human Rights Quarterly* 20, no. 3 (1998): 503–5.

59   Ibid., 506.

60   Paine, "Rights of Man," *Thomas Paine: Collected Writings* (New York: Library of America, 1995), 626–7.

61   Ibid., 627–8.

62   Ibid., 628.

63   Ibid., 630.

64   Ibid., 630–1.

65   Ibid., 632, 636–8.

66   Paine, "Agrarian Justice," *Thomas Paine: Collected Writings* (New York: Library of America, 1995), 400.

67   Harvey J. Kaye, *Thomas Paine and the Promise of America* (New York: Hill and Wang, 2005), 77.

68 E.P. Thompson, *The Making of the English Working Class* (New York: Vintage Books, 1966), 94.
69 Kaye, *Thomas Paine and the Promise of America*, 77–9.
70 Gross, *Fair Shares For All*, 5–6.
71 Quoted in Gillispie, *Science and Polity in France*, 47.
72 Ibid.
73 Ibid., 47–8.
74 Forrest, *The French Revolution and the Poor*, 29.
75 Gillispie, *Science and Polity in France*, 48.
76 Forrest, *The French Revolution and the Poor*, 27.
77 Notably, however, he also called for punishment for those who refused to work. Ibid.; Gross, *Fair Shares For All*, 5, 64; DiCaprio, *The Origins of the Welfare State*, ix, 38; Gillispie, *Science and Polity in France*, 48.
78 George Rosen, "Hospitals, Medical Care and Social Policy in the French Revolution," *Bulletin of the History of Medicine* 30 (1956): 134.
79 Weiner, "Introduction" in *Memoirs on Paris Hospitals*, by Jacques Tenon, xviii.
80 Rosen, "Hospitals, Medical Care and Social Policy in the French Revolution," 135–6; Gillispie, *Science and Polity in France*, 48.
81 Rosen, "Hospitals, Medical Care and Social Policy in the French Revolution," 135–6.
82 Ibid.
83 Forrest, *The French Revolution and the Poor*, 40–1.
84 DiCaprio, *The Origins of the Welfare State*, 37.
85 Gillispie, *Science and Polity in France*, 52.
86 Ibid., 55–6; Weiner, *The Citizen-Patient in Revolutionary and Imperial Paris*, 26–7.
87 Weiner, *The Citizen-Patient in Revolutionary and Imperial Paris*, 28; Gillispie, *Science and Polity in France*, 45.
88 "Health Committee Draft Legislation: A Plan for National Health Care," Appendix A of *Citizen-Patient in Revolutionary and Imperial Paris*, by Dora Weiner (Baltimore: Johns Hopkins University Press, 1993), 326–7.
89 Weiner, *The Citizen-Patient in Revolutionary and Imperial Paris*, 325n.
90 Forrest, *The French Revolution and the Poor*, 40–1.
91 Ibid.
92 DiCaprio, *The Origins of the Welfare State*, 39–40.
93 Gillispie, *Science and Polity in France*, 55–6.
94 Rosen, "Hospitals, Medical Care and Social Policy in the French Revolution," 139.
95 Ibid.
96 William Doyle, *The Oxford History of the French Revolution*, 2nd ed. (Oxford; New York: Oxford University Press, 2002), 424; Eric Hobsbawm, *The Age of Revolution: 1789–1848* (New York: Vintage Books; repr., 1996), 66.
97 Gross, *Fair Shares For All*, 200.
98 Ibid., 43.
99 Ibid.
100 Ibid., 44.
101 "Constitution of the Year I," in *The Constitutions and Other Select Documents Illustrative of the History of France 1789–1901* (Minneapolis: The H.W. Wilson Company, 1904), 173.
102 DiCaprio, *The Origins of the Welfare State*, 99; Rosen, "Hospitals, Medical Care and Social Policy in the French Revolution," 145–6.
103 Gross, *Fair Shares For All*, 174–5.
104 Although as Gross notes, metal workers had enjoyed a similar benefit *before* the Revolution. Ibid., 159–60.
105 Ibid., 177.
106 DiCaprio, *The Origins of the Welfare State*, 100–1.
107 Gross, *Fair Shares For All*, 26, 79, 96, 121, 185.
108 Ibid., 162.

109   Doyle, *The Oxford History of the French Revolution*, 399.

110   DiCaprio, *The Origins of the Welfare State*, 101.

111   Jones notes that the Jacobins held hospitals in low regard, and that their strategy aimed at "dehospitalizing" society. However, he also notes that hospital property produced only a minority of a hospital's income. Ibid., 107; Colin Jones, "Picking up the Pieces: The Politics and Personnel of Social Welfare From the Convention to the Consulate," in *Beyond the Terror: Essays in French Regional and Social History, 1794–1815* (Cambridge: Cambridge University Press, 1983), 57, 64.

112   Kaye, *Thomas Paine and the Promise of America*, 85.

113   Baker, "Introduction" in *Condorcet: Selected Writings*, xxxv.

114   For a discussion of social welfare in the Thermidorian and Directorial periods, see: Jones, "Picking up the Pieces: The Politics and Personnel of Social Welfare Form the Convention to the Consulate."

115   Ibid., 58–9.

116   Ibid., 66.

117   DiCaprio, *The Origins of the Welfare State*, 197.

118   Doyle, *The Oxford History of the French Revolution*, 401.

119   Rosen, "Hospitals, Medical Care and Social Policy in the French Revolution," 148–9.

120   Forrest, *The French Revolution and the Poor*, 30–1.

121   Colin Jones, *The Charitable Imperative: Hospitals and Nursing in Ancien Régime and Revolutionary France* (London: Routledge, 1989), 6, 22.

122   Gross, *Fair Shares For All*, 162.

123   DiCaprio, *The Origins of the Welfare State*, 205.

124   Weiner, *The Citizen-Patient in Revolutionary and Imperial Paris*, 10.

125   Or as Weiner puts it, the Committee on Mendicity failed in the sense that the American Bill of Rights failed—in the short-run. Ibid.

126   As Hobsbawm put it, Napoleon had killed only a single thing: the dream of liberté, égalité, and fraternité. Hobsbawm, *Age of Revolution*, 76.

127   Condorcet, "Sketch for a Historical Picture of the Progress of the Human Mind," 281.

3

Public Health, Social Medicine, and Industrial Capitalism

One day during the cold Scottish spring of the year 1838, three impoverished women—all out of work, all with young children—were seen by the physician William Pulteney Alison. Alison came from an established family and was a very prominent physician in Edinburgh. Yet throughout his career, Alison had also served as a physician to the poor.[1]

All of the women, he later recounted, were living in a "miserable state of destitution." There was little relief to be had from the public purse: the nineteenth-century Scottish Poor Law, even in comparison to the English Poor Law, was notable for its draconian frugality and largely voluntary system of funding.[2] And so, when the women were denied admission to the local workhouse, they—and their infants—were essentially left to their own meager resources. After several weeks of "severe suffering," as Alison noted, all of the children—presumably from some combination of cold and malnutrition—were dead.[3]

Alison told this story in his 1840 *Observations on the Management of the Poor in Scotland, and Its Effects on the Health of Great Towns.* In this book, he does not simply bemoan the inevitable sadness of life, but instead counters the establishment Malthusian notion that attempting to improve the condition of the poor through public aid would not be useful, and indeed would only worsen their moral condition. Alison seemed to find such arguments repulsive. Reflecting back on his encounter with the three women and their children, he thought the neglect of the poor was shameful, and that the resultant loss of life was as preventable as it was reprehensible. "If any one supposes," he wrote with more than justified acidity, "that the effect of this sacrifice of innocent life was to improve the morals of these women or their associates, I can only say, that he knows nothing of the effect of real destitution on human character and conduct."[4] What they deserved was neither moralistic rejection nor the unpredictable provision of voluntary charitable relief, but instead the supply of relief by public provision, by way of right.[5] Alison advocated a relatively more expansive system of welfare for Scotland, which would be supported by taxation and include medical staff to treat the sick poor.[6]

To be clear: the language of socioeconomic "rights" was mostly absent during the period of the Industrial Revolution.[7] Yet these events—and this period—is nonetheless crucial to the theme of this book. The great economic changes of the era, and its effects on health, pushed some—such as Louis-René Villermé, Edwin

Chadwick, Alison, Friedrich Engels, and Rudolf Virchow, all examined in this chapter—to freshly evaluate the relationship between poverty, health, healthcare, and individual rights. From such thinkers emerged the notion of the "social determinants of health," as they have come to be called. Indeed, it seems fair to argue that a public health discourse that centers on socioeconomic rights very much has its taproots in the nineteenth century.[8] And during the Revolutions of 1848, Virchow even went so far as to call for an (almost) explicit right to healthcare as part of a broader project of political justice.

Before turning to Virchow and 1848, however, this chapter will pick up where the last one left off—at the end of Enlightenment—to contextualize these developments in the changing political and economic dynamics of the time.

Economy and Public Health in the Post-Enlightenment

The last chapter began with the enormously ambitious health vision of the Marquis de Condorcet in the closing of his *Sketch for a Historical Picture*. However cheerful and heartening his prose, observed against the backdrop of the ensuing decades, his hopes seem momentously naïve. Though living standards in the industrial world would eventually rise, the impact of early industrial capitalism on the health and welfare of humanity was often no less than devastating. As E. P. Thompson has argued, even if we accept that the Industrial Revolution produced some improvement in average wages in the early nineteenth century, the rupture of traditional modes of living and the experience of economic dislocation and exploitation together produced a calamitous lived reality for the working classes.[9] The Enlightenment vision of a world where free enterprise was uninhibited and humankind lived in perpetual peace and prosperity could hardly be more at odds with the reality of the early Industrial Revolution, with the suffering and the *sickness* of the industrial city. Indeed, the early nineteenth century witnessed an actual deterioration in health in urban Britain, with a life expectancy at birth in the 30s in major British cities.[10] At the same time, there was also a recognition that existing modes of medical therapy were largely useless—so-called "therapeutic nihilism"—a fact that led some to turn to the field of public health instead.[11]

Indeed, public health as a scientific field is often traced back to the early industrial era in France.[12] Just as it is today, public health was an unavoidably and indeed intrinsically political undertaking, and its practitioners were clearly influenced by prevailing economic and political discourses.[13] As the historian Ann La Berge explains, the public health movement of this era was suffused by a "dialectic between liberalism and statism" that echoed a larger division between liberalism and what has become known as "social medicine."[14] The liberal approach had deep philosophical roots. The French liberal economist Jean-Baptiste Say (1767–1832), for instance, argued that the fundamental laws of economics were an unchanging and unchangeable fact, and that any form of charity—whether public or private—should not be extended to the working poor.[15] The era also saw the rise to prominence of the icy ideology of Thomas Robert Malthus (1766–1834). In his *Essay on the Principle of Population*, aimed explicitly at Enlightenment optimists like Condorcet, Malthus not only disputed the notion of the "perfectibility" of humankind, but also contended that suffering, want, famine, poverty, and so forth were the inevitable product of the laws of nature.[16] His thesis rested on the premise that the rate of population growth (if not contained) would always outpace the rate of growth of food production (given a fixed quantity of land).[17] However, various forces maintained equilibrium and prevented the poor from overpopulating the earth. One was the "preventive check," in which the poor, cognizant of their lack of food, prudently eschewed sex. If the preventive check failed, however, the "positive check" went into operation, which consisted of such necessities as "sickly seasons, epidemics, pestilence, and plague," with "gigantic inevitable famine" available as nature's last resort.[18]

Putting aside other aspects of this grim philosophy, from the perspective of policy, Malthus's theorem boiled down to the argument that government assistance to the poor was not only ineffective, but also frankly harmful, and so should be abolished.[19] The English Poor Law, after all, encouraged the poor to have families they could not support, and so in effect "create[d] the poor which they maintain . . ."[20] He disputed the notion that the poor had a "right to subsistence"—that right explicitly proposed by Liancourt, as described in the last chapter—when they were unable to find work, a false right that he argued conflicted with the real laws of nature.[21] Notably, his arguments were wielded against the poor's right to relief in both England and France, and he has been considered something of the "father of the new poor law," a harsher version of the English Poor Law that will be examined in the next section.[22]

The discourse of economic liberalism—including that of Malthus— permeated the thought of some of the public health reformers of the early nineteenth century.[23] Such an acceptance of the ideology of economic liberalism could very well neuter the capacity of some reformers to advocate for significant social change; as a result, the solutions of public health reformers could, all too often, amount to "the political analogue of therapeutic nihilism."[24]

The most famous exemplar of the liberal line of public health thought was Louis-René Villermé (1782–1863), who had served in the Napoleonic Wars as a surgeon.[25] Interestingly, none other than the duc de La Rochefoucauld-Liancourt, whose "Committee on Mendicity" was discussed at length in the preceding chapter, provided both patronage and crucial inspiration for Villermé.[26] Villermé is famous for his use of quantitative methods to demonstrate that poverty caused a substantial difference in mortality between the wealthy and the impoverished.[27] In his famous studies on mortality in Paris, published in the 1820s, he compared the mortality rates in each department of Paris, and found (by and large) that the richest departments had the lowest mortality and the poorest had the highest, and that the difference could not be explained by the various environmental and climatic factors that were then the prevailing explanations for differences in health.[28] He therefore concluded that "wealth . . . and misery are, for the inhabitants of the diverse arrondissements of Paris and under the conditions which these arrondissements impose upon them, the principal causes (we do not say the unique causes) to which must be attributed the great differences noted among the mortality rates."[29]

To some extent, one could interpret these findings as evidence that Malthus's "positive check" was at work on the poor. On the other hand, Villermé's findings implied that this increased mortality resulted not from the invisible hand of natural law, but from the particular socioeconomic environment of the poor. They were bold findings, with potentially broad-reaching policy implications, a fact, as historian William Coleman underscores, that makes the gelatinous timidity of Villermé's proposed solutions all the more jarring. His solutions to these various injustices was the old standby of individual responsibility, prudence, self-help, and hard work.[30] Like Say, Villermé ultimately argued that economic inequality and its sequelae were the inevitable "nature of things."[31] Apart from his support of a child labor law, Coleman shows, Villermé advocated nothing that would substantially affect what he had so clearly revealed: the great cost in human health and life that industrial poverty and inequality wrought.[32] Just as it was for Malthus, even the old English Poor Law was an object of his scorn (he called it "a legal premium to improvidence or sloth").[33] And the organization of labor—much less political change like that ushered in by the Revolutions of 1848—was simply out of the question.[34]

Before turning to the Revolutions of 1848—and the public health thought associated with them—it's worth first looking across the channel, where public health thinkers were grappling with similar issues.

Britain: New Poor Law, Health, and Socioeconomic Rights

The Industrial Revolution began in England, and it was not long before the deleterious health effects of early industrial capitalism became apparent. People flooded into the cities—looking for work and opportunity—but were mowed down by disease with terrifying efficiency in places like Manchester and Glasgow.[35] Was this the Malthusian "positive check" in action?

Many came to something of this conclusion: the Poor Law—the public system of poor relief examined in Chapter 1—was often blamed for the poverty and demoralization of the poor. Criticism of the Poor Law grew following the end of the Napoleonic Wars, and its lack of popularity among the ruling classes stemmed from a combination of its rising cost to taxpayers, its failure to contain working-class unrest, its deterrent effect on the mobility of labor, and an acceptance of Malthusianism and economic liberal ideology.[36] The Whig Parliament of 1832 appointed a Royal Commission, headed by "philosophic radical" and (later) public health thinker Edwin Chadwick (to whom we will return to shortly), to study how the Poor Law might be changed. The Commission's 1834 report made the point that the alleged generosity of the Old Poor Law (and especially the so-called "Speenhamland System" of wage supplementation) impoverished the able-bodied worker by tempting him with handouts.[37] This document became the basis of a "New Poor Law" that amounted to a historic change in the institution,[38] with important ramifications for public health and—as we will see—the right to health and healthcare.

First, a note about the ideological basis of the New Poor Law. At its heart was what has been termed an "automatic deterrence mechanism": by making the condition of those who relied on relief more wretched than that of the worst-off worker, you would (it was said) eliminate the temptation of poor relief.[39] Or as the Poor Law Commission put it, the position of the recipient of poor law relief "shall not be made really or apparently so eligible as the situation of the independent labourer of the lowest class."[40] This "principle of less eligibility" meant no more "outdoor" poor relief; instead, workers and their families would be confined to the brutal workhouses, wherein husbands and wives would be separated, work would be intense, and provisions meager.[41] As Esping-Andersen has noted, although the New Poor Law can be seen as a type of welfare system, it was a type of welfare system that had a commodifying effect that was designed to make "wage employment and the cash nexus the linchpin of a person's very existence."[42] And as T.H. Marshall notes, the New Poor Law forced those who needed relief to become legally *less than citizens*, and thus was tantamount to an abnegation of relief as a social right.[43]

Not surprisingly—and even though its provisions were by no means universally implemented, with many compromises made on the local level—the New Poor Law was despised and resisted by the poor and working classes.[44] Popular resistance to the New Poor Law would feed into—and be enveloped by—Chartism, a political movement that has been called the "first working-class political party."[45] The Chartist wave was also provoked by worsening economic conditions, climbing food prices, and rising urban unemployment in the late 1830s and early 1840s.[46] While the primary demands of the Chartists were predominantly political (e.g., expanded suffrage and a fairly elected Parliament), beneath them was outrage at socioeconomic conditions, including at the New Poor Law.[47]

Indeed, for some, the New Poor Law was tantamount to a violation of the historical socioeconomic rights of the English poor. The New Poor Law, as one scholar put it, was to some extent "seen as treating poverty as crime and robbing Englishmen of the rights and liberties that they had enjoyed for over two hundred years under the Old Poor Law."[48] Though this bygone era of social rights, invoked by Chartists and others, may have been largely mythical, it was nonetheless a powerful construct at a time of political turbulence and economic deprivation.[49] The radical journalist William Cobbett, for instance, explicitly attacked the New Poor Law as violating "the right, in case we fell into distress, to have our wants sufficiently relieved out of the produce of the land, whether that distress arose from sickness, from decrepitude, from old age, or from inability to find employment . . ."[50]

Some also explicitly critiqued the New Poor Law's effect on health. The New Poor law, contended radical John Knight, violated the traditional rights of British workers, and "deprives them of the free use of their lives and limbs, by shutting them up in a prison called a poor law workhouse, and as it endangers and jeopardizes their lives, when laboring under misfortunes over which they have no control, by compelling them to subsist upon food, so small in quantity, so impure, and so obnoxious in quality, as to produce disease and premature death ..."[51] The Chartist Reverend Joseph Rayner Stephens somewhat similarly argued that working men had a *right* to a reasonable quality of life and a quantity of work consistent with good health.[52] Some argued in favor of something more than a return to the Old Poor Law: the prominent Chartist Feargus O'Connor stated that "[i]f society were properly constituted, all the sick and infirm would be provided for by the government."[53]

Yet even outside the context of radical politics, the impact of the New Poor Law on *health* was a serious potential liability for its supporters, as some have noted. After all, if the principle of "lesser eligibility" pushed workers away from seeking aid *at the cost of causing starvation and disease*, it might actually be exacerbating the impoverishment of the masses. This question was, to some extent, subsumed within the larger one at the center of the battle over British public health of these decades, a story told by the historian Christopher Hamlin in his *Public Health and Social Justice in the Age of Chadwick*. Did, as some contend, poverty *cause* disease? Or, instead, did unsanitary conditions lead to disease, which in turn caused poverty? We can look back in hindsight and argue that both of these dynamics were at play at the same time (which, indeed, some contemporaries recognized). For proponents of the New Poor Law, however, the idea that destitution itself might be a cause of disease was a dangerous notion: it called into question the very framework of the New Poor Law, which relied on destitution as its basic deterrent. It also lent itself to the argument that improving population health required directly improving the economic condition of the poor. Conversely, if the unsanitary conditions in which the poor dwelled—the basic filthiness of what was viewed as a lower breed—were primarily responsible for the poor's illness and poverty, then the answer was simply more public health infrastructure: pipes and sewers and toilets and the like.[54]

Chadwick was the most famous and influential purveyor of the latter argument, as Hamlin argues. Following his work on the Poor Law Commission, Chadwick became interested in public health, and his efforts resulted in the famous *Report on the Sanitary Condition of the Labouring Population of Great Britain*. His survey includes quotations from various medical observers (including Villermé) intertwined with Chadwick's own observations and opinions, and it has typically been seen as a seminal document in public health history. Chadwick argued firmly that it was the environmental conditions of the poor—and not their poverty— that was the predisposing factor in illness. "In the great mass of cases . . . the attack of fever," he writes "precedes the destitution, not the destitution the disease."[55] Elsewhere, he refers to the "false opinions as to destitution being the general cause of fever ..."[56] Again and again, he attempts to untangle the *health effects* of industrial capitalism from the *political economy* of industrial capitalism itself. For instance, his skepticism as to the effects of occupational exposures on health is at times extraordinary (and directly contrary to that of Friedrich Engels, who will be discussed later). He does not believe that intense factory labor adversely affected the health of children, and elsewhere asserts that with respect to labor in the mills, there is "very little sickness that is *essential* to the occupation itself." [57] He does, however, contend that poor environmental conditions—dirty and crowded homes, poorly ventilated factories, and unclean water—led the working class not merely into poor health (and from there into destitution), but also to a degraded state of sexual depravity and inebriation.[58] As a result, he is not at all convinced that any sort of "pecuniary aid" would be helpful for the health of the poor: indeed, it may merely add "fuel to the flames" by allowing them to buy more alcohol.[59] The road to improve the health of the working class, in other words, is a technological one: "[t]he primary and most important measures, and at the same time the most practicable, and within the recognized province of public administration, are drainage, the removal of all refuse of habitations, streets, and roads, and the improvement of the supplies of water," as he writes in the book's conclusion.[60]

Thus, whatever public health innovations we may give Chadwick credit for, Hamlin argues that his work cannot be viewed through an apolitical and technocratic lens. As he contends, Chadwick's reforms were fundamentally conservative, intended as much to satisfy the political and economic concerns of elites as to clean the streets. Fundamentally, he suggests, Chadwick was fighting not only filth and the immorality and disease it caused, but also the errant political radicalism that emerged from this unclean *milieu*. In this sense, his *Report* was aimed as much against disease as it was against the mounting threat of democracy, Chartism, and indeed of revolution.[61] Or as Chadwick himself put it, "if a Chartist millennium were to be averted, the governing classes must free the governed from the sharp spur of their misery by improving the physical conditions of their lives."[62] Finally, it's worth noting that the basis of Chadwick's concern was the wage-earning male: women and children were at most derivative concerns in a public health calculus in which money mattered most.[63] Or as Chadwick wrote, "the public loss from the premature deaths of the heads of families is greater than can be represented by any enumeration of the pecuniary burdens consequent upon their sickness and death."[64]

Chadwick's, however, was not the only view on the matter. Aligned against him was a host of other public health thinkers—many of whom were doctors—who put forth a very different framework for understanding the intersection of public health, poverty, and disease.[65] In Scotland, William Pulteney Alison (1790–1859), with whom this chapter began, produced one of the most compelling competing visions to that of Chadwick.[66] Alison was based at Edinburgh University, an esteemed focus for medical research in this era, and he was also committed to the healthcare of the city's poor, whom he visited in their homes.[67] He was also a key participant in the fight over Scotland's Poor Law (which he thought should be expanded in an English direction), as well as in the fight over the public health of these decades.[68] In his landmark 1840 book *Observations on the Management of the Poor in Scotland, and Its Effects on the Health of Great Towns*, Alison makes the argument—contra Chadwick—that if disease springs from poverty, then it is "the grand evil of Poverty itself" that must be addressed to make headway against disease.[69] While he conceded that how exactly poverty caused disease was not entirely clear (something that investigators are still trying to elucidate today, though much has been learned), he argued that the relationship was nonetheless an empirical fact.[70] This was particularly evident in the case of typhus, which, he noted (like Villermé and others) disproportionately struck and spread among the economically and socially disadvantaged.[71] Although Alison sought to expand treatment for the sick poor, he acknowledged the therapeutic limits of contemporary medicine. He thus argued that society had to relieve not just the sick poor, but also *poverty itself*, and that this would go a long way in *preventing* the development of disease.[72]

In advocating for state welfare in order to alleviate and prevent sickness, Alison's approach significantly diverged from the ideas of Chadwick or Malthus and from economic liberalism more broadly, even if their notions of the structure of the Poor Law were similar.[73] "The general belief has been," as Alison summarized the standard position, "that ... the poor are most benefited by being left to themselves ... strengthened by the religious and moral feelings which have been inculcated in them ...."[74] Malthus, for instance, had argued that the Poor Law would only prompt the poor to recklessly procreate, as earlier noted. In contrast, Alison argued that "permanent relief to the miseries of the poor" would not lead to this endpoint.[75] Indeed, he found the Malthusian concept of "moral restraint" to be entirely wrongheaded, noting that severe misery rarely served to check imprudent reproduction or instill cautiousness.[76] Indeed, a guarantee of economic assistance provided the essential hope for the future that lay behind an effective "preventive check."[77]

And importantly, Alison advocated for such assistance to be given as a *right*. In this respect, like Villermé he seems to have been influenced by the duc de La Rochefoucauld-Liancourt and the "Committee of Mendicity," explored in the last chapter. Alison apparently had access to Liancourt's reports, as he quotes from them approvingly, and at length, in *Observations*. He questions how much suffering could have been avoided had the ideas of Liancourt been implemented.[78] Making relief a right, instead of an act of charity, would have the benefit of promoting the dignity of poor people. Would the independence of the poor be more "injured by *claiming that bounty as a right*," he asks, or by "*supplicating it as a boon*" to be obtained by seeking "the attention ... of their superiors"?[79] He cites Liancourt in support of his position in favor of the former; Liancourt had argued that private charity was unreliable insofar as it depended on the unreliable proclivities of the rich, and thus that a national needs-based system would be more conducive to the dignity and independence of the poor. [80]

Establishing a right to "relief" would thus, in his view, help ensure, or at least improve, the quality and longevity of life for the masses. Additionally, part of this relief would be in the form of medical care, e.g., building fever hospitals, or supporting fever patients and their families during sickness.[81] Alison's proposals were a rebuttal of both the moralistic economic liberalism of Malthus and the sanitary statism of Chadwick; he did not disagree with Chadwick's emphasis on environmental improvement so much as the limited scope of his proposed remedies and their failure to address the *lives* of the poor.[82] "Alison's writing in the early

1840s," argues Hamlin, "mark the epitome of a medical critique of industrialism and capitalism . . ."[83] For Alison, clinical medicine was inherently political, and should be centered around the "principle of delivering a health 'right' by comprehensively identifying and eliminating health 'wrongs'. . ."[84]

Ahead of the times he may have been, but it was Chadwick's vision, and not Alison's, that triumphed, as Hamlin notes. Chadwick's *Report* led to the 1848 passage of the historic Public Health Act. However, with few supporters either among the elite or the working class, this was to be a short-lived reform: an editorial in the *Times* famously whined about being "bullied into health" by Chadwick and his allies, and six years later, Parliament let the Act die.[85] Yet in the realm of the ideas, the debate between Alison (and like-minded thinkers) and Chadwick clearly underscores how the "right to healthcare" cannot be neatly disentangled from the political and economic inequalities that contribute to poor health, especially in an age when effective medical care was limited.

At the same time, the New Poor Law played an interesting role in the history of the "right to healthcare" in another respect: it helped give rise to a rudimentary yet flawed state system of medical care. As described in Chapter 1, the 1601 Poor Law Act had called for the support of the "lame, impotent, old, blind, and such other among them being poor and not able to work."[86] In subsequent years, many sick poor would indeed be cared for by parish medical officers, who were paid a salary in exchange for their treatment of the sick poor.[87] By the time of the enactment of the New Poor Law, medical officers were retained by roughly half of English parishes.[88] In line with this tradition, the Poor Law Amendment Act of 1834 included a line for the provision of medical care by Justices of the Peace.[89] In part as a result, over subsequent decades, thousands of district medical officers became responsible for the care and treatment of the sick poor, while workhouses gained infirmaries, effectively becoming state hospitals.[90] Some argue that the New Poor Law, despite its draconian intentions, created a new system of medical welfare.

Still, this all being said, the New Poor Law medical service was an absurdly underfunded, under-resourced, and understaffed operation: poor salaries, an unrealistically large patient population entrusted to the care of each physician, an absence of nurses, a lack of drugs, atrociously maintained workhouse infirmaries, and resistance from the bureaucracy created enormous hurdles for the New Poor Law physicians.[91] One physician, for instance, described a maternity ward as a "wretchedly damp and miserable room," where "[s]cores and scores of distinctly preventable deaths of both mothers and children took place. . . . "[92] The unique viewpoint some of these physicians gained from their experiences, however, led some to a critique of the healthcare status quo and to use various tactics to achieve better care for their patients.[93] Some even agitated to reform the Poor Law medical service in a fundamental fashion, proposing to rid it of the principle of less eligibility or even expanding it to all workers at public expense.[94] Hamlin underscores the boldness of some of these physicians and like-minded reformers: they "refused to make medicine a commodity," and at the same time "recognized, at least implicitly, a right to health that was being jeopardized by industrialization, urbanization, liberalism . . ."[95]

While the New Poor Law survived into the twentieth century, the New Poor Law physicians and other reformers succeeded, some argue, in significantly reforming the Poor Law medical service, improving its hospitals and reducing its stigma (to some extent), even if the more transformative proposals of reformers never became reality.[96] And by the early twentieth century, the Poor Law Board was contemplating the possibility of extending free medical care to all wage earners in England and Wales.[97] Although no such extension was to take place, some historians have made the argument that the Poor Law medical service was the seed that ultimately grew into Britain's universal system of healthcare—the National Health Service (NHS)—which essentially produced a legal right to free healthcare after the Second World War.[98]

Yet there is some irony to all of this. On the one hand, it may be true that there is a historical thread connecting the twenty-first century British welfare state—including its unique system of universal health care—with the often odious Poor Law. Indeed, Poor Law hospitals *became* some of the hospitals of the NHS. Yet on the other hand, the universalism of the NHS was an explicit rejection of the fundamental underpinnings of Poor Law medicine: the latter employed a *means test*[99] to provide a lower tier of medical service to an allegedly lower class of citizens in an authoritarian manner. The NHS, in contrast, was meant to provide a right to an equal quality of care to all, regardless of economic status, which is the essence of a decommodified healthcare benefit.

This leads us to a final individual who wrote about the politics of public health in nineteenth century England, the German Friedrich Engels. Engels inaugurates a new, more radical tradition of public health analysis, going beyond Chadwick but also Alison in his critique of how political economy could produce health, and sickness, in England.[100] In his *The Condition of the Working Class in England*—published in 1845 when he was only 24[101]— Engels excoriates the destructive effect of industrial capitalism on the health of English workers. Though he draws on and references the work of both Chadwick and Alison (among others), he is far more radical than these British writers in blaming the very political and economic infrastructure of England—not merely environmental filth (like Chadwick) or inadequacies in poor relief (like Alison)—for widespread sickness and premature death among the working class. "[W]hen society," he writes, "places hundreds of proletarians in such a position that they inevitably meet a too early and an unnatural death . . . when it deprives thousands of the necessaries of life, places them under conditions in which they *cannot* live . . . its deed is murder just as surely as the deed of the single individual . . ."[102] He delineates at great length the *health* effects—in careful medical detail—of various industrial occupations and environmental deprivations, and yet he goes beyond previous thinkers by laying blame for these effects at the doorstep of the capitalist system itself. In this respect, Engels provides an almost photographic negative of Chadwick's analysis. Indeed, he argued, "the industrial greatness of England can be maintained only through the barbarous treatment of the operatives, the destruction of their health, the social, physical, and mental decay of whole generations."[103] And although he was mainly concerned with the impact on health through economic circumstance, he also made reference to inadequacies in healthcare, of the "only too common lack of all medical assistance" among English workers.[104] "English doctors charge high fees," he notes, "and working men are not in a position to pay them. They can therefore do nothing, or are compelled to call in cheap charlatans, and use quack remedies, which do more harm than good."[105]

Yet what made Engels exceptional in comparison to the other writers we have examined was not merely his analysis of the social determinants of health, but his proposed solutions. As Howard Waitzkin has noted, Engels "implied that the solution to these health problems required basic political economic change . . ."[106] Indeed, Engels explicitly argued that such change must come from *below*: "Thus is the expulsion of the proletariat from State and society outspoken, thus is it publicly proclaimed that proletarians are not human beings, and do not deserve to be treated as such. *Let us leave it to the proletarians of the British Empire,*" he wrote "*to reconquer their human rights*" (emphasis added).[107]

While Engels' book wasn't translated into English until decades later,[108] it did have an immediate impact in the realm of public health thought in Germany: it influenced a German physician named Rudolf Virchow, and through him perhaps contributed to the emergence of a school of health thought—"social medicine"— that would have a significant impact on health rights ideas and practices in the twentieth century.[109]

The political context in which Virchow worked was critical: around this very same time, change—from below—was brewing on the continent.

Germany: Revolution, Medical Reform, and the Emergence of Social Medicine

In 1848—the same year that the British state brought the Chartist movement to heel and passed the Public Health Act—Europe exploded in revolution. The German state of Prussia was the birthplace of the pathologist Virchow, and it was in the revolutionary milieu of these years that Virchow would elaborate a theory of "social medicine" that became one important current feeding into the larger "right to health" stream of the twentieth century. Moreover, Virchow was to also embrace an explicit right to *medical care* within his larger highly politicized social medicine theory.

Virchow was an ambitious pathologist who quickly made a name for himself in the academic medical circles of Berlin.[110] Even before the Revolutions of 1848, something of his political leanings can be ascertained, as when he commented on the "awakening consciousness of the workers" in a letter to his father.[111] However, it was during the 1848 typhus epidemic in Upper Silesia—immediately preceding the outbreak of the revolution in Berlin—that his medical-political perspective was formed: He would hold throughout his life that his experience in Silesia was the turning point in the formation of his political beliefs.[112]

Typhus hit the impoverished region of Upper Silesia in 1848 with little mercy. Virchow—at that point a well-known physician—was appointed to the commission as a medical officer, and in February of 1847 he arrived to the region to investigate it.[113] In his letters, he described a wretched scene of misery, of "horrible, pitiable figures, moving barefoot in the snow . . ."[114] But he was also aghast at what he saw as the Crown's entirely inadequate response.[115] And his broader conclusion on the social and economic roots of the typhus epidemic were very similar to that of Alison, who also wrote about typhus. "No matter whether meteorological conditions, general cosmic changes and such are inculpated, never do these in themselves make epidemics," he later reflected, "they only induce them whenever, through poor social conditions, the people have lived under abnormal conditions for a long time." Further underscoring the role of poverty in this tragedy, he continued, "Typhus would not have grown to epidemic proportions in upper Silesia if the population had not been bodily and mentally neglected, and the devastation caused by cholera would be quite negligible if the disease claimed no more victims among the working classes than among the well-to-do."[116]

To Virchow, social conditions were the essential underpinning of the epidemic. Like Alison, he also rejected the blaming of poverty on the imprudent propensities of the poor.[117] And also like Alison (and unlike Chadwick), he argued that poverty itself was one of the primary determinants of the outbreak of epidemics such as typhus, though he went further in arguing that poverty *itself* was (in part) made by the powerful. Indeed, not far into his *Report on the Typhus Epidemic in Upper Silesia*, Virchow took aim at the exploitative aristocracy of the region, which repressed the destitute inhabitants of the region, who "always saw the fruit of their labors falling into the pockets of the landowners."[118] The government's response to the epidemic was in line with this longstanding pattern of exploitation and neglect. The Crown, Virchow charged, did little while the crisis was unfolding, and as a result, "the people died in their thousands from starvation and disease."[119] In essence, the epidemic, and scale of mortality it caused, was not merely a biological phenomenon, but a sociopolitical one. Medicine had, he argued, "led us into the social field," requiring the improvement of the overall condition of the people, and not simply individual treatment or government regulation.[120]

But how would this be accomplished? Here, Virchow goes well beyond Alison and is more akin to Engels in his argument for a *political* solution to disease. If one assumed the principle of "equality in the eyes of the law," then nothing less than political liberation—indeed "free and unlimited democracy"—was necessary, as he called for in his report.[121] "In a free democracy with general self-government," he contended, "such events [as famine and epidemic disease] are impossible."[122] Political repression led to economic and social inequality; these inequalities in turn led to starvation, deprivation, and disease. Simply addressing the second to last element in this string of causality, *deprivation*, through the palliative of charity would not suffice.

Notably, coincident with his investigation, revolution had spread from France to Germany. In March 1848, unrest broke out in Berlin, a turn of events that brought Virchow, eager to be involved, back to his city.[123] Indeed, soon after his return, Berlin was in full revolt, and he did not hesitate to join the barricades.[124] Following the initial success of the Berlin revolution, Virchow then became involved in the Prussian "medical reform" movement, and with a friend, Rudolf Leubuscher, started a journal of that name.[125] In the first issue of his journal, Virchow put forth the egalitarian aims of the movement. "Medical organization is to be reformed not so much for the benefit of physicians as for that of the patients," he wrote, and later continued with the argument that "physicians surely are the natural advocates of the poor and the social problem largely falls within their scope."[126] In subsequent issues, his articles dealt with a wide array of social and political issues connected to medicine. He argued against capital punishment, for the gradual end of war, and in favor of a variety of reforms ranging from social welfare and the regulation of working hours to periodic physician recertification.[127] He also touched poignantly on the notion of a *right to health and healthcare* that government is responsible to ensure, arguing that "the concept of *all having equal rights to healthful existence* follows from the definition of the state as the moral unity of its members, i.e. of individuals enjoying equal rights and obligated to act in solidarity. The endeavor of the state to implement these rights mainly falls to the Public Health Services" (emphasis added).[128]

Interestingly, Virchow almost seems to transform the Lockean notion of a "right to life" into a right to health, and *healthcare.* "As regards the scope of public health care, it is the community that has the obligation to safeguard the right of each individual to exist, i.e., to exist in health," he argued.[129] This strain of thought no doubt represents an interesting shift within the health care rights-commodity dialectic. Though it is admittedly impossible to guarantee health (much less eliminate death), "[i]t is possible to make provision for essential substances to be within everyone's grasp and to see to it that the very basis for living is not positively withdrawn or negatively withheld. This opportunity to live is the right of the individual, and the duty of the community . . ."[130] The right of an individual to life (and therefore health), in other words, generates a corresponding duty for the state to provide it. Indeed, these responsibilities are tied up, Virchow argues, in the very *definition* of the state: "When the state . . . allows its citizens to lapse into conditions in which they must starve to death, it ceases legally to be a state."[131]

Virchow proceeds from an acknowledgment that all have "equal rights to healthful existence" to a discussion of how healthcare should be provided to the poor in other issues of *Medical Reform.* He argued that the words " 'to everyone according to his needs,' nowhere applies more clearly and sharply as in public healthcare . . ."[132] This notion—of healthcare being available on the basis of needs, not means—is essential to the right to healthcare concept, and will emerge time and time again in coming chapters. He similarly argued that hospital admission should be based strictly according to need, not ability to pay, and that need should not be defined as already being on death's door: "Hospital admission must therefore be open to every patient that needs it, irrespective of whether he has money or not, whether he be Jew or heathen."[133]

The poor, however, needed access not only to hospitals, but also to physicians. Interestingly, Virchow opposed the formation of a separate corps of doctors designated for the poor. His argument was twofold. First, he argued that separate facilities only set the poor individual apart even further, stigmatizing his or her poverty:

> First a man had to become a pauper and only then was he given, in a bureau-cratic way, documents of legitimation which insured his poverty forever. The derelicts must not only taste their misery to the last drop, they must also carry it in their pockets in black and white. Only then were they taken care of, and a special physician for paupers was procured for them in advance.[134]

Second, he argued that a democratic society should be founded on the autonomy of the individual, and that the individual should be free to choose his or her own doctor: "Here everyone seeks the man of his confidence, each knows himself as the master of his body. Shall only the poor be precluded from this general right?"[135] Thus, the poor should not only have free access to healthcare, but also free choice of physician. In contrast, he envisions a public health service based on the "principle of equal rights for all . . ."[136] Virchow outlines a system of physician associations that would contract with municipalities and receive a lump sum to cover the cost of caring for all the poor in an area (somewhat akin to a modern non-corporate health maintenance organization, or HMO).[137] The poor would have free choice of physician within this association. Although such associations might not seem all that radically different from the pauper physicians he criticizes (and in rural areas, Virchow acknowledged, a single salaried charity physician might be unavoidable), the emphasis on the notion of healthcare equality is striking.[138] Broadly speaking, Virchow integrated the medical with the political in a novel manner: in his famous formulation, medicine had become a "social science," while "politics is nothing more than medicine on a large scale."[139]

In addition to writing and organizing under the medical reform banner, Virchow became involved in Berlin politics.[140] However, the window for political change was already closing. The middle class–working class alliance, as he wrote to his father, began to fracture.[141] In Paris, meanwhile, workers were soon dying in the streets in a fight against the very Republican government they had helped bring to power.[142] The tide soon turned against reform in Germany as well: the armies of reaction had bided their time, and now saw a chance to retake power. "For months the highest and noblest exaltation and now the most gruesome and wretched demoralization," Virchow wrote in a letter to his parents, later continuing: "In France, in Italy, in Austria and in our country the counter-revolution has conquered."[143] By the summer of 1849, the "springtime of peoples" was dead.

Although his immediate impact may have been limited, Virchow's work has inspired thinkers and activists ever since he published it. Many of the great historians of medicine—Henry Sigerist, George Rosen, and Erwin Ackerknecht, among others—wrote about Virchow's ideas, transmitting them to a whole new generation of scholars and activists. "Social medicine" in part arose from such thinking and analysis. While social medicine has been a heterogeneous movement, at its heart is a methodological approach to health like that used by Virchow in

Upper Silesia, i.e., through an examination of the myriad economic, political, environment, and cultural determinants of health and disease (and through seeking remedies along these same lines).[144] Virchow's influence also had an international reach. His ideas were influential on Latin American social medicine, which was in part the result of the emigration of some of his pupils to Latin America in the late nineteenth century.[145] One such individual, Max Westenhofer, became the director of the department of pathology at the University of Chile, where he influenced the future President of Chile, Salvador Allende, who in turn both wrote an influential social medicine text and introduced legislation that led to Chile's National Health Service (to be discussed in Chapter 6).[146] More recently, Virchow has had a direct impact on some notable individuals in the field of global public health, such as Paul Farmer, the infectious disease physician who has championed a human rights framework in the provision of global health and who has cited Virchow's influence and ideas.[147] Indeed, Theodore Brown and Anne-Emanuelle Birn have recently argued more broadly that the tradition of activist "health internationalism" in the United States very much emerged from the convergence of Virchowian social medicine thought with nineteenth-century currents of leftist internationalism.[148]

Returning to the nineteenth century, however, the straightforward truth of 1849 was one of outright defeat. Still, it was in Europe, many years later, that reformers first succeeded in *making* healthcare—if not health—a right, through the establishment of universal national health systems.

Conclusions

The public health movement of the early Industrial Revolution demonstrated a sociomedical fact that holds true today: class is a matter of life and death. Yet though many agreed that this was the reality, few agreed on the way forward. For many economic liberals, state aid would more likely hinder than help the poor. The especially harsh (and influential) line of Malthus even held that repressive traditions of state assistance such as the English Poor Law were simply an enticement to sloth and imprudent reproduction. Some, like Chadwick, believed that there was a clear—albeit narrow—role for the state: by improving the environmental *milieu* of the poor, the state could have a positive impact on their health, morality, and productivity.

However, this was not the only viewpoint on the issue. First, there was the more humanitarian critique of Alison, who found the argument that aid was counter-productive to be preposterous and cruel. Drawing (in part) on the ideas of Liancourt, Alison argued that if medical or economic aid was needed, it should be provided as of right. Both Engels and Virchow went further. Indeed, Virchow, in his writing, explicitly embraced the notion of the right to health: not only did men and women have rights, he argued, they had "*equal rights to healthful existence.*" Epidemics, in contrast, were in essence manifestations of *inequality*: not merely economic inequality, with some left in a state of terrible poverty, but political and social inequality.

1848 is an essential pivot in this book—a year when multiple strands of its story intersect. Chadwick's Public Health Act became law. The Chartists saw their final

68 · Health, Medicine, and Capitalism

year of potent protest: on April 10, 1848, one month after the Revolution had scattered the dictatorships of Continental Europe like so many bowling pins, 150,000 protestors assembled in Kennington Common in London in a massive rally.[149] It was only after the "June Days" in Paris, when the working classes were brought to heel, that the British government turned onto the Chartists, destroying their movement through heavy-handed repression.[150] Elsewhere in Europe, meanwhile, the forces of reaction were bringing an end to a short-lived era of revolutionary hope.

During this era, thinkers like Alison, Engels, and Virchow may very well have implicitly embraced the idea that working people had a "right to health," and perhaps also of healthcare. Clearly, however, it would remain for future generations to realize it.

Notes

1   Alison recounts this episode in a footnote: William Pulteney Alison, *Observations on the Management of the Poor in Scotland and Its Effects on the Health of the Great Towns* (Edinburgh: William Blackwood & Sons, 1840), http://id.lib.harvard.edu/aleph/007327085/catalog, 83,. (henceforth referred to as *Observations*). The biographical details in this paragraph are from Hamlin, *Public Health and Social Justice in the Age of Chadwick*, 74, 155. Hamlin also cites this passage of Alison's: Christopher Hamlin, *Public Health and Social Justice in the Age of Chadwick: Britain, 1800–1854* (Cambridge: Cambridge University Press, 1998), 82.

2   Rosalind Mitchison, "The Making of the Old Scottish Poor Law," *Past & Present*, no. 63 (1974), 58.

3   Alison, *Observations*, 83.

4   Ibid.

5   Ibid., 63–4.

6   The uniqueness of Alison's approach, which diverged from the "economic" consensus of his time, is central to the argument of Christopher Hamlin, who I return to later in the chapter. Hamlin, *Public Health and Social Justice in the Age of Chadwick*, 195; Christopher Hamlin, "William Pulteney Alison, the Scottish Philosophy, and the Making of a Political Medicine," *Journal of the History of Medicine and Allied Sciences* 61, no. 2 (2006): 144–86.

7   As Moyn puts it, rights talk was "strikingly abandoned" in the nineteenth century. Samuel Moyn, *The Last Utopia: Human Rights in History* (Cambridge, MA: Belknap Press of Harvard University Press, 2010).

8   Notably, Tobin's chapter on the historical roots of the right to health includes a discussion of how public health thought and the human right to health intersect. John Tobin, *The Right to Health in International Law* (Oxford: Oxford University Press, 2012), 34–41.

9   E.P. Thompson, *The Making of the English Working Class* (New York: Vintage Books, 1966), 177, 197–9, 209–12.

10 Szreter Simon and Graham Mooney, "Urbanization, Mortality, and the Standard of Living Debate: New Estimates of the Expectation of Life at Birth in Nineteenth-Century British Cities," *The Economic History Review* 51, no. 1 (1998), Table I page 88. Also see Flinn, introduction to *Report on the Sanitary Condition of the Labouring Population of Great Britain,* by Edwin Chadwick (Edinburgh: Edinburgh University Press, 1965), 4, 14.

11 E. H. Ackerknecht, "Hygiene in France, 1815–1848," *Bulletin of the History of Medicine* 22, no. 2 (1948): 144.

12 Ann Elizabeth Fowler La Berge, *Mission and Method: The Early Nineteenth-Century French Public Health Movement* (Cambridge: Cambridge University Press, 1992), 1, 25; Ackerknecht, "Hygiene in France, 1815–1848": 117–55.

13 La Berge, *Mission and Method*, 1–2.

14 Ibid., 2.

15 William Coleman, *Death Is a Social Disease: Public Health and Political Economy in Early Industrial France* (Madison: University of Wisconsin Press, 1982), 66, 72–3.

16 Condorcet had considered the possibility that the production of food would ultimately reach some limit, but somewhat vaguely suggests that enlightened men will consciously limit their reproduction. Marie-Jean-Antoine Nicolas Caritat de Condorcet, "Sketch for a Historical Picture of the Progress of the Human Mind," in *Condorcet: Selected Writings* (Indianapolis: Bobbs-Merrill, 1976), 270–1.

17 Thomas Malthus, *An Essay on the Principle of Population* (London: Penguin, repr. 1985), 71.

18 Ibid., 119.

19 Fraser, for instance, states that Malthus became the "high priest" of those seeking to abolish the British Poor Law. Derek Fraser, *The Evolution of the British Welfare State: A History of Social Policy since the Industrial Revolution*, 4th ed. (Basingstoke: Palgrave Macmillan, 2009), 46.

20 Malthus, *An Essay on the Principle of Population*, 97.

21 Both the overall point and the quote from Malthus are from Gaston V. Rimlinger, *Welfare Policy and Industrialization in Europe, America, and Russia* (New York: John Wiley and Sons, 1971), 40.

22 The quote is Rimlinger quoting James Bonar: Ibid., 38, 51.

23 Hamlin, *Public Health and Social Justice in the Age of Chadwick*, 194–5.

24 Roy Porter, *The Greatest Benefit to Mankind: A Medical History of Humanity* (New York: W. W. Norton, 1998), 407.

25 La Berge, *Mission and Method*, 1–3; Coleman, *Death Is a Social Disease*, 5. My brief summary of Villermé's large body of work is based on these two secondary sources.

26 Coleman, *Death Is a Social Disease*, 31, 101, 303.

27 I am greatly obliged here to Coleman's insightful book, which is the primary source for my discussion of Villermé. La Berge, *Mission and Method*, 60–1; Coleman, *Death Is a Social Disease*, 150.

28 Coleman, *Death Is a Social Disease*, 150–61; La Berge, *Mission and Method*, 59–66.

29 Quoted in Coleman, *Death Is a Social Disease*, 161.

30 Ibid., 231–45.

31 Ibid., 276.

32 Ibid., 241–2.

33 Quoted in ibid., 262.

34 Ibid., 237–42. Coleman notes that Villermé considered the February 1848 revolution to be "contrived by utterly corrupt interests." Ibid., 12.

35 Simon and Mooney, "Urbanization, Mortality, and the Standard of Living Debate."

36 Roy Lubove, *The Struggle for Social Security 1900–1935* (Pittsburgh: University of Pittsburgh Press, 1986), 182; Rimlinger, *Welfare Policy and Industrialization in Europe, America, and Russia*, 37–44; Fraser, *The Evolution of the British Welfare State*, 50–2.

37 Fraser, *The Evolution of the British Welfare State*, 50–2.

38 Ibid.

39 Hamlin, *Public Health and Social Justice in the Age of Chadwick*, 29; George Rosen, *A History of Public Health* (Baltimore: Johns Hopkins University Press, 1993), 173; Fraser, *The Evolution of the British Welfare State*, 53–5.

40 Quoted in Lesley Doyal and Imogen Pennel, *The Political Economy of Health* (Boston: South End Press, 1981), 143.

41 Fraser, *The Evolution of the British Welfare State*, 53–5; Hamlin, *Public Health and Social Justice in the Age of Chadwick*, 30–5; Thompson, *The Making of the English Working Class*, 267.

42 Gøsta Esping-Andersen, *The Three Worlds of Welfare Capitalism* (Princeton, NJ: Princeton University Press, 1990), 36.

43 T. H. Marshall, "Citizenship and Social Class," in *Citizenship and Social Class* (London: Pluto Press, 1992), 15.

44 Fraser notes, for instance, that the law did not force the new Poor Law Unions to construct workhouses, and that outdoor relief would continue in most unions in coming decades. Fraser, *The Evolution of the British Welfare State*, 58–64; John Knott, *Popular Opposition to the 1834 Poor Law* (London: Croom Helm, 1986), 7–8.

45 The quote is Hilton quoting John Belchem. Knott, *Popular Opposition to the 1834 Poor Law*, 129, 138–9; Boyd Hilton, *A Mad, Bad, & Dangerous People? England 1783–1846* (Oxford: Clarendon Press, 2006), 612.

46 Hilton, *A Mad, Bad, & Dangerous People? England 1783–1846*, 616.

47 Knott, *Popular Opposition to the 1834 Poor Law*, 129–42.

48 Ibid., 7.

49 Thompson, *The Making of the English Working Class*, 230.

50 Quoted in ibid., 761.

51 Quoted in Knott, *Popular Opposition to the 1834 Poor Law*, 5–6.

52 Ibid., 138.

53 Quoted in ibid., 141.

54 This paragraph relies throughout on Hamlin, who was a key source for this section overall. Hamlin, *Public Health and Social Justice in the Age of Chadwick*, for example, 90–1, 103, 140.

55 Edwin Chadwick, *Report on the Sanitary Condition of the Labouring Population of Great Britain* (Edinburgh: Edinburgh University Press, 1965), 210.

56 Ibid., 216.

57 Ibid., 223–4, 302.

58 Ibid. For example: 84, 164–7, 190, 197–8, 423. Hamlin makes this point as well: see Hamlin, *Public Health and Social Justice in the Age of Chadwick*, 167, 184.

59 Chadwick, *Report on the Sanitary Condition . . .*, 201.

60 Ibid., 423.

61 Hamlin, *Public Health and Social Justice in the Age of Chadwick*, 13, 157, 167, 171, 185.

62 Quoted in Doyal and Pennel, *The Political Economy of Health*, 145. For Chadwick on Chartism and radicalism, see also: Chadwick, *Report on the Sanitary Condition . . .*, 163, 267, 337.

63 Hamlin, *Public Health and Social Justice in the Age of Chadwick*, 207.

64 Chadwick, *Report on the Sanitary Condition of the Labouring Population of Great Britain*, 423.

65 Hamlin, *Public Health and Social Justice in the Age of Chadwick*, 90–110.

66 Hamlin discusses Alison in: Hamlin, *Public Health and Social Justice in the Age of Chadwick*; Hamlin, "William Pulteney Alison, the Scottish Philosophy, and the Making of a Political Medicine." I followed his lead to Alison's *Observations*.

67 Hamlin, "William Pulteney Alison, the Scottish Philosophy, and the Making of a Political Medicine," 152–5.

68 Ibid., 157–60.

69 Alison, *Observations on the Management of the Poor in Scotland and Its Effects on the Health of the Great Towns*, x.

70 Ibid., 10–11. I discuss some of the mechanisms and ideas here in Adam Gaffney, "The Politics of Health," review of *Beyond Obamacare: Life, Death, and Social Policy*, by James. S. House, *Los Angeles Review of Books*, October 26, 2015, accessed October 26, 2016, https://lareviewof books.org/review/the-politics-of-health.

71 Alison, *Observations*, 15. A number of physicians noted the connection between typhus and poverty. See Flinn, Introduction to *Report on the Sanitary Condition of the Labouring Population of Great Britain*, by Edwin Chadwick, 9–10.

72 Alison, *Observations*, 22.

73 Flinn emphasizes that Alison and Chadwick's views were not so very different, and that they both rejected Malthus. Conversely, Hamlin argues strongly for the uniqueness of Alison's "medical critique." Christopher Hamlin, *Public Health and Social Justice in the Age of Chadwick: Britain, 1800–1854* (Cambridge: Cambridge University Press, 1998), 81; M. W. Flinn, introduction to *Report on the Sanitary Condition of the Labouring Population of Great Britain*, by Edwin Chadwick (Edinburgh: Edinburgh University Press, 1965), 65–6.

74 Alison, *Observations*, 22.

75 Ibid., 53–4.

76 Ibid., 41, 50–7.

77 Ibid., 56–7.

78   Ibid., 57.
79   Ibid., 63.
80   Ibid., 57, 63–4.
81   Ibid., 109.
82   Flinn, introduction to *Report on the Sanitary Condition of the Labouring Population of Great Britain*, by Edwin Chadwick, 63–4; Hamlin, *Public Health and Social Justice in the Age of Chadwick*, 127.
83   Hamlin, *Public Health and Social Justice in the Age of Chadwick*, 81.
84   Hamlin, "William Pulteney Alison, the Scottish Philosophy, and the Making of a Political Medicine," 186.
85   Quoted in Rosen, *A History of Public Health*, 200.
86   Quoted in George Rosen, "Medical Care and Social Policy in Seventeenth Century England," *Bulletin of the New York Academy of Medicine* 29, no. 5 (1953):159.
87   M. W. Flinn, "Medical Services under the New Poor Law," in Derek Fraser (ed.), *The New Poor Law in the Nineteenth Century* (London: Macmillan, 1976), 47.
88   Ruth G. Hodgkinson, *The Origins of the National Health Service: The Medical Services of the New Poor Law, 1834–1871* (London: The Wellcome Historical Medical Library, 1967), 680. (I owe this citation to Hamlin.)
89   Flinn, introduction to *Report on the Sanitary Condition of the Labouring Population of Great Britain,* by Edwin Chadwick, 32; Flinn, "Medical Services under the New Poor Law," 48.
90   Flinn, "Medical Services under the New Poor Law," 48–59.
91   Ibid., 51, 53–9.
92   Ibid., 56.
93   Hamlin, *Public Health and Social Justice in the Age of Chadwick*, 92, 95. Hodgkinson discusses the complexities of the prescription of food and "extras," which was in reality a "recommendation" that could be blocked by the Board of Guardians. Hodgkinson, *The Origins of the National Health Service*, 35–43.
94   Hodgkinson, *The Origins of the National Health Service*, 60–2.
95   Hamlin, *Public Health and Social Justice in the Age of Chadwick*, 94, 96.
96   Flinn, "Medical Services under the New Poor Law," 59, 64–6; Hodgkinson, *The Origins of the National Health Service*, 5, 16–18, 63–6, 685–96.
97   Sidney Webb and Beatrice Webb, *The State and the Doctor* (London: Longmans, Green and Co., 1910), 7; Hodgkinson, *The Origins of the National Health Service*, 696.
98   Flinn, "Medical Services under the New Poor Law," 66; Hodgkinson, *The Origins of the National Health Service*, xv, 696.
99   The points made in this paragraph thus far draw on Fraser, *The Evolution of the British Welfare State*, 69.
100 Howard Waitzkin has previously emphasized the importance of Engels to public health/health rights thought. I follow the lead and the advice of Waitzkin to this source. Howard Waitzkin, *Medicine and Public Health at the End of Empire* (Boulder, CO: Paradigm Publishers, 2011), 11–13; Howard Waitzkin, personal communication to the author by e-mail, December 12, 2016.
101 David McLellan, Introduction to *The Condition of the Working Class in England* by Friedrich Engels (Oxford: Oxford University Press, 2009), ix.
102 Friedrich Engels, *The Condition of the Working Class in England* (Oxford: Oxford University Press, 2009), 106.
103 Ibid., 185.
104 Ibid., 113.
105 Ibid., 114.
106 Waitzkin, *Medicine and Public Health at the End of Empire*, 13.
107 Engels, *The Condition of the Working Class in England*, 297.
108 McLellan, Introduction to *The Condition of the Working Class in England* by Friedrich Engels (Oxford: Oxford University Press, 2009), xvi.
109 Waitzkin, *Medicine and Public Health at the End of Empire*, 13.
110 Erwin Heinz Ackerknecht, *Rudolf Virchow: Doctor, Statesman, Anthropologist* (Madison: University of Wisconsin Press, 1953), 5–13.

111   Ruldof Virchow, *Letters to His Parents: 1839–1864*, trans. L. J. Rather (Canton: Science History Publications, 1990), 60.

112   Ackerknecht, *Rudolf Virchow*, 14; Byron A. Boyd, *Rudolf Virchow: The Scientist as Citizen* (New York: Garland, 1991), 22.

113   Virchow, *Letters to His Parents: 1839–1864*, 76; Ackerknecht, *Rudolf Virchow*, 14.

114   Virchow, *Letters to His Parents: 1839–1864*, 77.

115   Rudolf Virchow, *Collected Essays on Public Health and Epidemiology*, trans. L. J. Rather (Canton, MA: Science History Publications, U.S.A., 1985), 1: 300–1.

116   Ibid., 117.

117   Successful efforts at enforcing abstinence from alcohol had merely, he thought, deprived the poor of one of their few remaining pleasures. Ibid., 217.

118   Ibid., 215–16.

119   Ibid., 308.

120   Ibid., 311.

121   Ibid., 315.

122   Ibid.

123   As he wrote, "the political uprisings that had in the meanwhile broken out made it mandatory for me to participate in the manifestations in the capital." Ibid., 206.

124   Virchow, *Letters to His Parents: 1839–1864*, 84; Ackerknecht, *Rudolf Virchow*, 15.

125   "Medical reform," as Boyd notes, was a heterogeneous movement that preceded 1848, with branches in many European countries (especially France), involving many individuals and producing a large mass of publications. Boyd, *Rudolf Virchow: The Scientist as Citizen*, 34–6.

126   Virchow, *Collected Essays on Public Health and Epidemiology*, 1, 4. Of note, only a selection of his articles is available in this translated volume.

127   Ibid., 18–20, 50.

128   Ibid., 16.

129   Ibid., 17.

130   Ibid.

131   Ibid., 15.

132   Ibid., 26.

133   Ibid., 26–7.

134   Ibid., 36.

135   Ibid., 39.

136   Ibid., 36.

137   Ibid., 44.

138   Ibid., 46.

139   Ibid., 33.

140   Boyd, *Rudolf Virchow: The Scientist as Citizen*, 42.

141   Peter N. Stearns, *The Revolutions of 1848* (London: Weidenfeld and Nicolson, 1974), 149; Virchow, *Letters to His Parents: 1839–1864*, 85–6.

142   Stearns, *The Revolutions of 1848*, 91–2.

143   Virchow, *Letters to His Parents: 1839–1864*, 98.

144   Theodore M. Brown and Anne-Emanuelle Birn, "The Making of Health Internationalists," in *Comrades in Health: U.S. Health Internationalists, Abroad and at Home*, ed. Anne-Emanuelle Birn and Theodore M. Brown (New Brunswick: Rutgers University Press, 2013), 15–20.

145   Howard Waitzkin, "One and a Half Centuries of Forgetting and Rediscovering: Virchow's Lasting Contributions to Social Medicine," *Social Medicine* 1, no. 1 (2006): 8.

146   Ibid., 8–9.

147   Tracy Kidder, *Mountains Beyond Mountains* (New York: Random House, 2003), 60–1.

148   Theodore M. Brown and Anne-Emanuelle Birn, "The Making of Health Internationalists," in *Comrades in Health: U.S. Health Internationalists, Abroad and at Home*, ed. Anne-Emanuelle Birn and Theodore M. Brown (New Brunswick: Rutgers University Press, 2013), 15.

149   Hilton, *A Mad, Bad, & Dangerous People? England 1783–1846*, 613.

150   Ibid.

4

Blood and Iron and Health Insurance

Towards the Modern Era

The eminent surgeon James Peter Warbasse should not have been surprised when in April 1918—with Great War jingoism drowning out rationale debate—he was abruptly expelled from his county medical society (which also, for good measure, took the liberty of forwarding some materials on the good doctor to the US Department of Justice).[1] Apart from Warbasse's affiliations with various left-wing political groups, his involvement in the labor movement, and his provocative social medicine-themed writings, he had now offended the society with a letter to the editor of a New York newspaper that was deemed insufficiently patriotic.[2] Perhaps he hoped that his prominent academic standing might have offered some protection: having trained with the best in Germany, Warbasse had authored scores of scientific papers as well as a multi-volume surgical text.[3] His views on healthcare, however, may have been working against him within his rather conservative medical society. Several years prior, for instance, Warbasse had forcefully argued for healthcare equity and rights in the pages of the preeminent *Journal of the American Medical Association*:

> Among the wealthy there now is a surfeit of doctors; among the poor, too few. . . . I believe that the wives of coal-miners and iron-workers are as worthy of the best scientific attention and the tenderest care in the hours of their need as are the wives of the rich. I believe that they should have it, not as a charity or welfare enterprise, but as a matter of social justice. It is their right.[4]

Such a striking sentiment about healthcare rights was, to put it delicately, problematic in the year 1918. Progressive reformers were working towards "compulsory health insurance" systems at the state level that would have created—to a quite limited extent—a right to healthcare for some workers for the first time. Throughout the state, physicians and reformers were engaged in hot political combat on this issue, complete with venomous red-baiting and charges of disloyalty.

This chapter deals with the creation (or attempted creation) of public health insurance systems: first in Germany, then in Britain, and finally in the United States. Simply stated, the actualization of a right to healthcare requires the creation of a system of universal healthcare. The period addressed by this chapter was when the right to healthcare moved from the realm of ideas to—at least to a limited extent in some places—that of laws and reality. At the same time, however, the very political and economic factors that underlay the emergence of these systems also shaped their contours and limited their scope. While these early healthcare systems may have ensured *some degree* of guaranteed access to healthcare for *some* of the working-class citizenry, they fell short of universalism. Though creating a legal right to medical services for some, in other words, they nonetheless failed to make healthcare itself a right for all.

Germany: The Beginnings of National Health Insurance

Today, universal health insurance is generally regarded—as it already was in 1918 when Warbasse stood accused of disloyalty—as a plank in the platform of the political Left. It may therefore seem ironic that what has been called "the first formal social health insurance system" arose in the late nineteenth century under the direction of Otto von Bismarck, the conservative, authoritarian chancellor of Germany (and a man not known for having a soft spot for socialism).[5] However, according to some historians and contemporary critics of Bismarck, his intention in pursuing social welfare was, in fact, to co-opt the Left: mollifying the masses with state pensions and health insurance, and thereby derailing the socialist movement which he so deeply despised.[6]

Things, of course, are never quite so simple, and historical shifts in governance are rarely due to the particular political stratagems of a single policymaker. Various systems can be seen as possible antecedents to German's welfare state (some going back to the Middle Ages), including the tradition of guild welfare and provident funds, the German Poor Law, and the Prussian Civil Code.[7] Additionally, as in England, some may have even seen state welfare as a way to shield taxpayers from what were seen as burdensome contributions to the Poor Law.[8] Other scholars have stressed the great economic transformation of the late nineteenth century. Germany made enormous strides in industrial growth following the Revolutions of 1848, but along with the rest of Europe, it faced a period of prolonged economic unease after the Depression of 1873: this critical epoch was characterized by deflation, a fall in profits, and a resurgence in protectionism, and has been considered a watershed in the history of capitalism.[9] Under such conditions of economic strain, "[t]he time was ripe," contends medical historian Henry Sigerist, "for social legislation."[10] The move away from laissez-faire liberalism, moreover, may have made some German industrial interests more open to the idea of state intervention in the social realm.[11] Indeed, some of the larger industrialists actually came to support some form of state social welfare during this period.[12]

Social stability, after all, can be crucial during times of political turmoil. From the ashes of the Revolutions of 1848, a new radicalism was on the rise in late nineteenth-century Germany. Ferdinand Lassalle—who had tried to start a socialist movement in the Rhineland with Karl Marx in 1848—founded Germany's first socialist party, the General German Workers' Association, in 1863.[13] Around the same time, another "48er, Wilhelm Liebknecht, returned to Germany at the direction of Karl Marx with a plan to initiate a socialist movement loyal to Marx's 'First International.'"[14] Liebknecht joined forces with former carpenter and labor activist August Bebel, and in 1869, Bebel's workers' organization combined with other socialist factions to found the Social Democratic Workers' Party, which later fused with Lassalle's General German Workers' Association to become the Social Democratic Party (SPD).[15]

Today, the SPD is the primary center-left party in Germany, the basic equivalent of the Democratic Party in the United States. Yet as it rapidly grew in strength and numbers in the late nineteenth century, the Marxist SPD was increasingly regarded as a revolutionary menace.[16] Bismarck saw in the SPD "a fundamental threat," as one historian has put it, "not only to the social and political order that he was establishing in Germany, but to the established order in Europe as a whole."[17] Before pursuing his social welfare laws, Bismarck moved against the socialist movement with the heavy scepter of state-power. On the pretext of two attempts at assassinating the Emperor, the Reichstag passed an anti-socialist law that outlawed freedom of assembly and of the press for any organizations with "social democratic, socialist, or communist activities . . ."[18] This had had an immediate and dramatic impact: the trade union movement was shattered, movement newspapers were outlawed, and prominent activists were expelled.[19]

Following these repressive measures, Bismarck proceeded to pass three milestone welfare laws, starting with his Sickness Insurance Law of 1883. Under this law—which was expanded upon in 1892, 1903 and 1911—industrial workers were insured through "sick funds" (*Krankenkassen*), which were administered and funded by both employees and employers, who contracted with doctors and hospitals. Medical benefits included doctor visits, surgical care, hospital care, drugs and supplies, and eyeglasses. Additionally, there was a benefit in cash of one half of wages for sick workers that began after four days of illness. Insured women would be eligible for a cash maternity benefit for eight weeks, though not for the actual costs of normal deliveries.[20] Subsequent expansions of this initial legislation delivered health insurance to more categories of workers in later years, for instance, to domestic and agricultural workers after 1911.[21] Two other pieces of legislation rounded out the fledgling German welfare state: industrial accident insurance (1884) and old age pensions (1889) for some workers lucky enough to live to age 70.

Many have contended that these social welfare laws, launched during years of political repression, were an attempt to undercut the appeal of socialism by combining subjugation with benefits. This "carrot and stick" explanation of the German welfare state—i.e., the carrot of welfare benefits, the stick of oppression—was in fact exactly how some in the SDP skeptically saw it.[22] Clearly, the government advertised its plans with anti-socialist rhetoric.[23] For instance, in 1881, the Kaiser argued in front of the Reichstag that:

> A remedy cannot alone be sought in the repression of Socialistic excesses; there must be simultaneously the positive advancement of the welfare of the working classes. And here the care of those workpeople who are incapable

of earning their livelihood is of the first importance . . . [the] insufficiency [of existing institutions] has to no small extent contributed to cause the working classes to seek help by participating in Social Democratic movements.[24]

In another instance, Bismarck stated that he intended "to bribe the working classes, or, if you like, to win them over to regard the State as a social institution existing for their sake and interested in their welfare."[25] Perhaps as a result of such rhetoric, the SPD had somewhat of an ambiguous orientation to Bismarck's proposals. The SPD Congress of 1883, for instance, declared that "so-called social reform is nothing but a tactical means designed to lure the workers away from the correct path."[26] Nonetheless, the SPD ultimately aligned itself with the overall thrust of Bismarck's welfare measures, while at the same time emphasizing its own more expansive versions of his bills.[27]

Yet some have argued that seeing Bismarck's health insurance law as nothing but a cynical ploy to buy off would-be revolutionaries and crush the SPD is too simplistic. According to historian E.P. Hennock, for instance, Bismarck's decisions about social welfare were made before the elaboration of his anti-socialist arguments; he therefore contends that anti-socialism was ultimately more of a "tactical device by a master tactician" that was used to push through a controversial package, and that the true motives of Bismarck lay more with the "high priority given . . . to industrial growth" and an understanding of its "technical dangers and social costs . . ."[28] Accident insurance, which covered industrial workers injured on the job, was, for instance, sold to Bismarck by one industrialist as "a reform to avoid industrial and political conflict, bringing greater productivity and political stability in its wake."[29] The German welfare state, according to this line of thinking, was an accommodation of—and not an anomaly in—the advance of industrial capitalism. By stabilizing the human strains within the industrial system, policymakers could allow industrial growth to continue unfettered. Others have emphasized the extent to which Bismarck's social welfare measures were an attempt to consolidate state power and strengthen the loyalty of the worker to the state, while maintaining the "traditional system of political inequality."[30] Less an attempt to lure workers away from a particular ideology, in other words, Bismarck's state welfare was intended to bring them into the fold of fidelity to an undemocratic state, or, as Esping-Andersen puts it, to "chain the workers directly to the paternal authority of the monarchy . . ."[31]

Perhaps all of these various factors played a role to some extent or another. Esping-Andersen, for instance, sees the underlying motives behind the conservative welfare state of Germany as "social integration, the preservation of authority, and the battle again socialism."[32] But putting aside the question of motives, it is worth considering the meaning of Bismarck's health insurance legislation from the perspective of rights. On the one hand, his health insurance law seems to represent a leftward shift within the healthcare rights-commodity dialectic. First, state health insurance took healthcare out of the commodities towards which a worker had to devote his or her disposable income. Second, health insurance was not simply another form of "Poor Law" charity, but instead the right of a worker. Social insurance, as one scholar has argued, "differed from the traditional care of the poor" insofar as it provided for the "insured person's individual legal right to claim benefits, free from any political or social discrimination."[33] In this sense, social health insurance, even if only to a limited extent, represented a shift away from a construction of healthcare as a commodity.

However, on the other hand, Bismarck's legislation neither intended nor achieved universalism. His plan covered predominantly industrial workers, and excluded those who were either unemployed or employed in a variety of non-industrial occupations, like casual laborers. In later years, it was expanded to various other categories of workers, and may have covered almost a third of the German population by the early twentieth century.[34] But in its design, it was simply not intended to create "a right to healthcare." Sickness insurance was aimed to ameliorate the rougher edges of industrial capitalism, and thus its primary beneficiary was the (usually male) industrial worker. Workers could pay extra to extend their benefits to their families, but again, these individuals received healthcare only as dependents, not as individuals in their own right.[35] Who else was excluded? The unemployed and their families, casual laborers, widows, much of the middle class, and many more.

So, while it is perhaps true, as Sigerist describes, that Bismarck's health insurance law "guaranteed medical care to the increasing army of wage-earners, not as a matter of charity but as a right that they acquired through their labor,"[36] this was effectively a legal right to some healthcare for a constricted segment of the population. In fact, the most marginalized parts of the population were the very ones excluded. Perhaps German health insurance was designed to cover the (relatively) better off workers because it was they—and not the very poor—who constituted a potential political threat.[37] Vicente Navarro takes this argument a step further, asserting that the corporatist organization of the German insurance scheme effectively split the working class itself:

> [W]hile the threat posed to the social order by the working class political party was the stimulus for the Act, the way in which the Act was developed, organized, and administered responded to the capitalist class aims of dividing the workers and weakening the class solidarity within the working class. By providing levels of benefits according to status and type of employment, and by having the state . . . administer the different health insurance programs, the capitalist and aristocratic classes tried to divide and control the working class.[38]

Whether or not that was its explicit aim, it seems fair to concede that it may have been, to some extent, its *effect*. Or, as Esping-Andersen puts it, "corporatist statist" welfare states (like that of Bismarck's) were designed to maintain social hierarchies: rights are therefore affixed to occupationally-defined class, with the resultant frequent exclusion of women.[39] They differ both from liberal welfare states—where benefits are meted out on the basis of a means test and associated with stigma (like under the New Poor Law)—as well as social democratic welfare states, which are based on the extension of the "principles of universalism and decommodification of social rights . . ."[40]

Indeed, around this time, a social democratic universalistic welfare alternative was laid out by the SPD, including for healthcare. In 1891—the year after the fall of Bismarck—the SPD proclaimed its "Erfurt Program," which, as historian Donald Sasson notes, established the essential principles and demands of social democracy for the next hundred years.[41] The Erfurt Program put forth a program for healthcare that went well went beyond that of Bismarck. In a few simple words, point eight of the Program calls for a right to healthcare: "Free medical care, including midwifery and medicines."[42] Critically, unlike the section of the document that dealt with "the protection of the working classes," this was to be a right enjoyed by all.[43] In this sense, Bismarck's health insurance law was ironically more distinctly focused on the specific interests of "labor" than the healthcare proposal of the party of labor itself, which envisioned a universal social right to healthcare.

Still, German sickness insurance nonetheless remains an important milestone—and a highly influential one—in the history of universal healthcare. Approximately a quarter century after the passage of the sickness insurance bill, the Liberal prime minister of Great Britain, David Lloyd George, toured Germany to investigate its social insurance system, and liked what he saw.[44] It would successfully serve as a model first for England, and then—less successfully—for the United States.

Britain: Poverty, Labor, and the Rise of New Liberalism

"[S]eething in the very centre of our great cities," warned a short pamphlet published in England in 1883, "concealed by the thinnest crust of civilization and decency, is a vast mass of moral corruption, of heart-breaking misery and absolute godlessness . . ."[45] So warned Andrew Mearns in his *The Bitter Cry of Outcast London*, an influential work that chronicled the worsening condition of London's lower classes, and that shocked Victorian sensibilities.[46] It was almost fifty years after Chadwick's New Poor Law, and apparently, the poor still had not been sufficiently scared out of poverty.

The recognition that existing institutions—in particular, the New Poor Law—had failed to solve the problem of deprivation was one factor that led to the creation of a new social welfare policy in Britain.[47] As in Germany, however, other concerns were at play, including an upsurge in working class agitation and a coalescing labor movement.[48] As it did elsewhere, the 1873 Depression exacerbated class tensions in England—and in the 1880s, they peaked.[49] In February 1886, a protest by unemployed workers led to the extraordinary "Trafalgar Square Riots."[50] These riots, it is argued, permanently changed elite perceptions of the working class: less an object of pity, they were now "a menace to be bought off . . ."[51] The government's response—the famous "March Circular"—directed local authorities to pay for public works to ameliorate unemployment, thereby all but admitting state responsibility for relieving unemployment separate from the action of the stigmatizing Poor Law.[52]

There were other factors, however. As in Germany, for instance, the pressure of a democratized populace and an enlarged franchise—achieved through various Reform Acts—had to be addressed.[53] The interplay between an expanded electorate and a mobilized working class contributed to the rise of a new political party, the Labour Party, in 1900. Though Labour remained a minority party for decades, it succeeded in pressing the Liberal Party from the left, pushing it into at least some action to avoid further electoral losses; in so doing, it contributed to the passage of new welfare laws.[54] Finally, a somewhat darker factor was the perception of imperial necessity: a strong world power, it was argued, needed strong, healthy young men to fight and die for it.[55]

The combination of these various pressures contributed to the 1905 passage of a comprehensive welfare program by the Liberal Party. This was the work of so-called "New Liberalism," [56] to be contrasted with the economic liberalism of the nineteenth-century Whigs. "In its social legislation," argues Gilbert, "it [New Liberalism] had ended the inviolability of personal wealth . . . Henceforth, society could call on a man's wealth not only to defend the realm or to promote the welfare of the nation, but to better the economic stratus and living conditions of specific individuals whom the donor himself did not choose."[57]

What did the New Liberals accomplish? Their first success was the passage of the Provision of Meals Act in December 1906, which enabled municipalities to provide meals to impoverished children (this was followed by legislation creating a "new school medical service" that provided healthcare for these children).[58] The gains of the Labour Party in the 1907 elections pushed the Liberals even further to the left.[59] The following year, they passed a "non-contributory" Old Age Pensions Act, which began operating in January 1, 1909, and which provided pensions for those over the age of 70.[60] The National Health Insurance Act came next. Great Britain by that point had something of a hodge-podge of provisions to provide healthcare to those who were unable to afford the services of a private physician, including the voluntary hospital, the outpatient dispensary (as Alison had worked for), and the Poor Law medical service (as described in the last chapter).[61] Of course, such provisions provided inadequate protection and excluded many.[62] The healthcare vision of the New Liberals, however, revolved less around the importance of providing medical benefits to the (usually male) worker for its own sake, and more around ameliorating the economic consequences of sickness for him and his family.[63]

Lloyd George was compelled to introduce various compromises into this "health insurance" bill after potent opposition arose from friendly societies, insurance companies, and the medical profession.[64] A contributory system—deemed more affordable than a tax-based one—was ultimately passed, and it covered manual laborers and all other workers earning less than a certain threshold between the ages of 16 and 70.[65] It provided five primary benefits: there was a medical benefit for doctors and drugs, coverage for care in a sanatorium, a maternity benefit (either for a worker or a worker's wife), a flat-rate sickness benefit for lost wages, and a disability benefit after the expiration of the sickness benefit.[66] Notably, however, there was no coverage for specialist care, hospital care, or funeral expenses, which had been covered by the German plan; even more striking was the complete absence of coverage for the dependents of the wage earner, thus that it was mainly adult men who were its beneficiaries.[67]

While the welfare legislation of this period was in some respects quite limited, in some respects it was a major departure in policy. Consider the issue of how these new programs were funded. Pensions were "non-contributory" and paid for through general taxation.[68] Additionally, unlike German sickness insurance—which was funded only by workers and employers—British National Health Insurance received a contribution from the government.[69] Existing revenues were insufficient to fund the new pension and insurance systems, thus making a new system of taxation necessary. This was accomplished by Lloyd George's "People's Budget" of 1909, which introduced a more progressive income tax together with other progressive taxes and duties on land.[70] This was a historical turning point, insofar as the "People's Budget" amounted to explicit economic redistribution for the purpose of social welfare.[71] In short, progressive taxation—and effective wealth redistribution—was utilized for the purpose of creating rights to new social programs, including medical care for the working class.

But how might these developments be viewed from the perspective of the healthcare rights-commodity dialectic? On the one hand, whatever the precise combination of motivations that historians have seen behind these early forays into the welfare state, an explicit concern for the individual *right* to healthcare seems absent. On the other hand, however, what made these social welfare programs different from the Poor Law or the medieval charitable hospital was that their benefits were provided as something of a legal *right*. After the passage of the Old Age Pensions Act, for instance, many of the elderly poor who had avoided the stigmatizing Poor Law were more than happy to come forward to receive its benefits.[72] Pensions were therefore "a new birthright of the British, a part of citizenship . . . State pensions were not charity and were paid as of right."[73] One scholar similarly credits the New Liberals with being "the first to begin articulating the principles of the welfare state itself, specifically the idea of state provision as a matter of right, based on ideals of equality and democracy, rather than the traditional idea that society should relieve extreme poverty."[74]

However, there is another side to this story. Like the German system, the British welfare state diverged from the universalism of modern human rights insofar as its scope was *not* universal. Again, this relates to political and economic interests, and is evidenced by the fact that health insurance benefits were for the (typically male) worker, not his spouse or children.[75] As a result, whereas a majority of adult men had health insurance coverage by 1914, less than a quarter of adult women were covered.[76] The ideological underpinning for this was bluntly revealed in one 1910 description of Lloyd George's sickness insurance proposal:

> Married women living with their husbands need not be included since where the unit is the family, it is the husband's and not the wife's health which it

is important to insure. So long as the husband is in good health and able to work, adequate provision will be made for the needs of the family, irrespective of the wife's health, whereas when the husband's health fails there is no one to earn wages.[77]

Societal economics, not human needs, were what mattered. Thus emerges another, and darker, side of New Liberalism: though it went beyond classical liberalism with respect to state involvement in social welfare, it did so, at least in part, in the interests of industrial capitalism. There was interest in treating illness, as Gilbert puts it, "only so far as it was desirable to put the breadwinner back to work as quickly as possible."[78] Thus, to again turn to Esping-Andersen's typology, healthcare in England in this period remained a mix of the corporatist-statist and liberal variety—it had not been decommoditized through the construction of a real social right.

The year 1915 saw the beginning of the First World War. The Liberal Party would be eclipsed by the Labour Party, which—after coming to power in the wake of the Second World War—would proceed to go well beyond "New Liberalism" and construct a system that very much guaranteed a decommoditized social right to healthcare. The United States, in contrast, did not. What lay behind the difference between the two English-speaking nations? For that matter, why does the United States still lack a "right to health?" The divergence actually began during these very same years, when the US—like Britain and Germany—sought to address the ills of industrialism through public health insurance.

The United States: Charity and the Health Politics of Progressivism

There has been a long, hard, and indeed ongoing discussion on why the United States is exceptional among high-income countries in its failure to create a system of universal healthcare. The unsuccessful campaign for a compulsory health insurance system that occurred around the time of the First World War—inspired by the German and English examples just examined—was perhaps the first suggestion that the US might diverge from the European model. This section, along with several sections of subsequent chapters, will explore why this divergence occurred, hopefully providing some sense of why the United States lacks a "right to healthcare" today.

Before turning to the early twentieth century, it is worth noting by way of background that in many respects, early America followed the European path with respect to social welfare. For instance, it relied on a system of poor relief like that of the English Poor Law, inclusive of regressive elements like the principle of "less eligibility."[79] For those who needed long-term care because of medical disability, for instance, relief went hand-in-hand with public humiliation.[80] The central problem with public relief, some believed, was that even if it was administered in a repressive fashion, its recipients might nonetheless come to regard it as a legal right. "The great defect in a state or city charity is that it must necessarily be more or less impersonal in its character and general in its relief," as the New York State

Charities Aid Association put it, "so that those who use it grow in time to feel that they have *the right to its aid . . .*" (emphasis added).[81] As seen again and again, this is the strange paradox at the heart of the Poor Law: it could simultaneously confer an economic right to the poor while also serving as a tool of state repression.

Charitable medical care for the poor took both public and private forms, and each was inadequate. In 1769, for instance, Samuel Bard, the personal physician to George Washington, decried the absence of a public charity hospital in New York City:

> . . . it is truly a reproach, that a City like this, should want a public Hospital.
> . . . The labouring Poor are allowed to be the support of the Community;
> their Industry enables the Rich to live in Ease and Affluence . . . how heavy
> a Calamity must Sickness be to such a Man, which putting him out of his
> Power to work, immediately deprives him and perhaps a helpless Family of
> Bread![82]

Even in the eighteenth century, many cities maintained public almshouses that functioned as de facto hospitals.[83] Towns and cities also frequently retained a physician to care for the poor, and fifteen had merchant marine hospitals, which had been created by Congress in 1798 in a unique act of public healthcare provision.[84] More generally, however, private voluntary hospitals, which might be either religious or philanthropic in origin, provided charitable care to a select group of the poor in the nineteenth century.[85] Workers, meanwhile, might rely on fraternal lodges, which sometimes provided basic and limited healthcare benefits, though often discriminated on the basis of race, sex, and age.[86] Trade unions also offered sickness plans, though these generally covered lost wages, not healthcare.[87]

Even put together, however, these various provisions were entirely insufficient. The turn of the nineteenth century saw a transformation in the role of the traditionally charitable voluntary hospital, which became more and more reliant on patients' fees.[88] By the 1920s, they had essentially become a "market-oriented institution," increasingly oriented to those with the resources to pay the bills.[89] Such facilities were clearly not meeting the needs of the working class, who might face financial ruin when they became ill. Concern about the rising costs to society of sickness—not necessarily of healthcare—grew in many circles.[90] The "costs" of sickness became an important rationale for a turn away from a reliance on public charity and towards a program of state-based social insurance after the turn of the century.[91]

Underlying this new concern, however, was also political pressure from below. As in Europe, these years saw the rise of left-wing political movements and trade unionism. Membership in the American Federation of Labor (AFL) multiplied in the first two decades of the century, while the Industrial Workers of the World began more radically confronting the economic status quo after its founding in 1905.[92] Union activists were not seeking more charity, however, which they fervently rejected: they were calling for more benefits and *rights*.[93] In fact, the Socialist Party appears to have been the first party in the US to include national health insurance in its platform.[94] While its 1900 platform called for "National Insurance of working people against accident, lack of employment and want in old age," its 1904 platform went further in calling for "insurance of the workers against accident, sickness and lack of employment; for pensions for aged and exhausted workers."[95]

The progressive movement also came to embrace social insurance. Lloyd George's 1911 National Insurance Act was no doubt one influence on progressives.[96] As in England, a key concern of Progressive Era reformers was addressing the economic hazard that would accompany sickness, though this was frequently combined with a genuinely humanitarian outlook. "The fear of losing one's job," Walter Lippmann wrote in his seminal text *Drift and Mastery*, "the necessity of being somebody in a crowded and clamorous world, the terror that old age will not be secured, that your children will lack opportunity—there are a thousand terrors which arise out of the unorganized and unstable economic system under which we live."[97] A system of health insurance, for some, was simply a rational step towards a better-ordered world. After the Socialists, the Progressive Party—founded in 1912 by former president Theodore Roosevelt—was the next to call for health insurance: its 1912 platform demanded for "[t]he protection of home life against hazards of sickness, irregular employment and old age through the adoption of a system of social insurance adapted to American use."[98]

Some progressive reformers pinned their hopes for change on the historic 1912 presidential election, a four-way contest between Progressive Party candidate Theodore Roosevelt, Republican William Howard Taft, Democrat Woodrow Wilson, and Socialist Eugene V. Debs.[99] In addition to social insurance, the Progressive Party's platform called for women's suffrage, labor rights, and an eight-hour workday.[100] Yet as historian Beatrix Hoffman notes, none of this was called for in the name of "rights": reforms would increase economic efficiency, while social insurance was to be funded, in part, by workers' contributions.[101]

Though progressive reformers were hoping for a win by Roosevelt and the Progressive Party, they nonetheless perceived that progress could be possible in the years of the Wilson administration.[102] The campaign for health insurance began after 1912, and was led by the American Association for Labor Legislation (AALL), a progressive think tank and advocacy organization established in 1906.[103] Though its founders had flirted with socialism in their earlier days, the AALL very much, as Hoffman puts it, "disavowed socialism and instead committed itself to preserving the capitalist system by curtailing its abuses."[104] Led by well-known progressive scholars, the AALL, whose stated goal was the "The Conservation of Human Resources,"[105] spearheaded a number of notable campaigns in the early twentieth century, initially with some success, such as with the federal prohibition on phosphorous in matches.[106] Notably, members of the AALL had helped ensure that the 1912 platform of Roosevelt's Progressive Party included a plank on social insurance.[107]

Not long after the election, the AALL set up a "Committee on Social Insurance," and subsequently convened a convention on the issue.[108] Its Committee on Social Insurance, though charged with the task of evaluating many forms of social insurance, started with health insurance, given the link between sickness and *destitution*, which was its primary concern.[109] Addressing the problem of sickness might, in the words of one proponent and authority (I.M. Rubinow, discussed shortly), break this "vicious cycle."[110] This half-economic, half-humanitarian argument was presented by the AALL itself in its "Brief for Health Insurance." The document acknowledges both the high levels of morbidity and mortality among American laborers, and the inadequacy of available and affordable medical facilities for workers, who are "unable to meet the expense of proper medical care." But even the charitable facilities that were available were avoided by many workers given the negative stigma of charity, it notes. The actual cost of medical care, moreover, was only one problem: the "wage loss due to illness" was just as important. As a result, a system of compulsory insurance covering both medical care and wage losses was the right solution.[111] Again, however, there was no mention whatsoever of the *rights* of laborers to decent healthcare: the emphasis was largely economic.

But as in both Britain and Germany, the case for health insurance appealed to different groups for different reasons. In addition to the economic and humanitarian arguments, a concern for "national efficiency" and "economic rationality" weighed prominently in the minds of some policymakers and academics.[112] Others supported social insurance on moral and redistributive grounds, such as Rubinow, a Russian-born physician, insurance advocate, Socialist party member, and prominent expert on the issue.[113] As it had done for William Pulteney Alison, Rubinow's time providing medical care for the poor (in New York), and his observations of his patients' living conditions, shaped his views on social policy.[114] "[W]age-workers must learn to see that they have a right to force at least part of the cost and waste of sickness back upon the industry and society at large," he wrote in his book *Social Insurance*, "and they can do it only when they demand that the state use its power and authority to help them, indirectly at least, with as much vigor as it has come to the assistance of the business interests . . . ."[115] Social insurance, for Rubinow, was "true class legislation," insofar as it was "an effort to readjust the distribution of the national product more equitably . . . ."[116] Unlike most of his contemporaries, however, Rubinow seemed to suggest that compulsory health insurance could also serve as a stepping-stone to a system of more fully socialized medicine.[117]

Rubinow was the only physician on the AALL's Committee on Social Insurance, and he was involved in preparing the organization's model bill.[118] His subcommittee issued an initial draft of the bill in November 1915, which would have provided a benefit to workers making below $100 a month (albeit excluding those working in domestic or casual roles) that included physician services, hospital care, surgical care, drugs, and both maternity and funeral benefits.[119] Notably, unlike English health insurance, it also provided coverage to workers' families.[120] Despite much initial enthusiasm, however, the subsequent health insurance campaign effort was to prove an utter failure.

In Europe, social insurance had been conceived, to some degree, as an attempt to co-opt radicalism, which earned it political support from quarters that might ordinarily have opposed its passage with violence. The political situation in the United States, however, was very different, and the organized left was far less threatening, at least in the electoral arena. The American Socialist Party (SP), for instance, running Eugene V. Debs, won only 6 percent of votes in the 1912 presidential election, which was to be its greatest success.[121] The relative weakness of the American Left may have contributed to the fact that health insurance advocates did not—or could not—wield social insurance as a political weapon, to placate the revolutionaries at the gates.[122] Nor did the advocates seek a more direct appeal to the laboring classes, instead turning to scholars, progressive employers, and public officials.[123]

Furthermore, although socialists supported health insurance,[124] organized labor was divided. Samuel Gompers, the president of the AFL, became a powerful foe of compulsory health insurance and the AALL.[125] Historian Alan Derickson has referred to the AFL's position as a "voluntarist view . . . [that] posited an overriding negative right of workers to be left alone . . ."[126] Some have noted, for instance, that some unions of this era were not interested in a public system of health insurance that would undercut their own benefit systems, and thereby perhaps weaken unions as a whole.[127] As a result, as sociologist Paul Starr puts it, "rather than pitting labor unions against capital," health insurance "pitted both of them against the reformers."[128]

In truth, however, the AALL itself deserves some of the blame, insofar as it made little effort to reach out to labor organizations or involve them in the development of its proposal.[129] Moreover, it would be too simplistic to portray labor as unanimously opposed to health insurance legislation. For instance, eighteen state labor federations, including that of New York, broke with the national AFL position against health insurance, as did twenty-one international unions.[130] On the national level, William Green of the United Mine Workers supported the model bill.[131] In New York, both the International Ladies' Garment Workers' Union and the Women's Trade Union League supported the health insurance movement *once* a maternity benefit was added to the bill, an understandably important inclusion for their female membership.[132] And some rare voices in labor circles, Derickson notes, went beyond the "period's preoccupation with productivity, responsibility, and need" and explicitly "spoke out for social rights."[133]

Yet if health insurance lacked powerful allies, it did not lack powerful enemies, and the failure of the campaign was in large part due to their effective mobilization.[134] Early on, however, there were some signs to suggest that organized medicine—in the form of the American Medical Association—might actually be amenable to progressive health insurance reform.[135] The insurance industry, on the other hand, appropriately came to regard compulsory health insurance as nothing less than an existential threat, and its aggressive propagandizing efforts may have helped to galvanize the opposition of physicians.[136] Meanwhile, industrial groups such as the National Association of Manufacturers and the National Civic Federation were soon joining the ranks of the health insurance opposition, as was the fledgling pharmaceutical industry.[137]

Hopes initially ran high. Yet, within a year, the tides had turned entirely against the ambitious and hopeful health insurance movement. The fight over health insurance was not being waged in a political vacuum: the United States would soon be at war with Germany, with great consequences for domestic politics. When health insurance bills were reintroduced into state legislatures in 1917, opponents of reform now had a distinct new ideological advantage. Physicians could now describe health insurance as not merely deleterious from a pecuniary perspective, but also distinctly anti-American.[138] "Coming straight from Germany," one physician testified to the New York State senate, health insurance was "devilish in principle and foreign to American ideals."[139] The National Association of Manufacturers asserted that insurance was "one of the vicious German ideas yet existent in this country."[140] Bolstering this counterstrike were the propagandizing efforts of the federal government: one bureau apparently even contracted articles that condemned social insurance.[141] Shortly before the US declaration of war, with warmongering rhetoric at a peak and health insurance cast as part of a German plot, the state council of the New York Medical Association reneged on its previously voiced support.[142]

Both health insurance and its supporters were denounced. One pamphlet, published by a conservative physicians group, described health insurance as a "dangerous device, invented in Germany, announced by the German Emperor from the throne the same year he started plotting and preparing to conquer the world."[143] The potential effect of such appeals at a time of bellicosity should not be underestimated. Indeed, in 1918, the President of the AMA argued that county medical societies should take an active role in helping the government hunt down and detain disloyal physicians.[144] These were not idle threats. As described at the beginning of this chapter, Warbasse was expelled from his medical society, which also forwarded its concerns to the Justice Department.[145]

Subsequent political developments—namely, the Russian Revolution—provided another ideological weapon to health insurance's opponents. In 1917, amidst military defeat and mass deprivation, revolution brought an end to the reign of the Tsar in Russia, and later that year Vladimir Lenin's Bolshevik Party took power and took Russia out of the war. The red-baiting of health insurance proponents came hard and fast. The leader of the Professional Guild of Kings County, for example, united fears of both Germany and Russia in a comically over-the-top denunciation of the New York bill, describing it as "MADE IN GERMANY," brought to the US "by a Russian disciple of Bolshevism and I WON'T WORKISM," and supported by the "disciples of Lenin and Trotsky . . ."[146] The guild not only labeled the AALL activists "pro-German" and "pro-Bolshevik," but also blamed them "in great measure for the negro race riots," thereby demonstrating a fusion of nationalistic fervor, anti-communist paranoia, and racism.[147]

The Red Scare ultimately brought the campaign for compulsory health insurance to a close. Although the health insurance bill actually made it through the New York State Senate in 1919, the red-baiting fervor of the Assembly Speaker allowed him to nix the bill without it even coming to the floor for a vote.[148] And in 1920, despite its prior tentative support, the AMA came out in full opposition. [149] The tide turned so far to the right that even the Sheppard-Towner bill of 1921, which set up prenatal care centers for the poor with federal support, was decried as the work of perverse radicals set to ruin the nation.[150]

And thus was the first campaign for health insurance in the US brought to a close. Wartime jingoism, xenophobia, and red-baiting were wielded by powerful health and business interests to create a toxic and indeed threatening *milieu* for reform. As a result, there was to be no leftward shift in the healthcare rights-commodity dialectic in the US during these years: on the contrary, subsequent decades would merely see an intensification of the process of healthcare commercialization. Moreover, the xenophobic streak of the anti-health insurance movement no doubt injected a noxious element of national chauvinism into the healthcare reform debate, the consequences of which proponents of universal healthcare continue to contend with today.

Conclusions

Many arguments were wielded, either implicitly or explicitly, to promote the creation of semi-universal health insurance systems during the period surveyed in this chapter: nations with imperial interests needed vigorous young men to fight for them; industrial production had to be protected; and a politically-activated working class had to be mollified, not merely subdued.[151] Moreover, the sequence of sickness, unemployment, and impoverishment was economically wasteful. This cycle, some argued, could be broken through social insurance, which would more fairly allocate the costs of illness between worker, capital, and state.[152] Yet, to some extent or another, it was most likely the rise of the working class as a powerful political force—whether represented in trade unions or mass-membership political parties like the SPD—that wonderfully concentrated the minds of policymakers, as the saying goes. It is clear that this political *milieu* was crucial; where labor and the Left were weaker and more divided—i.e., in the United States—the barriers to change were higher. And here, change did not come.

Thinking about these changes in terms of a healthcare rights-commodity dialectic sheds some additional light on the meaning of these new systems. Social insurance was premised on the idea that sickness, unemployment, or even poverty, were not the result of moral faults, but were consequent to a specific configuration of society and the economy. By creating a limited legal right to healthcare for some, such systems were a clear departure from the various systems of medical charity surveyed thus far: they represent an enshrinement in law, albeit in a limited sense and for particular political goals, of a socioeconomic right. For those eligible, they moved healthcare out of a basket of commodities to be purchased using the fruits of one's wage labor and into the realm of the semi-public good. And from this perspective, the advent of these systems represents a partial "leftward" shift along the rights-commodity healthcare dialectic.

Yet at the same time, in the case of all of these limited systems of health insurance, it is crucial to look at who was (or would have been) excluded, ranging from children to casual workers, from the unemployed to the very old, and all too often, most women.[153] These systems, in other words, simply did not create "a right to healthcare." The shift was partial; universalism was slighted, if not neglected altogether. This had little to do with the absence of "human rights" rhetoric, and everything to do with the fact that benefits were only provided to select groups of the population, that they were limited to (or centered around) male heads of household, and that they left behind some of the most marginalized groups and individuals. The historian Colin Gordon summarizes the shortcomings of this era's "social insurance" ideology well:

> [T]hey . . . drew a clear boundary between the worthy poor (industrial poor) and others. The needs of women and children were subsumed by the family-wage logic of 'workingman's insurance.' Social provision reflected and reinforced patterns of occupational and racial segregation. And farmers, farm laborers, domestics, and the self-employed would claim uneven access to a welfare state provided or paid for at the workplace.[154]

Hoffman makes some similar points. For instance, although the proposed legislation did not formally discriminate on the basis of race, leaving both domestic and agricultural laborers out of the AALL labor legislation resulted in the de facto racist marginalization of black workers.[155] And the AALL's failure to consider the interests of blacks likely contributed to the lack of support among black physician groups for the health insurance campaign.[156] The unemployed and the impoverished were also excluded. All of these individuals would thereby be forced to rely (if they were fortunate) on private and public charity care, leading to a tiered and inherently unequal system.

Why did these systems evolve in this way? In part, because they were aimed more at the unstable fault lines of industrial capitalism than they were at any goal of a social right to health. As a result, industrial workers, and not the public at large, were the primary target of this new era of healthcare policy.[157] Then, as now, it was the distribution of political and economic power that would draw the confines of change.

In contrast, the daring surgeon Warbasse favored a rather more fundamental shift in the right-commodity dialectic of healthcare. "In the place of our commercialized organization," he wrote, "we should have a more equable and humane distribution of health forces."[158] He was, however, but one voice amidst many. He was outnumbered. And he would no doubt be dismayed at where things would stand a full century later.

Notes

1   "Expelled Doctor to Fight," *The New York Times*, April 18, 1918, http://query.nytimes.com/mem/archive-free/pdf?res=9F01E7DD103BEE3ABC4052DFB2668383609EDE, accessed November 10, 2016; Theodore M. Brown, "James Peter Warbasse," *American Journal of Public Health* 86, no. 1 (1996): 109–10.

2   Frank L. Babbott, "James P. Warbasse," *New England Journal of Medicine* 258, no. 6 (1958): 287–8; Theodore M. Brown and Anne-Emanuelle Birn, "The Making of Health Internationalists," in *Comrades in Health: U.S. Health Internationalists, Abroad and at Home*, ed. Anne-Emanuelle Birn and Theodore M. Brown (New Brunswick: Rutgers University Press, 2013), 19.

3   Babbott, "James P. Warbasse," 287–8; Theodore M. Brown, "James Peter Warbasse," 109–10.

4   James P. Warbasse, "The Socialization of Medicine," *Journal of the American Medical Association* LXIII, no. 3 (1914): 266. I owe this citation to Brown, "James Peter Warbasse."

5   Quote from Uwe Reinhardt in an interview with Underwood. Anne Underwood, "Health Care Abroad: Germany," *New York Times Prescription Blog*, September 29, 2009, http://prescriptions.blogs.nytimes.com/2009/09/29/health-care-abroad-germany/.

6   This interpretation appears everywhere. For example: Paul Starr, *The Social Transformation of American Medicine* (New York: Basic Books, 1982), 239; Henry E. Sigerist, "From Bismarck to Beveridge: Developments and Trends in Social Security Legislation. I. The Period of Bismarck," *Bulletin of the History of Medicine* 13 (1943), 375–6.

7   E. P. Hennock, *The Origin of the Welfare State in England and Germany, 1850–1914: Social Policies Compared* (Cambridge: Cambridge University Press, 2007), 26, 151–4, 331; I. M. Rubinow, *Social Insurance: With Special Reference to American Conditions* (New York: Holt, 1916), http://catalog.hathitrust.org/api/volumes/oclc/747412.html, 14; Gaston V. Rimlinger, *Welfare Policy and Industrialization in Europe, America, and Russia* (New York: Wiley, 1971), 94–5; Sigerist, "From Bismarck to Beveridge: Developments and Trends in Social Security Legislation. I. The Period of Bismarck," 369–70; Jurge Tampke, "Bismarck's Social Legislation: A Genuine Breakthrough?" in *The Emergence of the Welfare State in Britain and Germany, 1850–1950*, ed. Wolfgang J. Mommsen (London: Croom Helm, 1981), 72–3, 78.

8   Hennock, *The Origin of the Welfare State in England and Germany, 1850–1914*, 331.

9   E. J. Hobsbawm, *The Age of Empire, 1875–1914* (New York: Vintage, 1989), 34–9; E. J. Hobsbawm, *The Age of Capital, 1848–1875* (New York: Vintage Books, 1996), 303–8.

10 Sigerist, "From Bismarck to Beveridge: Developments and Trends in Social Security Legislation. I. The Period of Bismarck," 372.

11 As Holburn puts it: "After 1873 the depression naturally raised questions about the cause of the crash and its aftermath, and liberal economic policies came under fire." Rimlinger, *Welfare Policy and Industrialization in Europe, America, and Russia*, 108–9; Hajo Holburn, *A History of Modern Germany, 1840–1945* (Princeton, NJ: Princeton University Press, 1982), 267.

12 Hans-Peter Ullmann, "Germany Industry and Bismarck's Social Security System," in *The Emergence of the Welfare State in Britain and Germany, 1850–1950*, ed. Wolfgang J. Mommsen (London: Croom Helm, 1981), 143; Rimlinger, *Welfare Policy and Industrialization in Europe, America, and Russia*, 109; Tampke, "Bismarck's Social Legislation: A Genuine Breakthrough?" 74–6.

13 Holburn, *A History of Modern Germany, 1840–1945*, 284.

14 Ibid., 285.

15 Ibid., 286–7; Gordon A. Craig, *Germany, 1866–1945* (New York: Oxford University Press, 1978), 94.

16 In the 1877 elections, for instance, the SPD was taking half a million votes; though perhaps not so threatening in absolute terms, this represented a five-fold increase over six years (compared to the combined votes of the workers' parties in 1871). Rimlinger, *Welfare Policy and Industrialization in Europe, America, and Russia*, 111; Craig, *Germany, 1866–1945*, 95.

17 Craig, *Germany, 1866–1945*, 93.

18 Quoted in ibid., 146.

19 Ibid., 146–7.

20 The preceding facts in this paragraph about these benefits are drawn from Henry J. Harris, "Appendix C: Sickness Insurance in Germany," in *Health, Health Insurance, Old Age Pensions: Report, Recommendations, Dissenting Opinions*, ed. Ohio Health and Old Age Insurance Commission (Columbus, OH: The F. J. Heer Printing co., 1919), https://books.google.com/

books?vid=HARVARD:HNP1W2&printsec=titlepage#v=onepage&q&f=false, 342–7. Also, see Ronald L. Numbers, *Almost Persuaded: American Physicians and Compulsory Health Insurance, 1912–1920* (Baltimore: Johns Hopkins University Press, 1978), 10–11.

21   Numbers, *Almost Persuaded*, 10.

22   Hennock, *The Origin of the Welfare State in England and Germany, 1850–1914*, 94; Craig, *Germany, 1866–1945*, 151.

23   Hennock, *The Origin of the Welfare State in England and Germany, 1850–1914*, 94–5.

24   Quoted in William Harbutt Dawson, *Bismarck and State Socialism: an Exposition of the Social and Economic Legislation of Germany since 1870* (London: S. Sonnenschein & Co., 1890), https://books.google.com/books?vid=HARVARD:32044088882691&printsec=titlepage#v=onep age&q&f=false, 110–11. A different translation of this quote also appears in Gaston V. Rimlinger, *Welfare Policy and Industrialization in Europe, America, and Russia* (New York: Wiley, 1971), 112.

25   Quoted in Numbers, *Almost Persuaded*, 10.

26   Quoted in Rimlinger, *Welfare Policy and Industrialization in Europe, America, and Russia*, 124–5.

27   Craig, *Germany, 1866–1945*, 151.

28   E. P. Hennock, "Social Policy under the Empire—Myths and Evidence," *German History* 16, no. 1 (1998): 69.

29   Hennock, *The Origin of the Welfare State in England and Germany, 1850–1914*, 89.

30   As Rimlinger explains, Bismarck first focused on foreign policy, and strengthening the empire against other nations. Subsequently, however, he sought the "internal consolidation" of the state against the insurgent socialists. Rimlinger contends that welfare programs would bind workers to the state. Hennock emphasizes that Bismarck could suppress the Socialists with force alone, but that he was more "concerned to further the industrial development of Germany and the power of the *Reich*." Rimlinger, *Welfare Policy and Industrialization in Europe, America, and Russia*, 9, 112, 116. Also see: Holburn, *A History of Modern Germany, 1840–1945*, 290–1; Hennock, *The Origins of the Welfare State in England and Germany, 1850–1914*, 95–6.

31   However, as Esping-Andersen notes, what Bismarck got was less state-centric than he had hoped, based as it was on occupationally separate schemes. Gøsta Esping-Andersen, *The Three Worlds of Welfare Capitalism* (Princeton, NJ: Princeton University Press, 1990), 59.

32   Esping-Andersen, *The Three Worlds of Welfare Capitalism*, 40.

33   Gerhard Albert Ritter, *Social Welfare in Germany and Britain: Origins and Development* (Leamington Spa: Berg, 1986), 4.

34   Numbers, *Almost Persuaded*, 10.

35   Ibid., 11.

36   Sigerist, "From Bismarck to Beveridge: Developments and Trends in Social Security Legislation. I. The Period of Bismarck," 384.

37   A point made by Hennock. E. P. Hennock, "The Origin of British National Health Insurance and the German Precedent 1880–1914," in *The Emergence of the Welfare State in Britain and Germany, 1850–1950*, ed. Wolfgang J. Mommsen (London: Croom Helm, 1981), 95.

38   Vicente Navarro, "Why Some Countries Have National Health Insurance, Others Have National Health Services, and the United States Has Neither," *International Journal of Health Services* 19, no. 3 (1989): 394.

39   Esping-Andersen, *The Three Worlds of Welfare Capitalism*, 26–7.

40   Ibid.

41   Donald Sasson, *One Hundred Years of Socialism* (London: I.B.Tauris & Co. Ltd, 2014), 24–5.

42   "The Erfurt Program," *German History in Documents and Images*, accessed March 8, 2015, http://www.germanhistorydocs.ghi-dc.org/sub_document.cfm?document_id=766.

43   Sassoon makes note of the division of the document into rights that were to be enjoyed by all, and into reforms explicitly geared to the working class. Sasson, *One Hundred Years of Socialism*, 24.

44   Hennock, "The Origin of British National Health Insurance and the German Precedent 1880–1914," 87.

45   Andrew Mearns, *The Bitter Cry of Outcast London* (Boston: Cupples, Upham, 1883), 1.

46 The impact of the *Bitter Cry* is discussed in: Gilbert, *The Evolution of National Insurance in Great Britain: The Origins of the Welfare State* (London: Michael Joseph Ltd., 1966), 28–32.

47 Rimlinger, *Welfare Policy and Industrialization in Europe, America, and Russia*, 58–60; Gilbert, *The Evolution of National Insurance in Great Britain*, 235–7.

48 Rimlinger, *Welfare Policy and Industrialization in Europe, America, and Russia*, 57.

49 Fraser, *The Evolution of the British Welfare State*, 160; Gilbert, *The Evolution of National Insurance in Great Britain*, 24, 32.

50 Gilbert, *The Evolution of National Insurance in Great Britain*, 32–5.

51 Ibid.

52 Fraser, *The Evolution of the British Welfare State*, 169; Gilbert, *The Evolution of National Insurance in Great Britain*, 38–9.

53 Rimlinger, *Welfare Policy and Industrialization in Europe, America, and Russia*, 57.

54 Gilbert, *The Evolution of National Insurance in Great Britain*, 247; Fraser, *The Evolution of the British Welfare State*, 175–7, 182.

55 Esping-Andersen also emphasizes a new awareness among liberals that the structure of the economy had changed, away from smaller scale enterprises towards larger and consolidated enterprises. Gilbert, *The Evolution of National Insurance in Great Britain*, 76–7, 84–7; Esping-Andersen, *The Three Worlds of Welfare Capitalism*, 42, 63.

56 Moon discusses how New Liberalism grew out of a "sustained critique of 'classical' liberalism"— in particular its laissez-faire economic approach—and came to embrace welfare state protections. Donald Moon, "The Idea of the Welfare State," in *The Oxford Handbook of the History of Political Philosophy* (Oxford: Oxford University Press, 2013), 662–3.

57 Gilbert, *The Evolution of National Insurance in Great Britain*, 447.

58 Fraser, *The Evolution of the British Welfare State*, 177–9.

59 Ibid., 182.

60 Ibid., 182–3.

61 Gilbert, *The Evolution of National Insurance in Great Britain*, 303–13.

62 As Gilbert notes, for those with low incomes, there was essentially no "'system' of medical care at all." Ibid, 303.

63 Ibid., 314–15.

64 Ibid., 290, 365.

65 Edith Abbott, "Appendix B: Health Insurance in Great Britain," in *Ohio Health and Old Age Insurance Commission: Health, Health Insurance, Old Age Pensions*, 312–17.

66 Ibid., 317–18; Roy Lubove, *The Struggle for Social Security 1900–1935* (Pittsburgh: University of Pittsburgh Press, 1986), 68–9.

67 Nick Bosanquet, "Health Economics: Finance, Budgeting, and Insurance," in *Companion Encyclopedia of the History of Medicine*, ed. W. F. Bynum and Roy Porter (London: Routledge, 1997), 2: 1379; Lubove, *The Struggle for Social Security 1900–1935*, 68–9; Doyal and Pennel, *The Political Economy of Health*; 165, 172.

68 As Esping-Andersen notes, the non-contributory nature of these pensions was not consistent with the usual liberal ideology of welfare benefits, wherein they should be tied to contributions in an actuarial and contractual manner. He notes that this was similar to Social Security, which initially was supposed to be based on actuarial principles but which came to be both mandatory and redistributive. Esping-Andersen, *The Three Worlds of Welfare Capitalism*, 64.

69 Edith Abbott, "Appendix B: Health Insurance in Great Britain," 312–17.

70 Fraser, *The Evolution of the British Welfare State*, 186–8.

71 A point made by ibid., 187–8. Also: Gilbert, *The Evolution of National Insurance in Great Britain*, 9.

72 Fraser, *The Evolution of the British Welfare State*, 183–4.

73 Ibid., 184.

74 Moon, "The Idea of the Welfare State," 663.

75 Gilbert, *The Evolution of National Insurance in Great Britain*, 314–15; Fraser, *The Evolution of the British Welfare State*, 198.

76 Edith Abbott, "Appendix B: Health Insurance in Great Britain," 315.

77 Quoted in Gilbert, *The Evolution of National Insurance in Great Britain*, 315n.

78 Ibid., 314–15.

79 Hace Sorel Tishler, *Self-Reliance and Social Security 1870–1917* (Port Washington: Kennikat Press, 1971), 4–8; Lubove, *The Struggle for Social Security 1900–1935*, 183–5.

80 David Barton Smith and Zhanlian Feng, "The Accumulated Challenges of Long-Term Care," *Health Affairs* 29, no. 1 (2010): 29–30.

81 Quoted in Tishler, *Self-Reliance and Social Security 1870–1917*, 33.

82 Quoted in Henry Ernest Sigerist, "An Outline of the Development of the Hospital," *Bulletin of the Institute of the History of Medicine* 4 (1936), 574.

83 John Duffy, *The Sanitarians: A History of American Public Health* (Urbana: University of Illinois Press, 1990), 31–2.

84 Ibid., 31–2; Numbers, *Almost Persuaded*, 6–7; Beatrix Rebecca Hoffman, *Health Care for Some: Rights and Rationing in the United States since 1930* (Chicago: University of Chicago Press, 2012), xxvi–xxvi.

85 Hoffman, *Health Care for Some*, xxiv–xxviii.

86 Colin Gordon, *Dead on Arrival: The Politics of Health Care in Twentieth-Century America* (Princeton, NJ: Princeton University Press, 2005), 51; Beatrix Rebecca Hoffman, *The Wages of Sickness: The Politics of Health Insurance in Progressive America* (Chapel Hill: University of North Carolina Press, 2001), 10.

87 Numbers, *Almost Persuaded*, 6.

88 Rosemary Stevens, *In Sickness and in Wealth: American Hospitals in the Twentieth Century* (New York: Basic Books, 1989), 10–11

89 Bosanquet, "Health Economics: Finance, Budgeting, and Insurance," 1376. See also Hoffman, *The Wages of Sickness*, xxxii.

90 Tishler, *Self-Reliance and Social Security 1870–1917*, 164–5.

91 Ibid., 92, 164–5.

92 Robert H. Zieger, Timothy J. Minchin, and Gilbert J. Gall, *American Workers, American Unions: The Twentieth and Early Twenty-First Centuries*, fourth ed. (Baltimore: Johns Hopkins University Press, 2014), 18–19.

93 Tishler, *Self-Reliance and Social Security 1870–1917*, 35, 64–5, 83.

94 Numbers, *Almost Persuaded*, 14.

95 Quoted in John R. Commons and A. J. Altmeyer, "The Health Insurance Movement in the United States," in *Health, Health Insurance, Old Age Pensions* (Columbus, OH: 1919), 310.

96 Numbers, *Almost Persuaded*, 33; Hoffman, *The Wages of Sickness*, 1.

97 Walter Lippman, *Drift and Mastery* (Madison, WI: University of Wisconsin Press, 1985), 138.

98 Quoted in Commons and Altmeyer, "The Health Insurance Movement in the United States," 310.

99 Tishler, *Self-Reliance and Social Security 1870–1917*, 160.

100 Eric Foner, *The Story of American Freedom* (New York: W.W. Norton; repr., 1999), 160.

101 Hoffman, *Health Care for Some*, xxxiii.

102 Tishler, *Self-Reliance and Social Security 1870–1917*, 160; Daniel S. Hirshfield, *The Lost Reform: The Campaign for Compulsory Health Insurance in the United States from 1932–1943* (Cambridge, MA: Harvard University Press, 1970), 13.

103 Lubove, *The Struggle for Social Security 1900–1935*, 29–31.

104 Hoffman, *The Wages of Sickness*, 25.

105 Tishler, *Self-Reliance and Social Security 1870–1917*, 92; Hoffman, *The Wages of Sickness*, 24.

106 Numbers, *Almost Persuaded*, 16.

107 Hirshfield, *The Lost Reform*, 13.

108 Starr, *The Social Transformation of American Medicine*, 244.

109 Numbers, *Almost Persuaded*, 19.

110 Quoted in Starr, *The Social Transformation of American Medicine*, 245.

111 American Association for Labor Legislation, "Brief for Health Insurance," *American Labor Legislation Review* 6, no. 2. (1916): 155–216, quotes 155 and 163. I owe this citation to Lubove, *The Struggle for Social Security 1900–1935*, 219.

112 Starr, *The Social Transformation of American Medicine*, 244.

113 Numbers, *Almost Persuaded*, 18; Lubove, *The Struggle for Social Security 1900–1935*, 34–5. Rubinow also strongly stressed the economic arguments, however.

114 Lubove, *The Struggle for Social Security 1900–1935*, 34.

115 Rubinow, *Social Insurance*, 298.

116 Ibid., 491.

117 Ibid., 271–2.

118 Numbers, *Almost Persuaded*, 17–20.

119 Ibid., 25; Lubove, *The Struggle for Social Security 1900–1935*, 71; Hoffman, *The Wages of Sickness*, 29.

120 Lubove, *The Struggle for Social Security 1900–1935*, 71.

121 Michael Kazin, *American Dreamers: How the Left Changed a Nation* (New York: Alfred A. Knopf, 2011), 111–13. Kazin argues that the typical explanations for the weakness of Progressive-era socialism fail to take into account that it wasn't a single movement—but instead three.

122 Hoffman notes that Bismarck's notion of using health insurance as a weapon against socialism was "entirely disregarded" in the American context. Hoffman, *The Wages of Sickness*, 66–7.

123 Rimlinger, *Welfare Policy and Industrialization in Europe, America, and Russia*, 71.

124 Hoffman, *The Wages of Sickness*, 37.

125 Numbers, *Almost Persuaded*, 60; Hoffman, *The Wages of Sickness*, 36, 130–4; Rimlinger, *Welfare Policy and Industrialization in Europe, America, and Russia*, 83.

126 Alan Derickson, "'Take Health from the List of Luxuries': Labor and the Right to Health Care, 1915–1949," *Labor History* 41, no. 2 (2000): 172.

127 Rimlinger, *Welfare Policy and Industrialization in Europe, America, and Russia*, 80; Tishler, *Self-Reliance and Social Security 1870–1917*, 189; Hoffman, *The Wages of Sickness*, 124; Hirshfield, *The Lost Reform; the Campaign for Compulsory Health Insurance in the United States from 1932–1943*, 20.

128 Starr, *The Social Transformation of American Medicine*, 251.

129 Hoffman, *The Wages of Sickness*, 34.

130 Hoffman, *The Wages of Sickness*, 120; Derickson, "'Take Health from the List of Luxuries': Labor and the Right to Health Care, 1915–1949," 176.

131 Hirshfield, *The Lost Reform*, 19.

132 Hoffman, *The Wages of Sickness*, 120.

133 Derickson, "'Take Health from the List of Luxuries'": Labor and the Right to Health Care, 1915–1949," 177.

134 On the role of physicians, see Numbers, *Almost Persuaded*.

135 Ibid., 29–36.

136 Hoffman, *The Wages of Sickness*, 106; Hirshfield, *The Lost Reform*, 21–2.

137 Rimlinger, *Welfare Policy and Industrialization in Europe, America, and Russia*, 76–7; Tishler, *Self-Reliance and Social Security 1870–1917*, 177; Starr, *The Social Transformation of American Medicine*, 252.

138 Hoffman, *The Wages of Sickness*, 86.

139 Quoted in Numbers, *Almost Persuaded*, 68.

140 Quoted in Rimlinger, *Welfare Policy and Industrialization in Europe, America, and Russia*, 76.

141 Starr, *The Social Transformation of American Medicine*, 253.

142 Numbers, *Almost Persuaded*, 67.

143 Quoted in Starr, *The Social Transformation of American Medicine*, 253.

144 Numbers, *Almost Persuaded*, 76.

145 "Expelled Doctor to Fight," *The New York Times*, April 18, 1918; Theodore M. Brown, "James Peter Warbasse," *American Journal of Public Health* 86, no. 1 (1996).

146 Quoted in Numbers, *Almost Persuaded*, 87.

147 Quoted in Lubove, *The Struggle for Social Security 1900–1935*, 89.

148 Hirshfield, *The Lost Reform*, 23–4.

149 Numbers, *Almost Persuaded*, 108.

150 Ibid., 107.

151   Gilbert, *The Evolution of National Insurance in Great Britain*, 60, 72; Hennock, *The Origin of the Welfare State in England and Germany*, 332. See earlier discussion and citations on the threat of socialism as the source of Bismarck's reforms.

152   Or as two AALL progressives themselves put it, "Underlying the agitation for compulsory health insurance is the belief that there exists an excessive amount of sickness; that such sickness is one of the principal causes of poverty; and that existing agencies are inadequate either to prevent or distribute equitably the cost of such sickness." Commons and Altmeyer, "The Health Insurance Movement in the United States," 294.

153   Hirshfield, *The Lost Reform*, 14–15; Gordon, *Dead on Arrival*, 92.

154   Gordon, *Dead on Arrival*, 92.

155   Hoffman, *The Wages of Sickness*, 30–1.

156   Ibid., 74.

157   As early described and cited, this is a point made by many. For instance, Hirshfield, *The Lost Reform*, 15.

158   Warbasse, "The Socialization of Medicine," 266.

5

The Rhetoric and Reality of Health Rights in Depression and War

"We stand today," Eleanor Roosevelt proclaimed to the General Assembly of the newly formed United Nations on December 9, 1948, "at the threshold of a great event both in the life of the United Nations and in the life of mankind, that is the approval by the General Assembly of the Universal Declaration of Human Rights . . ."[1] Roosevelt, who had played a crucial role in the production of this historic, sweeping document, proceeded to draw hopeful analogies between the impact of the Universal Declaration of Human Rights (UDHR) and that of other rights documents, stretching from the Magna Carta to the Declaration of the Rights of Man and Citizen. Yet if the UDHR was, to some extent, part of a lineage in continuity with earlier "rights" documents, it went well beyond them in both scope and content.[2] In particular, it boldly proclaimed fundamental human rights to social and economic goods like healthcare.

The 1948 Declaration thus occupies a central place in histories of human rights, as well as in the history of the right to healthcare. Indeed, the history of "healthcare as a right," and sometimes of socioeconomic human rights more generally, is often told as if it begins around the time of the hopeful and grandiose promises of 1948.[3] Yet at the same time, the meaning of the rise of healthcare rights rhetoric in this era should not be simplistically viewed as a triumphant moment of egalitarian global cohesion. The gap between soaring rights rhetoric and reality was obvious from the beginning, in nations both rich and poor. Nor has it shrunk.

This era—often seen as the beginning of the modern age of human rights— is nonetheless pivotal to the history of the human right to healthcare, but perhaps not in the way that it is usually discussed. Talk of healthcare rights did not necessarily correspond with the realization of the right to healthcare. Despite an emerging rights discourse, and in spite of an increasing appreciation of the inadequacies of commercialized healthcare, a right to healthcare was not to be constituted during the New Deal era in the United States (or, indeed, thereafter). In contrast, in the wake of the Second World War, the Labour Party in the United Kingdom succeeded in transferring healthcare from the realm of commodities to that of rights, as described in the next chapter. Moving from the rhetoric of healthcare rights to the reality of universal healthcare was, ultimately, a question less of philosophy and proclamations than of the balance of political power.

This chapter begins by turning back to the United States, following the rise and fall of healthcare reform in the era of the Great Depression. It will then turn to the international arena, and trace the hope, the possibilities, but also the profound disappointments of this first stage in human rights history.

Healthcare Costs and Commercialization at the Dawn of the New Deal

The First World War, as described in the last chapter, spelled the end of the first campaign to achieve a system of semi-universal healthcare in the United States. The prospects for healthcare progressives, however, did not improve with the coming of peace. On the contrary, the pro-corporate, laissez-faire prosperity of the 1920s proved frankly inhospitable for those who sought to expand the role of the government in healthcare policy.[4] "If the Federal Government should go out of existence," President Calvin Coolidge dryly commented, "the common run of people would not detect the difference in the affairs of their daily life for a considerable length of time."[5] The AMA was sufficiently emboldened during these years to (successfully) pursue the repeal of the Sheppard-Towner Act, a Progressive Era achievement that had provided federal funding to state programs for poor mothers.[6] In such an environment, universal healthcare fell off the governing agenda entirely.

This was not, however, a stable economic or political status quo. The prosperity of the era was built upon the thin film of swollen speculative bubbles; the collapse of the stock market in 1929 would unleash the greatest challenge that American capitalism had yet faced. As the human and economic disaster of the Great Depression unfolded, the inadequacies of American healthcare were only amplified, while at the same time, a window for reform was reopened.

Yet much had changed since the Progressive Era. In particular, more and more Americans were susceptible to the rising costs of care in a fragmented and commercialized healthcare system. No doubt, the vulnerability of industrial workers and the poor to the potentially disastrous costs of sickness persisted. But at the same time, the middle classes were increasingly threatened by rising healthcare costs during these years of evolving healthcare technology and emerging new modalities of treatment.[7] By the 1930s, the primary policy concern was less the economic loss of missed wages, and more the *costs of medical care itself*.[8] Furthermore, the problems of healthcare commercialization were becoming more apparent. Hospitals had come some way from their charitable roots: they could now be a source of bankruptcy for even the reasonably well-off.[9] Chapter 3 traced the ramifications of industrial capitalism on *health*. Now, in the twentieth century, capitalism was increasingly encroaching upon the realm of *healthcare*. A shift in the healthcare rights-commodity dialectic was underway.

The formation and work of the Committee on the Costs of Medical Care (CCMC), a group assembled in the late 1920s, shed some important light on these developments, and on the tension in this dialectic.[10] For five years, this committee—composed of experts in healthcare, public health, and social policy—investigated the inadequacies of US healthcare, an effort that culminated in an influential proposal for reform.[11] The final recommendations of the committee, issued in 1932, give a sense of the spectrum of healthcare policy—and healthcare rights thought—at the dawn of the New Deal era. One striking aspect of these reports—including both the committee's majority report and the dissenting minority reports—is the extent to which they recognized the fundamental flaw in treating healthcare as a commodity.

The majority report, for instance, criticized the maldistribution of healthcare facilities in the country, as evidenced by the surplus of healthcare resources in some regions and the scarcity in others.[12] This was the inevitable consequence of the fact that healthcare resources were deployed not on the basis of need, but instead "according to real or supposed ability of patients to pay for service."[13] Likewise, a family's income determined the adequacy of healthcare that it obtained.[14] The underlying problem here was the "fee-for-service" system—not so much because it encouraged doctors to provide more care than was necessary (a ubiquitous argument today), but because it discouraged those with limited means from seeking healthcare when they needed it.[15] Two problems therefore had to be addressed: first, the "sometimes crushing burden" of healthcare costs had to be more equitably *distributed*, and second, the provision of healthcare had to be better *organized*.[16] Meeting the first requirement required a system of health insurance of some type (perhaps subsidized with taxation), while the second aim would be best met by organizing healthcare delivery around integrated "community-medical centers."[17] These centers would optimally be centered on a hospital, and would provide the full spectrum of medical, dental, and nursing care for the local population.[18]

In many ways, the recommendations of the majority report countered the ethos of healthcare commodification. For instance, the community-medical centers were to be strictly non-profit affairs, with the report contending that "*lay groups organized for profit have no legitimate place in the provision of this vital public service.*"[19] The majority proposal likewise strictly precluded the "participation by commercial insurance companies" as part of the system, which, it argued, would simply raise costs without improving quality.[20] Interestingly, even the conservative minority report, though it diverged from essentially all of the recommendations of the majority, joined in denouncing the commercialization of healthcare. Medical ethics, the conservative minority report contended, were not consistent with advertising for patients or "a corporation running a clinic," and was concerned that the insurance schemes could lead to the "commercialization of the practice of medicine . . ."[21] Practices, should not, moreover, "pay out dividends or engage in any form of profit-making."[22] (At the same time, the authors of the conservative minority proposed doing little in the way of expanding access to healthcare for those with limited means.)

But did the recommendation of the majority amount to an implicit endorsement of *a right* to healthcare? In some respects, the answer may be yes. Through its criticism of a system of out-of-pocket healthcare financing, the CCMC was acknowledging the inadequacies of a consumerist model of healthcare.[23] More broadly, by proposing a largely decommodified form of healthcare, and by additionally proposing that the "indigent" be provided care predominantly with public funds, the recommendations of the majority would have constituted a step towards universal healthcare.[24] However, in one crucial respect, the proposal of the CCMC fell well short of a "right to healthcare": it did not propose a universal system. It called for "voluntary cooperative health insurance," a plan to be bought by those who wanted it (and could afford it), with the very poor covered through special funding.[25] However, as a subset of committee members in the majority argued (together with the two progressive dissenters, who went even further), this scheme would have still excluded many. Voluntary insurance, these members contended, "will never cover those who most need its protection," especially the "low-paid working group who are not indigent but live on a minimum subsistence income." Voluntary insurance would therefore "not solve the fundamental problems of providing satisfactory *medical service to all* . . ." (emphasis added).[26]

The two progressive dissenting reports went even further. One of these was written by Walton Hamilton, a scholar and former member of the American Association for Labor Legislation (AALL) (notably, many of his students played important roles in the New Deal).[27] In his dissent, Hamilton joined in the denunciation of the commodification of healthcare. However, unlike those who drafted the conservative minority report—which contended that health insurance would usher in the commercialization of the profession—Hamilton argued that the "importation" of the "medical business enterprise" from the "commercial world" was *already* underway.[28] To make medicine a public service, Hamilton argued, would require the "complete elimination of the aims and the arrangements for profit-making from the practice of the art."[29] He instead proposed a more fully universal system, based on what he calls the "venerable principle of medicine"—in fact traceable back to nineteenth-century socialism—of "to each according to his needs, from each according to his ability to pay."[30] Compulsory health insurance, he contended, was actually *the least* that the CCMC should have advocated. Healthcare should be made available to all, funded by a graduated income-based tax.[31]

Hamilton thereby went further in declaiming healthcare commodification, but at the same time, he more directly called for healthcare to be treated *as a public good.* "The plain truth," he put it, "is that, rich as the country is in potential wealth, the haphazard system of private medical enterprise is a luxury we cannot afford. In a society in which the lives and fortunes of all are mutually interdependent, the maintenance of the physical welfare of the people must be a public function."[32] Such a proposal—unlike the majority report and the conservative minority reports—indeed seems consistent with a rights-based conceptualization of healthcare. Together, these conflicting reports thus demonstrate a tension in the interpretation of healthcare along a rights-commodity divide in this era. But would such thinking translate into the legislation of a new social right?

Not in the short term, at least. Hamilton's ideas, for instance, were well outside the political mainstream, even in the pre-McCarthy era. Even the recommendations of the far more moderate majority report were considered radical, and the specter of communism was again wielded against even this incremental reform.

An article in the *New York Times* on the CCMC's report, for instance, was headlined "Socialized Medicine is Urged in Survey" (which was, in fact, not the case).[33] The majority report won a hysterical rebuke from the AMA, which called it an "incitement to revolution" and the result of "socialism and communism": indeed, it was a document that raised the very question of "Americanism versus Sovietism for the American people."[34] With the AMA's takedown of the AALL's compulsory insurance proposal still a recent memory, such accusations no doubt had teeth. The response of the AMA to a report that mainly endorsed *voluntary* health insurance may have served as a warning to would-be reformers that healthcare reform would be better sidestepped altogether.[35]

Yet these were changing times. The report of the CCMC was adopted on October 31, 1932; the following month, Franklin Roosevelt took the presidency, and the Democrats swept Congress. The new administration had to contend with an unhappy populace being squeezed to its limits by the Great Depression, together with a historic labor mobilization. Much that was once unfeasible again entered the realm of political possibility. At the same time, a novel discourse of socioeconomic rights was emerging. For some, the New Deal represented a unique opportunity to legislate a right to healthcare in America.

Rights and Healthcare in the New Deal

A bursting stock market bubble, the callous contagion of bank failures, soaring unemployment, and a coalescing radical opposition meant that laissez-faire inaction was less and less a feasible policy option in the early days of the Great Depression. This was likewise true in the realm of healthcare, particularly as the economic strains of the Depression amplified the inadequacies of American medicine. Traditional charitable facilities were overwhelmed by the growing needs and swelling numbers of the unemployed and the poor.[36] Even where it was available, care at charity clinics could involve formidable barriers, intrusions, and indignities for those who needed it.[37] During the New Deal, however, efforts were made at both the private and the public level to extend the availability of healthcare to the poor and unemployed.[38] In response to rising need, for instance, some municipalities provided publicly funded medical relief, while welfare agencies would sometimes reimburse private hospitals for charity care.[39]

Some New Deal programs also functioned to expand access to healthcare. The Federal Emergency Relief Administration (FERA), for instance, briefly helped to pay for the basic medical needs of some of the needy. Other New Deal agencies were involved in various public health efforts, such as building hospitals or expanding public health services in poor areas. The Tennessee Valley Authority included a Medical Service and Health Section that provided health centers for employees and funded some health services. Perhaps most pioneering was the Farm Security Administration (FSA). The drought of 1936–7 had devastated Midwestern farming families, leaving them unable to afford basic medical care. To meet their needs, the FSA sponsored a pre-paid cooperative system of health insurance, in which families paid an annual sum in exchange for access to medical, surgical, and hospital care. Hundreds of thousands of individuals were covered by this system, and the concept was to prove influential as a model in later years.[40]

These efforts, nonetheless, amounted to a vastly insufficient patchwork in light of the extent of unmet medical needs. The FSA and the FERA, for instance, may have expanded access to healthcare for the poor, but only partially, incrementally, and temporarily. However, viewed collectively, some argue that these programs—however limited or imperfect—amounted to much more: because of them, many people received free publicly provided medical care for the first time.[41] The increased availability of some free healthcare was, of course, by no means tantamount to any sort of social right to healthcare itself.

But at the same time, as Daniel Hirshfield notes in his seminal study of the healthcare reform efforts of this period, by the middle of the decade, some were indeed calling for a move *beyond* the existing system, and towards such a right: "Gradual public acceptance of the theory that adequate medical care was a right of every citizen," he argues, "and the massive economic and social dislocations caused by the depression had undermined this traditional system of medical relief by the mid-1930s."[42] Nor is Hirshfield's reference to a public belief in a "right" to healthcare an anachronism: during this period a discourse about social and economic rights—including to healthcare—was emerging.

The notion of the "liberal" economic right—whether the right to do business, to "truck, barter, and exchange" (in Adam Smith's words) or to own and enjoy property—goes back centuries, for instance with Locke's fundamental inclusion of a right to property in his *Second Treatise*.[43] This ideal was even enshrined in the Declaration of the Rights of Man and Citizen. Yet running alongside the notion of the "liberal" economic right (to property) has been what one might term a "left" economic right (to social goods). As discussed in Chapter 1, the theoretical right of the poor to the property of the rich in the Middle Ages might be described as the philosophical antecedents of the latter. But by the 1930s and 1940s, a more explicit articulation of rights to specific universal socioeconomic goods—education, healthcare, and social security in old age—was emerging on both the national and the international stage.

The right to property might even be contextualized as—to some extent—incompatible with these other economic human rights. FDR, for instance, noted in a famous speech to the Commonwealth Club in 1932 that Jefferson had recognized that the property rights of some could conflict with the individual rights of others, necessitating government intervention.[44] Government was responsible not only for the protection of property, but also for "an economic declaration of rights, economic constitutional order," as FDR put it in this speech.[45] Although he did not mention healthcare at that point, a right to healthcare was common among the various proposals and declarations of the Second World War era, and would be later embraced by FDR himself. Even during the New Deal, however, some were calling for health rights. One sociologist, for instance, referred to "adequate medical service as a social necessity," and maybe even a "social right" at a 1934 conference, while a journalist labeled medical care "The Fifth Human Right" (following some other necessities of life).[46] The notable black intellectual

Kerry Miller justified a right to healthcare on the basis of the Declaration of Independence: Jefferson's right to life, he argued, necessitated good health.[47] And later, in his 1944 State of the Union address, Roosevelt himself famously delineated a specific economic bill of rights that included healthcare.

However, it is also important to recognize that a discourse of economic rights was not a major factor in the expansion of the welfare state during the New Deal. The broad, potent, and (for some) menacing labor mobilization of the 1930s probably played a much larger role. From the quantitative perspective, organized labor tripled its membership during these years, hitting a historic peak.[48] Qualitative changes in the composition of the labor movement, however, were equally critical. The historically conservative American Federation of Labor (AFL)—which, as described in the last chapter, had worked against health insurance during the Progressive Era—was not up to the task of organizing the massive armies of workers in the big industries.[49] The Committee for Industrial Organization (CIO) split off from the AFL, and its unions were soon leading—and winning—historic, larger-than-life victories in the colossal steel and automobile industries.[50] They accomplished this through the powerful weapon of the sit-down strike, which by "directly encroaching upon the sanctity of corporate property" and bringing production to a standstill, constituted a particularly political (and perhaps revolutionary) form of industrial confrontation and perhaps even a "group ethos that valued human rights over property rights."[51] In contrast to the AFL, which for some time held firm to an ideology of "voluntarism" that precluded support for the welfare state, the CIO strongly embraced social legislation, including a national health insurance system.[52] It seems fair to assume that FDR's economic bill of rights was intended to meet—at least to some extent—the demands of this growing and powerful social force.

And indeed, by the mid-1930s, Roosevelt—facing an increasingly emboldened Left, evaporating support from business, and an ascendant labor movement that increasingly embraced the idea of social rights—was calling for more change.[53] In his 1936 speech to the Democratic National Convention, for instance, he drew on the language of social rights. He criticized those "royalists of the economic order" who "denied that the government could do anything to protect the citizen in his right to work and his right to live."[54] And indeed, the administration secured the passage of key social welfare legislation during these years of the "Second New Deal." At least in theory, the benefits of the Second New Deal were not conceived as public charity, but as the "universal rights of citizenship . . ."[55] Social security represented one of the key achievements of the New Deal, while some hoped that a system of national health insurance would be another.

However, the New Deal was to prove another moment in which a right to healthcare was again deferred in America. This was not for lack of interest or need. Indeed, Roosevelt, in 1934, announced the creation of a Committee on Economic Security—which was to be headed by Secretary of Labor Frances Perkins—to study and develop a social security proposal. Many of the commissioners in the CES saw health insurance as "equally important" as old age insurance: it was even, as they put it, "the most immediately practicable and financially possible form of economic security."[56] And early on, there were hopeful signs that this could be achieved. The CES created a subcommittee on medical care, which was led by Walton Hamilton, the CCMC member whose progressive dissent was earlier discussed.[57] It also appointed a "Technical Committee on Medical Care" that was led by Edgar Sydenstricker, a healthcare reform advocate who had served on the CCMC and who had provided the second progressive dissent (like Hamilton, he thought the majority report did not go far enough, though his dissent amounted to a single sentence).[58] With these men at the helm, the inclusion of health insurance into a social security program might have seemed assured.

However, the positions of the powerful medical stakeholders had not changed since the Progressive Era. In particular, the potent political power of the medical profession—organized within the AMA—was both respected and feared by the administration.[59] The very appointment of Sydenstricker to the Technical Committee produced a firestorm at the AMA.[60] In light of this hostile environment, the administration requested that the CES delay issuing a legislative proposal, and healthcare reform was put on the back burner.[61] Aware that such a delay could prove fatal, Sydenstricker fought to ensure that the CES's general report of early 1935 did not entirely neglect the issue.[62] However, its eventual statement on healthcare was basically a call for further research into a system of compulsory health insurance, outlining certain principles that would underlie its approach.[63] Even this statement, however, alarmed the AMA, which called an emergency special session—only the second in its history—that condemned compulsory insurance.[64] Though the CES completed its report on medical care in June 1935, the administration feared that the controversy it provoked could endanger Social Security altogether, and so did not even release it until after passage of the Social Security bill.[65] The Social Security Act that was signed into law that August was therefore bereft of the guarantee for medical care that was, for so many, absolutely fundamental to true "social security."[66]

That said, this did not signify that national health insurance was dead on arrival: many insiders remained hopeful that it could still be achieved in coming years.[67] Yet for somewhat similar reasons, the second stage of New Deal healthcare reform was also to prove a failure. This time, reformers turned to the amenable Interdepartmental Committee for the Coordination of Health and Welfare Activities (ICHWA), set up by the administration in 1935 to organize the government's scattered social welfare and healthcare-oriented programs.[68] The ICHWA set up its own Technical Committee on Medical Care, with I.S. Falk serving as spokesman, to devise a proposal for a national health program.[69] Its final report, issued in February 1938, called for an increase in Social Security spending on health, an increase in federal and state health spending, and (most contentiously) a deprioritized and weakened proposal for federally aided, state-based compulsory health insurance.[70] Nonetheless, the AMA again saw this as little less than a frontal assault on the medical profession.[71] Its worries were amplified even further after the "National Health Conference" in July 1938, which had been set up at Roosevelt's suggestion to discuss the ICHWA's recommendations.[72]

The National Health Conference unnerved the AMA even as it emboldened reform enthusiasts. The Conference was attended not only by academics and health professionals, but also by a broader spectrum of society, including activists from labor unions and farmers' groups.[73] As Hoffman notes, "[t]he most explicit demands for a right to healthcare came from the labor movement, including a refusal to define health as a market good."[74] A representative from the AFL, for instance, argued not only that health was "not a commodity," but also that it was actually "within the realm of human rights . . ."[75] A steel unionist boldly proclaimed, "My people are asking that our Government take health from the list of luxuries to be bought only by money and add it to the list containing the 'inalienable rights' of every citizen."[76] A physician named Joseph Slavit, who led the leftist "American League for Public Medicine," argued in favor of an even more radical system of state medicine, with services free at the point of care.[77] And agitation sometimes took place outside the conference hall as well. In 1939, for instance, a Bronx Democrat succeeded in introducing a piece of legislation, supported by Slavit's League, that would have created an entirely public health service in New York, with the "goal of providing free medical and dental care to all" through a "State Civil Service," as the *New York Times* noted at the time.[78] Labor's changing orientation during this historic moment clearly constituted a crucial turning point: "Commencing in the thirties and continuing through the following decade," notes Derickson, "labor and its allies in the New Deal coalition vigorously pressed the claim that U.S. citizens had a right to medical services."[79]

However, in response to the "apparent public support" generated by the National Health Conference, the AMA started a new aggressive stage in its anti-health reform campaign, and around the same time, the administration's enthusiasm for health reform began to wane.[80] In part, this reflected a larger turn in the political tides. Apart from the intransigence of the medical lobby, interrelated political and economic developments had taken the wind out of the sails of the reformers. Roosevelt, having not fully embraced Keynesian thinking on the continued importance of fiscal and monetary stimulus during times of economic contraction, prematurely aimed to reduce the budget deficit during the apparent recovery of 1937. The resulting recession and spike in unemployment proved extremely damaging for New Deal Democrats in the 1938 election.[81] The resultant Congress had enough votes between Republicans and conservative Democrats to sink any bold progressive legislation, and the "Second New Deal" was soon brought to a close.

Still, for a brief period, however, many still hoped that a bold health insurance reform could be made a reality. Roosevelt sent the program of the National Health Conference to Congress, but only for study.[82] Senator Robert Wagner of New York saw a window of opportunity, and drew on the ICHWA's National Health Program proposal for his "Wagner Health Bill" of 1939.[83] But between the gathering clouds of war on the one hand, and the mobilization and red-baiting of the AMA on the other, it is perhaps not surprising that Roosevelt all but abandoned the Wagner bill.[84] One persistently optimistic reformer contended that only US entry in the

Second World War could forestall legislative success on the issue of health insurance.[85] With Hitler already on the march in Europe, however, that was only a matter of time. By the time of the Japanese bombing of Pearl Harbor, the National Health Program movement was all but dead.[86]

In assessing this period, it seems reasonable to ask—from a more theoretical perspective—why Social Security and the New Deal failed to achieve the social welfare program—national health insurance—that was at the center of the British and German systems outlined in the last chapter. Scholars have described a number of factors that together likely played a role, but to some extent, the failure of the New Deal health reform movement parallels that of the Progressive Era. On the one side of the battle was a powerful, headstrong, and united opposition—business, insurance companies, and the physician lobby. On the other were well-meaning reformers who lacked powerful allies, both "above" and "below." FDR, for instance, was not at this point eager to take on a politically hazardous issue that could endanger his other goals. At the same time (and despite the expression of enthusiasm at the National Health Conference), the reformers failed to fully join forces with labor and other popular mobilizations from "below."[87] Healthcare reform remained an excessively technocratic solution lacking a popular base. Ultimately, the failure of the Roosevelt administration to create a system of national health insurance reflects the balance of power within both American politics and medicine.

This is not to say that the reformers accomplished nothing. Hirshfield argues that, at the very least, their efforts helped to broaden the public's conceptualization of healthcare rights. They "put forth plans based on the assumption that the government had a duty to guarantee adequate medical care to all its citizens," and in so doing "helped the public see that medical care was as much a basic human right as unemployment compensation or a decent income in old age."[88] Indeed, FDR himself came to describe healthcare as a human right, articulating this forcefully in his 1944 State of the Union Address. But at this point, the nation was at war. The window of opportunity for major social legislation had been closed, and FDR did not live to see it reopen.

An International Right to Health?

The Second World War era saw the rapid rise in rights rhetoric from a position of obscurity to one of international prominence. Considering how marginal the whole discourse of universal rights—and the specific phrase "human rights"— had previously been,[89] it is in some respects rather surprising how quickly the rhetoric of human rights was used to justify both the war against fascism and the socioeconomic rights of the welfare state.[90] For although the emergence of the "human right" in these years is sometimes described as a reaction to the atrocities of the Second World War (especially the Holocaust),[91] "human rights" were used to promote and defend the Allies' aims throughout the war. For instance, the 1942 "Declaration of the United Nations"—which put forth the goals of the Allied powers—called for the protection of "human rights and justice" among them.[92]

It is also important to stress how central socioeconomic rights were to the human rights framework *from the outset.* For instance, British author H. G. Wells, who did a great deal to mainstream the idea of "human rights" on the international stage during the war years, wrote a draft Declaration of Human Rights inclusive of both civil-political rights and a number of socioeconomic rights, including food, education, and medical care (his declaration was published throughout the globe and denounced by the fascist powers).[93] FDR's famous and extremely influential "Four Freedoms" speech in June 1941 can be interpreted in a similar light, and was perhaps meant to provide a common ideological foundation for both his welfarist New Deal domestic policy and his anti-fascist foreign policy.[94] In this speech, though he begins by discussing the threat of fascism and the importance of war readiness, he argues that democracy also required "[j]obs for those who can work" and "[s]ecurity for those who need it." In addition to expanding social security and unemployment insurance, he also notably called for "widen[ing] the opportunities for adequate medical care."[95] The fourth freedom—"freedom from want"—became a sort of rallying cry for those who sought to expand the welfare state. Indeed, the speech is sometimes regarded as a critical "turning point" in the acceptance and advancement of the socioeconomic right.[96] Its rhetoric was incorporated into the Atlantic Charter, the Beveridge Report, and the United Nations' Universal Declaration of Human Rights.[97] For instance, the Beveridge Report—a pivotal document that helped to usher in the post-Second World War British welfare state, including its universal National Health Service—described "The Way To Freedom From Want."[98] The Atlantic Charter, which declared the war goals of the Allied powers and which was the production of a clandestine meeting between Roosevelt and Churchill, clearly drew on "Four Freedoms" phraseology, and included an endorsement of socioeconomic rights, albeit vaguely phrased as "improved labor standards, economic advancement and social security . . ."[99]

Human rights rhetoric, however, was by no means only an Anglo-American development. Individuals and groups from many countries called for—and frequently drafted—postwar bills of human rights, generally inclusive of both civil-political rights and "socialist" rights like social security, work, and healthcare. These included statements from the American Law Institute, the "Pan American" declaration, and a bill from the International Labor Organization, all of which were highly influential in the drafting of the UDHR.[100] And in the US, the enormously ambitious draft of the New Deal organization, The National Resources Planning Board (NRPB)—which included a right to "medical care" among other socioeconomic rights—was to be the inspiration for Roosevelt's famous "Second Bill of Rights."[101] These were not isolated efforts. The French sociologist Georges Gurvitch, who produced his own draft of an international bill, credited the various antecedents to his own draft, among which he included Roosevelt's "Four Freedoms" address, the NRPB's Bill of Rights, and a draft from the ILO.[102] He also describes the French League of Rights of Man's 1936 "Additions to the Declarations of Rights of Man and Citizen," which contended that a variety of social and economic guarantees be added to the political and civil guarantees of the 1789 Declaration, such as "the right of old men, sick men and invalids to the surroundings necessitated by their condition," as he approvingly quoted.[103] In his draft *Bill of Social Rights*, published in 1944, Gurvitch used Roosevelt's "four freedoms" phraseology, arguing for "a social right to a minimum of economic security, guaranteed by a system of social insurance against poverty, sickness, incapacity to work, and old age, granting him freedom from fear."[104]

The law professor Hersch Lauterpacht also called for socioeconomic rights in his own proposed international bill. He preceded his draft with a discussion of the historical roots of human rights. He noted that "natural law" had historically been used for various goals, including the defense of "vested interests" (as when the US Supreme Court struck down minimum wage or child labor laws),[105] but he drew on a variety of other sources to identify a different strain of rights thinking, which instead identified socioeconomic rights with "economic freedom." Among the influences he includes in this historical tradition are many of the sources discussed so far in this book, including Thomas Paine, the Convention of the French Revolution, the English Poor Law, Roosevelt's Second Bill of Rights, various national constitutions, and H. G. Wells's Declaration.[106] Lauterpacht argued that economic rights were essential to the realization of political rights: "[T]he value of political freedom," as he put it, "is impaired by the absence of substantive economic freedom, by economic insecurity, by undeserved want, and by absence of educational opportunity."[107] Not surprisingly, Lauterpacht's proposed international bill contained a range of socioeconomic rights, including to public assistance during sickness.[108]

To summarize, a novel discourse of "rights" emerged during the years around the Second World War, and within this discourse, socioeconomic rights (usually including a right to healthcare) had an important place. Socioeconomic rights—from a policy perspective—were not anything new. The European Left, as described in previous chapters, had argued for the delivery of such socioeconomic goods—including healthcare—since the nineteenth century, such as with the previously discussed Erfurt Program of the SPD. But faced with the cataclysm of the Great Depression and the Second World War, many closer to the political center came to embrace these social rights, like FDR. In 1944, FDR delivered his State of the Union Address to the nation via radio. In advocating a "Second Bill of Rights," FDR joined the chorus of voices calling for the acceptance of a broad spectrum of socioeconomic rights. He contended in his address (like Lauterpacht) that socioeconomic rights, rather than undercutting political rights, were actually essential to guaranteeing them. A "Second Bill of Rights" was needed to guarantee for all the right to a "useful and remunerative job," the right "to earn enough to provide adequate food and clothing and recreation," the right to a "decent home," and the "right to adequate medical care and the opportunity to achieve and enjoy good health."

Roosevelt would not, however, live to see the end of the war. Yet even as he lay dying on the floor of his vacation home from a cerebral hemorrhage, Allied forces were closing in on Germany, and planning for the postwar world had begun. Indeed, partially through Roosevelt's influence, Britain and the USSR had been reluctantly persuaded to accept a single mention of human rights in the draft charter produced at the Dumbarton Oaks conference for the future United Nations.[109] And by the time of Germany's surrender on May 7, the famous San Francisco United Nations conference was already underway.

Postwar: Human Rights Enshrined

Despite all of the human rights talk of the war years, the fate of a "human rights" mission within the United Nations—much less a postwar commitment to the "right to healthcare"—was by no means preordained. The importance of the "human rights" cause was simply not an issue of particular importance to the great powers.[110] Nor was the American delegation itself particularly enthusiastic about acknowledging social and economic rights in the UN charter.[111] Yet through a variety of pressures—perhaps most importantly the role played by developing nations, especially from Latin America as well as nongovernmental advocacy groups[112]—the San Francisco conference was to pave the path to both the Universal Declaration of Human Rights (UDHR) and the World Health Organization (WHO), each of which proclaimed a human right to health or healthcare.

The Charter delegated the establishment of a human rights commission to the UN Economic and Social Council, and in June 1946, the Commission on Human Rights, charged with drafting the international bill of human rights, was created.[113] This Commission on Human Rights, some note, was to some extent a "concession" to smaller nations and interest groups.[114] Additionally, a request from the Brazilian delegation—which included a line from the Archbishop of New York arguing that "Medicine is one of the pillars of peace"—led to a commitment to an international health organization in the UN Charter, leading to the establishment of the WHO.[115] However, despite the importance of socioeconomic rights within the rights discourse of the 1940s, the prominent inclusion of such rights as medical care in the UDHR was by no means inevitable. Scholars have supplied a variety of explanations for how, and why, the UDHR came to prominently include socioeconomic rights, including "medical care," and they might be divided into two categories.

The first was the role played by particular delegates or states. As many have noted, the human rights documents of this era are commonly assumed to be the work of the West. However, Western nations like the US and UK were in fact fairly hesitant when it came to social and economic rights to goods such as healthcare.[116] On the contrary, many less powerful nations, particularly from Latin America, aggressively advocated that socioeconomic rights have a place in the UDHR.[117] A surge of democratization in the interwar period in the region may in part explain this development.[118] Many of these new governments wrote constitutions that included social and economic rights, such as Mexico's Revolutionary 1917 Constitution (which included articles on working hours, child labor, and unemployment insurance, the "first of their kind," as Carozza notes "in any constitutional document") and Chile's 1925 Constitution (which included a state duty on public health).[119] Chile's delegate Hernán Santa Cruz, a leftist aristocrat and friend of later Chilean president Salvador Allende (who will be revisited in the next chapter), played an important role in advocating for the inclusion of social and economic rights in the UDHR.[120] Indeed, he supplied an influential model, inclusive of social and economic rights, to the Canadian John Humphrey, who wrote the first draft of the UDHR.[121] This declaration was the American Law Institute's (ALI) rights statement, which was heavily indebted to the constitutions of various states, including some from Latin America, and held that states had "a duty to maintain or insure that there are maintained comprehensive arrangements for the promotion of health, for the prevention of sickness and accident and the provision of medical care . . ."[122] Humphrey—a socialist, international lawyer, and later Director of the UN's Human Rights Division—relied heavily on such rights documents, and was especially influenced by the submissions of the Latin American delegation.[123] In particular, he called the ALI document the "best of the texts from which I worked . . ."[124] In many instances, such as with the right to healthcare, Humphrey even relied on the wording from these sources.[125] Finally, the role of Eleanor Roosevelt, the chair of the committee, was important. She was both personally sympathetic towards the idea of social and economic rights and successful in convincing an unenthusiastic State Department to go along with their inclusion in the document.[126]

A second factor, advanced by Stephen P. Marks, sees the social and economic rights of the UDHR as the culmination of successive expansions in rights thought driven by the European revolutionary tradition, beginning with 1789.[127] There is no doubt some justice in this view, in the more specific case of the right to health. As seen in Chapter 2, for instance, the work of the Committee on Mendicity advanced thinking about rights into the arena of welfare and healthcare. Labor and left-wing thought and action in the nineteenth century, as described in Chapters 3 and 4, expanded on the Revolutionary agenda of 1789. An important "medical reform" movement, for instance, accompanied the Revolution of 1848, while the SPD's Erfurt Program of 1891 proclaimed demands for a comprehensive welfare state that included "free medical care." The declarations of the post-Second World War period, as Marks describes, drew on 150 years of revolutionary tradition. "Socialist and social democratic ideas galvanized the revolutions of 1848, 1871, and 1917," as he puts it, "and economic, social and cultural rights have since been included in numerous European and Latin American constitutions."[128] Although he is speaking of social and economic rights generally, the relevance to the right to healthcare is clear.

Regardless, the final document, adopted by the General Assembly on December 10, 1948, declared a long list of fundamental social and economic rights. However, in some respects, as some have noted, the right to "medical care" is one of the less robust socioeconomic rights in the UDHR. It declares a right "to a standard of living adequate for the health and well-being of himself and of his family, including food, clothing, housing and medical care and necessary social services . . ."[129]

However, so phrased, the right to medical care seems contingent on belonging to the family of a male "breadwinner."[130] To some extent, this reveals the influence of the "social insurance" model of healthcare, in which workers receive certain social benefits together with wages in exchange for their labor. Others saw other limitations. An Indian Commission member, for example, contended that the phrasing of a right to "medical care" was inadequate, and that a broader "right to health" would better address the fact that much more than medical care was needed.[131] The proposal of the Indian delegation was simpler and more universal: "every human being has the right to health."[132] At one point, the Second Session of the Committee adopted a broader right to health, using the "highest attainable standard" language of the World Health Organization's 1946 Constitution.[133] However, the Third Session would later omit this more sweeping language, and instead simply added "medical care" to a list of other social welfare benefits as opposed to giving it its own article.[134]

The newly formed WHO, in contrast, had already proclaimed a much more ambitious human right to healthcare. The UN Charter had called for the establishment of an international health organization, and in the spring of 1946, a Technical Preparatory Committee for the organization held a meeting in Paris. The committee drafted a constitution for the future WHO that included a truly sweeping declaration of the "right to health." At the International Health Conference held in New York City that summer, sixty-one states signed the Constitution of the World Health Organization, which used this language in its preamble.[135]

The preamble begins with the listing of a number of principles, the first of which is an extraordinary definition of health as a state of "complete physical, mental and social well-being and not merely the absence of disease or infirmity." And instead of a right to "medical care" or even to "healthcare," the document proceeds to call for a right to health itself: "The enjoyment of the highest attainable standard of health is one of the fundamental rights of every human being without distinction of race, religion, political belief, economic or social condition." Furthermore, the final principle makes the guarantee of a right to health a public charge: "Governments have a responsibility for the health of their peoples which can be fulfilled only by the provision of adequate health and social measures."[136] Together, these principles demand much more than a social insurance benefit to certain medical services that workers had already won in countries like Great Britain: they were tantamount to a call for a fully universal and global right to health that governments were responsible for delivering. In her *The Right to Health as a Human Right in International Law*, Brigit Toebes is correct to call the WHO definition "a breakthrough in the field of international health and human rights law," even though the implementation of this right left much to be desired.[137]

There can be little doubt that this era saw the articulation of a grandly expansive and still inspiring right to health and healthcare. However, as will be described in the next chapter, its realization would still largely depend on the balance of political power on both the national and international stage.

Conclusions

In the wake of a war of truly cataclysmic horror, some enormously ambitious statements of rights—including rights to health and healthcare—were made on the world stage. These documents, in particular the UDHR, harkened back to the heritage of Enlightenment rights declarations, incorporating their notions of human equality and even echoing some of their wording. However, they went further in their declaration of rights to a broad array of socioeconomic goods, including healthcare. In this respect, such documents might be seen as achieving a pivotal shift in the healthcare rights-commodity dialectic. Yet the UDHR has proven similar to the rights statements of the Enlightenment era in another sense: it proclaimed rights that it did not realize. The UDHR was, of course, just a declaration, and was intended to be followed by a legally binding covenant; together, these documents would constitute the international bill of rights. However, as will be described in the next chapter, under Cold War pressures the covenant was split in half, with socioeconomic rights separated from civil and political rights. Moreover, progress was slow, and the fate and potential impact of the socioeconomic covenant remained unclear—particularly in light of opposition from the US.

Even as Eleanor Roosevelt proclaimed the historic launch of the UDHR in 1948, the future of the US orientation towards international human rights—especially socioeconomic rights—remained unclear. In the same celebratory statement quoted at the outset of the chapter, Roosevelt hinted at this, noting that her "[g]overnment has made it clear . . . that it does not consider that the economic and social and cultural rights stated in the declaration imply an obligation on governments to assure the enjoyment of these rights by direct governmental action."[138] But what is the meaning of a right if a government takes no responsibility to guarantee it? In the absence of "direct governmental action," in truth, a right to healthcare is degraded to an aspiration, or an inspiration, only.

In 1945, Hersch Lauterpacht had cautioned against a statement that promised rights that it did not protect, for such a declaration "would purport to solve the crucial problem of law and politics in their widest sense by dint of a grandiloquent incantation whose futility would betray a lack both of faith and of candour."[139] To those who find the UDHR inspirational, Lauterpacht's judgment might seem harsh. For all those who continue to live under conditions of unnecessary sickness and poverty—conditions that contravene the provisions of the UDHR—it would no doubt also ring true. In the postwar era, for much of the world's population, healthcare was not a right, but instead remained in the basket of commodities, to be purchased at potentially great cost—if it was available at all.

Notes

1   Eleanor Roosevelt, "Statement to the United Nations' General Assembly on the Universal Declaration of Human Rights," *The Eleanor Roosevelt Papers Project*, accessed January 20, 2015, http://www.gwu.edu/~erpapers/documents/displaydoc.cfm?_t=speeches&_docid=spc057137. This address is cited by Mary Ann Glendon, *A World Made New: Eleanor Roosevelt and the Universal Declaration of Human Rights* (New York: Random House, 2001), 166.

2   Morsink notes that parallels in wording between the UDHR and the rights documents of the eighteenth century demonstrate the intellectual influence of the French Enlightenment on the drafters of the UDHR. Johannes Morsink, "The Philosophy of the Universal Declaration," *Human Rights Quarterly* 6, no. 3 (1984): 310–11.

3   The first chapter of Jonathan Wolff's recent book on the human right to health, for instance, is entitled "The Universal Declaration of Human Rights," though his discussion is much broader. Jonathan Wolff, *The Human Right to Health* (New York: W.W. Norton & Company, 2012), 1–12.

4   Starr notes that the movement "slept through the 1920s." Paul Starr, *The Social Transformation of American Medicine* (New York: Basic Books, 1982), 257.

5   Quoted in David M. Kennedy, *Freedom from Fear: The American People in Depression and War, 1929–1945* (New York: Oxford University Press, 1999), 30.

6   Starr, *The Social Transformation of American Medicine*, 260–1.

7   Ibid., 258–60; Daniel S. Hirshfield, *The Lost Reform: The Campaign for Compulsory Health Insurance in the United States from 1932–1943* (Cambridge, MA: Harvard University Press, 1970), 28–9.

8   A point made by Starr. Starr, *The Social Transformation of American Medicine*, 258.

9   For instance, as Starr points out, for some families, medical bills could equal as much as half of their annual income. Ibid., 258–60.

10 A number of writers discuss the CCMC, including, among others: Colin Gordon, *Dead on Arrival: The Politics of Health Care in Twentieth-Century America* (Princeton, NJ: Princeton University Press, 2005), 15, 181, 262–3; Starr, *The Social Transformation of American Medicine*, 261–6; Roy Lubove, "The New Deal and National Health," *Current History* 72 (1977): 198.

11 Committee on the Cost of Medical Care, *Medical Care for the American People: The Final Report of the Committee on the Costs of Medical Care, Adopted October 31, 1932* (Chicago: Chicago University Press, 1932), vi.

12 Ibid., 4–5.

13 Ibid.

14 Ibid., 7.

15 Although the majority report also noted the potential for incentivizing physicians to provide unnecessary care. Ibid., 12, 19, 24.

16 Ibid., 31–4, 44 (quote on 34).

17 Ibid., 48, 59, 68, 110, 120.

18 Ibid., 110.

19 Ibid., 47–8.

20 Ibid., 50.

21 Ibid., 162–4.

22 Ibid., 197.

23 A point made by Timothy S. Jost, *Health Care at Risk: A Critique of the Consumer-Driven Movement* (Durham: Duke University Press, 2007), 53.

24 Committee on the Cost of Medical Care, *Medical Care for the American People*, 123–4.

25 Ibid., 121–4.

26 Ibid., 130–1.

27 Malcolm Rutherford, "Walton H. Hamilton and the Public Control of Business," *History of Political Economy* 37, no. supplement 1 (2005): 235.

28 Committee on the Cost of Medical Care, *Medical Care for the American People*, 193–4.

29 Ibid., 195.

30 Ibid., 196.

31 Ibid.

32 Ibid., 199–200.

33 Headlined noted and quoted in Starr, *The Social Transformation of American Medicine*, 266.

34 Quoted in Lubove, "The New Deal and National Health," 198.

35 This point is made by Starr, *The Social Transformation of American Medicine*, 266.

36   Beatrix Rebecca Hoffman, *Health Care for Some: Rights and Rationing in the United States since 1930* (Chicago: University of Chicago Press, 2012), 4–7.

37   Ibid., 13–15.

38   Hirshfield, *The Lost Reform*, 71–2.

39   Starr, *The Social Transformation of American Medicine*, 271.

40   The facts in this paragraph are drawn from: Lubove, "The New Deal and National Health," 199; Hirshfield, *The Lost Reform*, 81–6; Hoffman, *Health Care for Some*, 17–19.

41   A point made by Hoffman, *Health Care for Some*, 20. See, also Hirshfield, *The Lost Reform*, 71–2, 97.

42   Hirshfield, *The Lost Reform*, 81.

43   "The great and chief end, therefore," as Locke put it, "of men's uniting into commonwealths, and putting themselves under government, is the preservation of their property." John Locke, *Two Treaties of Civil Government* (London: J.M. Dent & Sons, 1949), 180.

44   A point made by Sunstein, who traces the significance of the Commonwealth Club Address with respect to FDR's later elaboration of a "Second Bill of Rights." Cass R. Sunstein, *The Second Bill of Rights: FDR's Unfinished Revolution and Why We Need It More Than Ever* (New York: Basic Books, 2004), 26–7, 67–71; Franklin Roosevelt, "The Commonwealth Club Address," accessed March 23, 2015, https://Online.Hillsdale.Edu/Document.Doc?Id=282.

45   Franklin Roosevelt, "The Commonwealth Club Address."

46   Quoted in Hoffman, *Health Care for Some*, 23–4.

47   Ibid., 24.

48   Anthony J. Badger, *The New Deal: The Depression Years, 1933–40* (New York: Hill and Wang, 1995), 118.

49   Robert H. Zieger, Timothy J. Minchin, and Gilbert J. Gall, *American Workers, American Unions: The Twentieth and Early Twenty-First Centuries*, fourth ed. (Baltimore: Johns Hopkins University Press, 2014), 84–5.

50   Ibid., 87, 110.

51   The quote is from Mike Davis. Mike Davis, *Prisoners of the American Dream: Politics and Economy in the History of the US Working Class* (London: Verso; repr., 1991), 61; Badger, *The New Deal: The Depression Years, 1933–40*, 124; Zieger, Minchin, and Gall, *American Workers, American Unions*, 87.

52   Zieger, Minchin, and Gall, *American Workers, American Unions*, 62, 94–5; Kennedy, *Freedom from Fear*, 25; Eric Foner, *The Story of American Freedom* (New York: W.W. Norton; repr., 1999), 200.

53   Davis argues that the "mass desertion" of corporate interests from FDR's camp during these years of industrial unrest prodded Roosevelt into the arms of the CIO. Davis, *Prisoners of the American Dream*, 63.

54   The speech is discussed by Sunstein (also the source of this quotation): Sunstein, *The Second Bill of Rights*, 73–7, quotation on 76–7.

55   Foner, *The Story of American Freedom*, 205–6.

56   Quoted in Gordon, *Dead on Arrival*, 16.

57   Starr, *The Social Transformation of American Medicine*, 267.

58   Hirshfield, *The Lost Reform*, 45; Starr, *The Social Transformation of American Medicine*, 267; Committee on the Cost of Medical Care, *Medical Care for the American People*, 201.

59   Gordon, *Dead on Arrival*, 17; Starr, *The Social Transformation of American Medicine*, 279.

60   Starr, *The Social Transformation of American Medicine*, 268.

61   Ibid.; Hirshfield, *The Lost Reform*, 50.

62   Hirshfield, *The Lost Reform*, 52.

63   Ibid., 52 and 175–6; Lubove, "The New Deal and National Health," 82.

64   Lubove, "The New Deal and National Health," 200.

65   Starr, *The Social Transformation of American Medicine*, 269; Lubove, "The New Deal and National Health," 224.

66   As Lubove explains, however, it did contain some important health-related provisions, such as funding for healthcare for disabled children and maternal health. On the basis of these

provisions, he concludes that the medical implications of the act were "profound," insofar as they "established a permanent machinery to distribute federal funds for health and medical purposes . . ." Lubove, "The New Deal and National Health," 200.

67 Gordon, *Dead on Arrival*, 17–18.

68 Hirshfield, *The Lost Reform*, 102; Starr, *The Social Transformation of American Medicine*, 275; Gordon, *Dead on Arrival*, 17–18.

69 Starr, *The Social Transformation of American Medicine*, 275.

70 Lubove, "The New Deal and National Health," 225–6; Hirshfield, *The Lost Reform*, 105–7; Paul Starr, *Remedy and Reaction: The Peculiar American Struggle over Health Care Reform*, revised ed. (New Haven, CT: Yale University Press, 2013), 38.

71 Hirshfield, *The Lost Reform*, 123–4.

72 Lubove, "The New Deal and National Health," 225–6; Hirshfield, *The Lost Reform*, 124.

73 The National Health Conference is discussed by many others, including: Hoffman, *Health Care for Some*, 26–9; Daniel M. Fox, *Health Policies, Health Politics: The British and American Experience, 1911–1965* (Princeton, NJ: Princeton University Press, 1986), 89; Alan Derickson, "'Take Health from the List of Luxuries': Labor and the Right to Health Care, 1915–1949," *Labor History* 41, no. 2 (2000): 171–87.

74 Hoffman, *Health Care for Some*, 28.

75 Quoted in ibid.

76 Quoted in both: Derickson, "'Take Health from the List of Luxuries': Labor and the Right to Health Care, 1915–1949," 172; Hoffman, *Health Care for Some*, 28.

77 Hirshfield, *The Lost Reform*, 113.

78 "Public Medicine Asked at Albany," *The New York Times*, January 27, 1939, accessed January 15, 2015, http://search.proquest.com.ezp-prod1.hul.harvard.edu/docview/102866228?accountid =11311.

79 Derickson, "'Take Health from the List of Luxuries'": Labor and the Right to Health Care, 1915–1949," 172.

80 Hirshfield, *The Lost Reform*, 116–17, 120–1.

81 The discussion of the economic and political trends of 1937–1938 in this paragraph relies on Kennedy, *Freedom from Fear, 1929–1945*, 337–55, 363, 376.

82 Fox, *Health Policies, Health Politics: The British and American Experience, 1911–1965*, 91.

83 Hirshfield, *The Lost Reform*, 136; Monte M. Poen, *Harry S. Truman Versus the Medical Lobby: The Genesis of Medicare* (Columbia: University of Missouri Press, 1979), 22.

84 Fox notes that Roosevelt stated that he approved only the provisions of the bill providing for hospital construction, and that his lack of support was a factor in the bill's failure to even be voted on in the House of Representatives (notably, it was passed by the Senate). Lubove, "The New Deal and National Health," 226; Hirshfield, *The Lost Reform*, 135–6; Hoffman, *Health Care for Some*, 30; Poen, *Harry S. Truman Versus the Medical Lobby*, 22–8; Fox, *Health Policies, Health Politics: The British and American Experience, 1911–1965*, 91.

85 Gordon, *Dead on Arrival*, 18.

86 Hirshfield, *The Lost Reform*, 160; Poen, *Harry S. Truman Versus the Medical Lobby*, 27.

87 My interpretation in this paragraph draws on my reading of the work of the scholars that I cite throughout this section, but also more specifically from the conclusions of Hirshfield and Hoffman. Hirshfield, *The Lost Reform*, 43–4, 66; Hoffman, *Health Care for Some*, 25, 30.

88 Hirshfield, *The Lost Reform*, 165.

89 Pre-war human rights efforts were few and far between, and the meaning of these rights could be highly contradictory. The proposals that did exist sparked little mainstream interest, as Burgers' research documents. Jan Herman Burgers, "The Road to San Francisco: The Revival of the Human Rights Idea in the Twentieth Century," *Human Rights Quarterly* 14, no. 4 (1992): 449–64. Also see: Samuel Moyn, *The Last Utopia: Human Rights in History* (Cambridge, MA: Belknap Press of Harvard University Press, 2010), 49–50; Kenneth Cmiel, "The Recent History of Human Rights," *The American Historical Review* 109, no. 1 (2004): 128.

90 Elizabeth Borgwardt, *A New Deal for the World: America's Vision for Human Rights* (Cambridge, MA: The Belknap Press of Harvard University Press, 2005), 53–5.

91 Moyn states that the notion that human rights emerged in reaction to revelations of Nazi atrocities is "inaccurate and depoliticized." Moyn, *The Last Utopia*, 82–3.

92 Burgers, "The Road to San Francisco: The Revival of the Human Rights Idea in the Twentieth Century," 448; Borgwardt, *A New Deal for the World*, 55.

93 His impact on Franklin Roosevelt or the UDHR is unclear. See: A. W. Brian Simpson, *Human Rights and the End of Empire: Britain and the Genesis of the European Convention* (Oxford: Oxford University Press, 2004), 163–4; Glendon, *A World Made New*, 57; Burgers, "The Road to San Francisco: The Revival of the Human Rights Idea in the Twentieth Century," 464–8.

94 On the roots of the four freedoms, see: Simpson, *Human Rights and the End of Empire: Britain and the Genesis of the European Convention*, 172–3.

95 Franklin Roosevelt, "Annual Message to Congress on the State of the Union," *Franklin D. Roosevelt Presidential Library and Museum*, accessed March 8, 2015, http://docs.fdrlibrary. marist.edu/od4frees.html.

96 Brigit C.A. Toebes, *The Right to Health as a Human Right in International Law* (Antwerpen: Intersentia/Hart, 1999), 14.

97 Additionally, Britain, as Simpson emphasizes, in seeking to associate itself with the rhetoric of the United States (a potential and powerful ally), attempted to incorporate the "four freedoms" into its own rhetoric. Regarding the role of the Four Freedoms Speech see: Elizabeth Borgwardt, *A New Deal for the World*, 48–9; Wolff, *The Human Right to Health*, 3; Simpson, *Human Rights and the End of Empire*, 174–5.

98 Inter-departmental Committee on Social Insurance and Allied Services, *Social Insurance and Allied Services: Report by Sir William Beveridge* (New York: The Macmillan Company, 1942), 7.

99 The significance and impact of the Atlantic Charter with respect to the history of human rights is disputed, and no doubt, the document was read in different ways by different individuals. See: Borgwardt, *A New Deal for the World: America's Vision for Human Rights*, 29, 34, 53–4; Simpson, *Human Rights and the End of Empire*, 180–2; Moyn, *The Last Utopia*, 88–9, 93; "The Atlantic Charter," *The Avalon Project: Documents in Law, History, and Diplomacy*, accessed January 10, 2015, http://avalon.law.yale.edu/wwii/atlantic.asp.

100 Simpson notes, however, that there were significant differences of opinion with respect to the inclusion of socioeconomic rights in the bill of rights produced by the American Law Institute. Burgers provides a compendium of the pre-Dumbarton Oaks statements. Glendon, *A World Made New*, 57; Simpson, *Human Rights and the End of Empire: Britain and the Genesis of the European Convention*, 187–91, 196–8; Burgers, "The Road to San Francisco: The Revival of the Human Rights Idea in the Twentieth Century," 471–4; Johannes Morsink, *The Universal Declaration of Human Rights: Origins, Drafting, and Intent*, (Philadelphia: University of Pennsylvania Press, 1999), 1–2.

101 Sunstein, *The Second Bill of Rights*, 85–8; Simpson, *Human Rights and the End of Empire: Britain and the Genesis of the European Convention*, 187–8.

102 Georges Gurvitch, *The Bill of Social Rights* (New York, NY: International Universities Press, 1946), 12–14. I owe this citation to Simpson.

103 Quoted by ibid., 17.

104 Ibid., 85.

105 Hersch Lauterpacht, *An International Bill of the Rights of Man* (New York: Columbia University Press, 1945), 37–8.

106 Ibid., 156–9.

107 Ibid., 156.

108 Ibid., 155.

109 M. Glen Johnson, "The Contributions of Eleanor and Franklin Roosevelt to the Development of International Protection for Human Rights," *Human Rights Quarterly* 9, no. 1 (1987): 24. See also: Glendon, *A World Made New*, 6 and 9; Burgers, "The Road to San Francisco: The Revival of the Human Rights Idea in the Twentieth Century," 474.

110 Moyn, *The Last Utopia*, 60; Glendon, *A World Made New: Eleanor Roosevelt and the Universal Declaration of Human Rights*, xv.

111   Johnson, "The Contributions of Eleanor and Franklin Roosevelt to the Development of International Protection for Human Rights," 26–7.

112   Mary Ann Glendon, "The Forgotten Crucible: The Latin American Influence on the Universal Human Rights Idea," *Harvard Human Rights Journal* 16 (Spring 2003): 27–30; Susan Eileen Waltz, "Universalizing Human Rights: The Role of Small States in the Construction of the Universal Declaration of Human Rights," *Human Rights Quarterly* 23, no. 1 (2001): 44–72; Morsink, *The Universal Declaration of Human Rights*, 2; Burgers, "The Road to San Francisco: The Revival of the Human Rights Idea in the Twentieth Century," 475–6; Glendon, *A World Made New*, 17–18; Moyn, *The Last Utopia*, 60.

113   Wright-Carozza, "From Conquest to Constitutions: Retrieving a Latin American Tradition of the Idea of Human Rights," *Human Rights Quarterly* 25, no. 2 (2003): 285.

114   Glendon, *A World Made New*, xv; Waltz, "Universalizing Human Rights: The Role of Small States in the Construction of the Universal Declaration of Human Rights," 52.

115   Toebes, *The Right to Health as a Human Right in International Law*, 15.

116   John Tobin, *The Right to Health in International Law* (Oxford: Oxford University Press, 2012), 68

117   While some have pointed to the essentially socialist strain of the Latin American contribution, others—namely Wright-Carozza—have argued that the Latin American human rights discourse incorporated a greater diversity of elements, including (1) the activist strand of thought of Bartolomé de Las Casa (who—and here Wright-Carozza relies on the work of Brian Tierney, discussed in Chapter 1—went past Aquinas in using "natural rights" to defend the rights of Indians); (2) the unique Latin American assimilation of both the North American and the French Revolutionary "rights" tradition of the late eighteenth century; and (3) the highly influential Constitution and rights tradition of "social liberalism," for instance as found in the Mexican Constitution of 1917. Glendon, "The Forgotten Crucible," 27–40; Wright-Carozza, "From Conquest to Constitutions: 281–313.

118   Morsink, *The Universal Declaration of Human Rights*, 130.

119   Ibid.; Wright-Carozza, "From Conquest to Constitutions: Retrieving a Latin American Tradition of the Idea of Human Rights," 304; Toebes, *The Right to Health as a Human Right in International Law*, 79–80.

120   Waltz, "Universalizing Human Rights: The Role of Small States in the Construction of the Universal Declaration of Human Rights," 60; Glendon, "The Forgotten Crucible," 35–6.

121   Glendon has argued that the Latin American proposals provided a sort of third way between US/UK and Soviet proposals, thereby making its general acceptance by a broader array of UN member nations possible. Glendon, "The Forgotten Crucible: The Latin American Influence on the Universal Human Rights Idea," 39; Waltz, "Universalizing Human Rights: The Role of Small States in the Construction of the Universal Declaration of Human Rights," 60.

122   This point and the quote from the draft are from: Tobin, *The Right to Health in International Law*, 26.

123   Morsink, *The Universal Declaration of Human Rights*, 130–3; Glendon, *A World Made New*, 57–8; Glendon, "The Forgotten Crucible: The Latin American Influence on the Universal Human Rights Idea," 30–2; Waltz, "Universalizing Human Rights: The Role of Small States in the Construction of the Universal Declaration of Human Rights," 58.

124   Quoted in Tobin, *The Right to Health in International Law*, 26.

125   Morsink, *The Universal Declaration of Human Rights*, 130–3.

126   Glendon, *A World Made New*, 43; Johnson, "The Contributions of Eleanor and Franklin Roosevelt to the Development of International Protection for Human Rights," 36.

127   Stephen P. Marks, "From the 'Single Confused Page' to the 'Decalogue for Six Billion Persons': The Roots of the Universal Declaration of Human Rights in the French Revolution," *Human Rights Quarterly* 20, no. 3 (1998): 459–514.

128   Ibid., 506.

129   The United Nations, "The Universal Declaration of Human Rights," http://www.un.org/en/documents/udhr/.

130   A point made by Morsink, *The Universal Declaration of Human Rights*, 198.

131   Brigit C. A. Toebes, *The Right to Health as a Human Right in International Law*, 37.

132   Quoted in Morsink, *The Universal Declaration of Human Rights*, 192.

133   Ibid., 194.

134   Toebes, *The Right to Health as a Human Right in International Law*, 39–40.

135   This paragraph relies on Toebes, *The Right to Health as a Human Right in International Law*, 29–31.

136   The World Health Organization, "The Constitution of the World Health Organization," http://www.who.Int/governance/eb/who_constitution_en.pdf.

137   Toebes, *The Right to Health as a Human Right in International Law*, 36.

138   Roosevelt, "Statement to the United Nations' General Assembly on the Universal Declaration of Human Rights."

139   Lauterpacht, *An International Bill of the Rights of Man*, 9.

6
Postwar
Health and Death in the Cold War

Nestled in the foothills of the stunning Trans-Ili Alatau mountain range, Alma-Ata—the capital of the Kazakh Soviet Socialist Republic—had some practical advantages as the host city of an international conference on health. For one, it was home to the Lenin Convention Center, which housed a capacious 3,000-seat auditorium. Nor were accommodations in the city an issue: in order to house delegates from the 134 nations in attendance, the Soviets rapidly erected a hotel with a thousand beds. And although the auditorium's audio system lacked (in the Soviet fashion) the capacity for audience participation, this was easily fixed by some re-rigging performed by a company from Italy.[1]

Ultimately, the Soviet Union had its wish, and in September 1978, the week-long "International Conference on Primary Healthcare," jointly sponsored by the WHO and the United Nations Children's Fund (UNICEF), was held on its grounds in modern-day Kazakhstan. Now, on the one hand, Soviet efforts to ensure that the conference was held on their turf might make Alma-Ata seem like little more than one especially small skirmish in the Cold War.[2] Cold War politics no doubt suffused the lead-up to the conference at Alma-Ata as well as the debate about healthcare policy of this period more generally. On the other hand, the conference at Alma-Ata can be seen as a transcendence of the politics of the Cold War. From it came the path-blazing "Declaration of Alma-Ata," an international proclamation of health principles, embraced by developing nations, and by no means a piece of Soviet health propaganda. The declaration both drew on, and went beyond, the health rights statements examined in the last chapter, and the conference remains one of the seminal moments in the history of the human right to health.

The Declaration of Alma-Ata began by reasserting the WHO's broad 1946 definition of health: "[H]ealth, which is a state of complete physical, mental and social well-being, and not merely the absence of disease or infirmity, is a fundamental human right . . ." It went beyond the WHO definition, however, by highlighting the critical importance of socioeconomic development, community participation, and attention to the national and local health needs of developing countries. A broadly and ambitiously conceived system of "primary healthcare," it asserted, could help undo the deadly legacy of colonialism and under-development, and allow all to live healthy lives by the year 2000.[3]

It had a powerful, immediate, and inspirational impact. "[A]fter Alma-Ata in 1978," WHO director-general Halfdan Mahler reflected decades later, "everything seemed possible."[4] Indeed, there were many reasons to be hopeful at that moment. Many "Third World" nations around the globe had emerged from colonial dominance, often with ambitious plans for the advancement of their health systems and a desire to confront the serious health problems their nations faced.[5] Observers, meanwhile, were reporting sweeping improvements in health from nations of the Communist bloc, especially China and Cuba. In much of the developed world, meanwhile, de facto "rights" to healthcare had crystallized through the expansion of the welfare state. And with Alma-Ata, the emphasis on limited "vertical" disease-specific programs of both the WHO and the larger "global health" community seemed to be shifting to a much more ambitious agenda of universal primary care, based on the idea of a right to health. "The immediate impact of the Declaration was tremendous," recalled Mahler, "because people left Alma-Ata with the conviction that they had participated in a health revolution."[6]

This chapter will trace the history of the human right to healthcare (and to some extent, health more broadly) throughout the decades of the Cold War, starting around the time of the Universal Declaration of Human Rights and concluding in the period shortly after Alma-Ata. The number of developments in both international human rights law and national health systems during this period would make any attempt at exhaustiveness impossible. Rather than endeavoring to describe developments along the rights/commodity dialectic in nation after nation (a daunting project indeed), this chapter will focus on a limited number of illustrative cases where the right to healthcare was advanced, stalled, or thwarted. As these examples will show, the rise (or fall) of health rights in this era was largely divorced from the absence or presence of rights thought and rhetoric. Instead, the interplay of political dynamics both within the nation-state and between states critically determined how, why, and where health rights emerged.

This chapter will discuss case studies from three groups of nations—the "First," "Second," and "Third Worlds"—to illustrate these themes. In the "First World," a de facto legal right to healthcare emerged in Great Britain, but noticeably did not in the United States. Two "Second World" examples—the Soviet Union and China—illustrate the mixed legacy of communism with regard to advancing a right to healthcare.[7] After surveying some developments in international law on the right to health in the post-Second World War era, this chapter will then focus on several "Third World" examples in Latin America—Chile, Cuba, and (after a discussion of Alma-Ata) Nicaragua—to comparatively explore how the tides of global political change affected the emergence and/or rollback of health rights in these nations. Efforts to create social rights—including to healthcare—could easily be caught in the crossfire of the high-casualty conflicts of the Cold War. The year 1948 may have seen a great proclamation of the human right to health, but it was state power, not any international rights regime, that made—and unmade—the right to healthcare during the sometimes heady, frequently deadly decades of the Cold War.

Great Britain: The National Health Service and a De Facto Right to Health

With the end of the Second World War and the coming of peace came a bold desire for a better future. The Western European political left—which had previously played a role in the advent of universal healthcare systems from a position *outside* of power—emerged from the ashes of the Second World War with political power and a willingness to wield it. As the historian Tony Judt notes, the discrediting of fascism meant that only those pre-war parties with strong "anti-Fascist credentials" thrived in the postwar years, and that predominantly meant parties of the Left.[8] And though these left-wing (predominantly socialist though non-communist) parties did not usually dominate the parliaments of the postwar European world, they were nonetheless among its "major political forces," elected with a mandate to produce social change.[9]

This was not, however, a homogeneous development. In many nations, the parties of the Left shared power, but only in a few did they truly dominate.[10] Great Britain—where the Labour Party swept Winston Churchill from power in a landslide victory in 1945—was perhaps the most famous example of the latter, with great consequences for the right to healthcare. When Labour took power, it had a large "mandate for change" from the public. As the historian Donald Sassoon explains,

> [T]here can be no disputing that the Labour Party was expected to introduce a fairer society . . . where excessive inequalities would be removed, and in which those which persisted . . . would not deprive anyone of certain basic social rights, such as employment, healthcare and education . . . the citizenship rights which had been the rallying cry of the liberal-democratic tradition—the juridical equality of all—would be supplemented by new socio-economic rights.[11]

No doubt, new socioeconomic rights were created, even if not articulated in the nascent language of "human rights." The Labour Party succeeded along these lines with the passage of the National Health Act of 1946, which created a system of universal free healthcare, equally available to all. Though this law was an extension of an earlier generation of incremental reforms (as Judt notes of the welfare reforms of this era more generally), it was also a "genuinely radical departure."[12] It created one of a new "array of [social] rights" that reinvigorated the meaning of equality and citizenship, as T. H. Marshall described shortly after its inception.[13]

Of course, like all major historical events, the creation of the NHS had many roots. First, one might emphasize its various possible antecedents: the Poor Law medical service;[14] Welsh health systems for miners;[15] public hospitals, themselves sometimes the outgrowth of Poor Law infirmaries;[16] and the voluntary charity hospitals, with their origins in the Middle Ages.[17] But most importantly, there was the 1911 National Health Insurance Act, explored in Chapter 4. This bill significantly expanded healthcare for the mostly male workforce, but it also excluded many from care (e.g., workers' families) and failed to cover many key healthcare services (e.g., hospital care and specialist care).[18] Indeed, with the Second World War coming to a close, National Health insurance left approximately half of the population of Britain uncovered.[19] Nonetheless, the 1911 Act arguably helped to pave the way for the later reforms, insofar as it both "acclimated the public to state intervention" in healthcare and generated "public pressures for the expansion of coverage."[20] However, by the Second World War, a consensus had emerged that this fragmented "system" was neither acceptable nor adequate.

Second, one might emphasize the proposals for universal healthcare that emerged in the interwar years. The "Dawson Report" of 1920, for instance, proposed a system of "primary health centres," revolving around general practitioners, that would—reflecting social medicine thought—integrate both "curative and preventive" health services; however, the Dawson Report largely fell by the wayside until the years of the war.[21] In 1930, the British Medical Authority abandoned its previous resistance to state intervention in healthcare and produced a proposal of its own. Although the BMA proposal would have expanded the reach of the 1911 National Health Insurance Act (for instance, to workers' families), it would have maintained its fundamentally non-universal scope, with coverage depending on income.[22] Such reform proposals, however, were still essentially incremental visions, and they were soon trumped by more expansive and universalist proposals.

Critically, it was during these years that a new "Left health policy" began to crystallize. Proposals for universal medical care had been part of the political program of the Left since the nineteenth century, as seen in the Erfurt Program of the German SPD (described in Chapter 4). This was not a universal phenomenon among socialist groups in Britain, however. The Fabians and the early Labour Party, for instance, emphasized public health and sanitary and environmental measures over what one would think of as a "socialized" healthcare.[23] However, partially as a result of the work of the Labour-affiliated Socialist Medical Association (SMA), this changed.[24]

The program of the SMA, "A Socialized Medical Service," published in 1931, did emphasize public and preventive health alongside curative medicine. However, it went beyond earlier proposals for expanded insurance coverage by calling for a truly universal public health system—one not limited to the poor or the working class, but for the entire population. The *universalism* of this vision set it apart from the various corporatist systems already in existence, whether in Britain or Germany. Instead of a tiered system of private care for the rich and public care for the poor, the SMA proposed a system that would provide high-quality, world-class medicine to *all*: "The object of the Medical Service of the future," the document reads, "will be to put every advance of modern medical science and specialist treatment as well as skilled nursing freely within the reach of all. The Service must be so efficient and so well organized that everyone, rich and poor alike, will be ready to take advantage of it."[25] Additionally, "the Service must be free for all," with "no economic barrier between the doctor and his patient."[26] Finally, it proposed that this "free and all-embracing" service be staffed by salaried state physicians.[27] This program was adopted into the Labour Party's platform in 1934, and was thereafter its official healthcare policy.[28]

The years of the war made other actors and parties more amenable to the SMA's radical vision than one would expect. The impact of the war itself—ranging from aerial bombardment to the rationing of basic goods to the common experience of fighting at the front—was, to some extent, a communalizing experience across class lines.[29] As Derek Fraser explains, "The war was to have a decisive influence in producing a common experience and universal treatment for it . . . in its wake the spirit and practice of universalism affected the course of social policy."[30] In fact, the diffuse desire for fundamental postwar welfare reforms pushed even the wartime Conservative Party into tentatively supporting an expansion of healthcare.

This sentiment was reflected in the widespread acclaim that met the 1942 publication of *Social Insurance and Allied Sources* (commonly known as the Beveridge Report), one of the key documents in the history of the British welfare state. William Beveridge was a Liberal economist, social worker, and writer who, in 1941, was selected to chair a committee tasked with performing a survey of social insurance in Britain. Given the provocative conclusions of the committee, the report ultimately bore his signature alone.[31] Drawing on Roosevelt's important phraseology of "freedom from want," the Beveridge Report famously outlined a proposal for a comprehensive system of social insurance, covering unemployment, retirement, maternity, education, sickness, and—importantly—healthcare. The report acknowledged the shortfalls of the existing system of healthcare, both in terms of who was covered and what treatments were available "as of right."[32] To address this, it proposed—like the SMA—not merely an expansion of the existing corporatist system of insurance, but a health service that was both *universal* and *free at time of use.* "All classes," the report reads, "will be covered for comprehensive medical treatment and rehabilitation," which (it later notes) would generally be available "without a charge on treatment at any point."[33] The service was intended to cover not only basic healthcare, but also—like the proposal of the SMA—the full gamut of modern medical treatment. According to the report, a "comprehensive national health service" would "ensure that for every citizen there is available whatever medical treatment he requires, in whatever form he requires it, domiciliary or institutional, general, specialist or consultant, and will ensure also the provision of dental, ophthalmic and surgical appliances, nursing and midwifery and rehabilitation after accidents."[34]

The report was met with mass approval: approximately 635,000 copies were sold,[35] and the sheer popular groundswell behind it essentially precluded a retreat from Beveridge's principles by either the Conservatives or Labour. Indeed, as one scholar has argued, the Government's initial "lukewarm reception" was met by a "popular and parliamentary outcry" so intense as to drastically transform "perceptions of what was politically possible," forcing Churchill to "publicly . . . commit himself to a major programme of economic and social reform. . . ."[36] The Coalition Government's "White Paper," published two years later, embraced the principles of a comprehensive and free health service, causing much consternation among the conservative leaders of the British Medical Authority, who campaigned against it.[37] Yet it is important not to overemphasize the extent of consensus: the parties diverged in central ways on issues of organization, ownership, and financing.[38] The Conservatives, indeed, sought to take a step back from the 1944 White Paper, while Labour ultimately went beyond it.[39]

And it was Labour's vision—which was to a large extent that of the SMA—that emerged triumphant. After Labour came to power in the historic 1945 elections, Aneurin Bevan, an "abrasive and militantly class conscious" former miner, was appointed Minister of Health.[40] Bevan skillfully crafted a bill that was quickly passed by the Labour government in November 1946 despite vociferous opposition from the medical profession. As historians have emphasized, Bevan made some crucial contributions to the form of the NHS. First, he became committed to the nationalization of hospitals. Second, because he conceived of a health service of high quality that would be used by all, he opposed imposing any upper income threshold that would disqualify individuals from using it.[41] This notion of a health service based on an "explicit egalitarian commitment and a first-class standard of treatment" very much took Bevan a step beyond earlier reformers.[42] His vision was the antithesis of charity medicine, however well-funded and widely available such care might be: "[S]ociety," Bevan stated, "becomes more wholesome, more serene and spiritually healthier, if it knows that its citizens have at the back of their consciousness the knowledge that not only themselves, but all their fellows, have access, when ill, to the *best that medical skill can provide*" (emphasis added).[43] T. H. Marshall similarly emphasized a few years after the passage of the Act that—unlike Poor Law-type welfare systems which provided a *minimum* to the poor—the NHS was intended to provide a "reasonable maximum" for the great majority of society, and thus aimed to become "the norm of social welfare."[44] Financed primarily through general taxes, the National Health Service—rather amazingly—was ready to launch in the summer of 1948.

Shortly before its onset, a four-page leaflet was mailed to every house and apartment to announce the new system, and the text of this document speaks to its comprehensiveness and universality. The NHS, its first page reads, "will provide you with all medical, dental, and nursing care. Everyone—rich or poor, man, woman or child—can use it or any part of it. There are no charges, except for a few special items. There are no insurance qualifications."[45] The document proceeds to describe how, from age 16 and up, everyone can select the doctor of her choice, and how the NHS would cover maternity services, "all forms of treatment in general or special hospitals," mental healthcare, surgical care, prescription drugs, dental care, eye care, and "home health services"—all without charge. "From then on," as historian Rudolf Klein puts it in his history of the service, "everyone was entitled, as of right, to free care—whether provided by a general practitioner or by a hospital doctor—financed by the state."[46]

What, ultimately, made this possible? Historians differ here, with early accounts downplaying the role of socialist ideas and even of the Labour Party. For instance, in his 1958 book, Harry Eckstein disputes what he calls the "obvious" and "popular" account of the NHS's origins, namely, that it was the unsurprising outcome of a socialist government pursuing socialist policies, or of the especially "egalitarian"

Bevan.[47] He conceives it instead as a long-in-the-making attempt to rectify the structural inadequacies of the "old medical service" of Britain, which needed new sources of funding and administrative reorganization.[48] Indeed, he contends that the previous medical service was a particular failure from the perspective of the *middle* classes, who, by his account, were the primary beneficiaries of the NHS (they now got free care that they previously had paid for).[49] Klein, on the other hand, emphasizes the importance of a bipartisan consensus, while Daniel Fox stresses how the NHS facilitated a regionalized reorganization of hospitals in Britain.[50] Such interpretations, however, erase the role of class conflict or labor mobilization in the advent of universal healthcare, as Webster notes. He, in contrast, argues instead that Labour, and the workers' mobilization underlying it, played key roles in the developments that eventually culminated in the creation of the NHS.[51] This is not to say that there was not also an element of political consensus, but rather that the universalist impulse within this consensus *originated* from, and advanced under the banner of, Labour ideology. Government bureaucrats ultimately adopted Labour's unique "conception of the health service" as a universal good that was founded on the principles of "universalism, comprehensiveness, and funding from central taxation."[52] The resultant "alliance" helped secure the success of this vision.

Setting aside the issue of how the NHS came to be, how did its emergence relate to the "human right to health"? These events, after all, preceded the Universal Declaration of Human Rights, and there is no evidence that the human rights rhetoric of the United Nations Charter played any significant role in British social policy at this stage.[53] Although, as seen in the last chapter, ideas about socioeconomic rights were flourishing (to some extent) during the war years, there is little reason to think that an explicit *ideology* of human rights played any role in the foundation of the NHS.

Nevertheless, it seems impossible to avoid the conclusion that, in many senses, the NHS indeed *created* a social right to healthcare. As Moyn notes, FDR's "breakthrough" was to label these post-Beveridge social programs as "rights" in his 1944 State of the Union address.[54] Yet the "rights" label seems less important, from a certain perspective, than the actual *content* of a given social program or protection. At the end of the day, the NHS was founded on the *universalism* of Labour's vision of healthcare, and as Webster puts it, "[h]ealth care thus became an inalienable right rather than a benefit dependent on the vagaries of the market."[55] It was tantamount to a profound shift in the rights/commodity dialectic and, indeed, "a major step towards the decommodification of welfare" itself.[56] The NHS physician and scholar Julian Tudor Hart similarly praised the NHS's track record of providing "non-commercial health for every citizen as a human right . . ."[57] Although this right did not arise from a written constitution or the dictates of international law, it nonetheless exists in statutory form.[58] Thus, as one scholar argues, the right to health proclaimed by Article 25 of the UDHR "finds relatively full expression in the operation and scope of the NHS."[59]

The NHS was, to a very real extent, a pioneering advance in health rights, even if few people involved in its creation said much—or, for that matter, thought much—about the idea of health rights. But it was tantamount to a social right to health nonetheless, albeit one forged out of political mass struggle. Yet this "right to health" was by no means an inevitability. Across the Atlantic, around this same time, there was much hope that the United States would follow a similar path: not that it was set to nationalize its hospitals or create a salaried medical service *per se*, but rather that there was a growing consensus for a universal national health insurance system that would, in its own way, create a right to health. That right to health in the US was not, however, to be forged in this era. But why?

The United States: Cold War Politics and the Fall of Universal Healthcare

In May 1946, the same year that saw the passage of the National Health Service Act, the prominent editor of the *Journal of the American Medical Association* (*JAMA*) Morris Fishbein, a public figure in his own right, addressed the annual meeting of the New Hampshire Medical Society. Turning to unfolding developments across the Atlantic, he said, "As I look over at what is happening in Great Britain, I shudder for the future of medicine there. The nation proposes to take over—in the old sense in which Al Capone used to 'take over'—the medical profession and the hospitals, which will be administered as state institutions."[60] Fishbein was no less worried about domestic developments, however. Before Congress was the Wagner-Murray-Dingell (WMD) bill, which he deemed "an unfortunate piece of legislation."[61] His opposition should come as no surprise, for the WMD bill shared significant common ground with British developments. One historian, for instance, has described it as "an American answer to the Beveridge plan."[62] Like the Beveridge plan, it proposed a comprehensive expansion of the welfare state, which would have significantly expanded on the welfare provisions of the New Deal, extending the reach of social security, unemployment insurance, and public assistance programs.[63] Critically, it would have gone beyond Wagner's 1939 bill, which was described in the last chapter, and established a *national* health insurance program.[64]

The Beveridge plan, in fact, had helped to inspire developments not only in Britain, but also in the United States. The drafting of the first WMD bill during the years of the Roosevelt administration was reportedly encouraged, at least to some extent, by the release of the report.[65] When Beveridge came to visit and lecture in the United States during the war, Roosevelt was reported to have whined to Secretary of Labor Frances Perkins about being robbed of credit: "Why does Beveridge get his name on this? . . . It is not the Beveridge plan. It is the Roosevelt plan."[66] And yet, as seen in the last chapter, Roosevelt never really embraced the cause of national health insurance. The initial WMD bill, floated in 1943, was neither impeded nor championed by Roosevelt.[67] But the elections of 1944 brought new hope to the New Dealers, who expected a national health insurance proposal from FDR in spring of the following year.[68]

Though FDR died that April, Truman picked up the baton of national health insurance. Yet WMD would never come into existence, in no small part because of the exertions of the American Medical Association, supported by the pages of Fishbein's *JAMA*. As a result, a right to healthcare failed to emerge in the United States in the post-Second World War era. Why was this the case? One can approach the question in two ways. The first is to look at the history of these years, and the sequence of events and balance of forces that ultimately produced failure. The second is to frame this as a subquestion within a larger dilemma: What is it about the United States that has made it, for so long, essentially unique among industrialized, developed nations in failing to create a system of universal healthcare?

It is worth beginning with an examination of the role of labor in the United States. In Britain, a long period of working-class mobilization helped both to produce the ideology of universalism behind the NHS and to advance its creation and implementation through the election of an overtly working-class-oriented Labour Party. Similarly, in the United States, the years of the New Deal and the Second World War saw a moment of labor mobilization unique in the nation's history. However, unlike in Britain, where there was a "third" party of the working class (the Labour Party), in the US, the fate of organized labor was intimately tied to that of the Democratic Party, which was not an explicit working-class party.[69] Nonetheless, and in spite of the early "voluntarism" of the AFL, the labor movement in the US, like that of Britain, had gradually come to embrace healthcare as a socioeconomic right by the Second World War.

For instance, as the historian Alan Derickson describes, from 1930 onward, "without much assistance from political philosophers and policy intellectuals," the labor movement sought to "recast the question of health reform as one of social justice and positive human rights."[70] Similar to their fellow workers in the UK who were in and allied with the Labour Party, labor activists "sought a concept of citizenship that encompassed social as well as civil and political rights," among them healthcare.[71] In 1947, the Teamsters union even did this using the global language of rights, announcing that "adequate medical care is a basic human right."[72] At the 1949 convention of the AFL, President William Green similarly went beyond the typical discourse and "globalized the issue," by arguing that the "poorest . . . in the world" deserved medical care, which only the "Welfare State" could provide.[73] In his writings, Green similarly sought to "universalize the issue," arguing against narrow health services that only catered to the poor, or occupationally based plans provided by employers.[74]

A second factor to be considered is the role of leadership. Truman, like Labour Prime Minister Clement Attlee, was supportive of expanding healthcare access. Some stress Truman's personal, long-standing interest in healthcare reform, while others have argued that Truman took on health reform because he appreciated the role that labor had played in his selection as Roosevelt's vice presidential candidate.[75] Whatever the case may be, soon after the surrender of Japan, Truman began calling for Congress to deliver a national health program, drawing on the language of FDR's famous "Second Bill of Rights" speech: "Our new economic bill of rights," Truman said in a message to Congress in November 1945, "should mean health security for all, regardless of residence, station, or race—everywhere in the United States."[76] Finally, in both nations, there was a popular mandate for change. Indeed, in 1945, some *three-quarters* of Americans favored a program of health insurance for the nation.[77] To summarize, the labor movement, the president, and a large majority of the country wanted to see a program of national health insurance. What could possibly have gone wrong?

As mentioned earlier, there is no question that the influence of the American Medical Association—with Fishbein at the helm of its pre-eminent journal—played a critical role in defeating a national health program. However, the failure of the health insurance battle cannot simply be attributed to the interest group politicking of the AMA. A much larger political shift took place in these years, part of which was mediated by the onset of the Cold War and the domestic political repression that it enabled. The targets of McCarthyism included organized labor itself, progressive groups within the medical community that might have more successfully pushed back against the AMA, and key government administrators and policy experts working on health reform. On the other side of the equation, business and nascent corporate health interests added muscle and money to the AMA's campaign against national health insurance (NHI).[78]

The opening day of the Senate hearings on WMD in the spring of 1946 gives a sense of how critical a role red-baiting would play. While the chairman of the hearings was still in the middle of his opening statement, Robert A. Taft, a Republican senator from Ohio, butted in and declared, "I consider it [WMD] socialism. It is to my mind the most socialistic measure that this Congress has ever had before it."[79] After a short verbal altercation, he then stormed out. Officials testifying from the big unions were treated with particular harshness, attributable (in part) to rising anti-union public opinion.[80]

Larger political trends, however, also diminished the chance of victory. Republicans performed strongly in the 1946 midterm elections, taking both the House and the Senate. The wave of strikes of the postwar years instigated an anti-labor backlash, which culminated in the passage of the Taft-Hartley Act of 1947 over Truman's veto.[81] The new Congress, moreover, sought to cast support for NHI as part of a communist plot.[82] Still, particularly in light of the popularity of NHI, there were grounds for optimism. Truman continued to push for it, both in Congress and on the campaign trail, and his victory in the fall of 1948 put it back on the agenda.[83]

In 1949, Truman again appeared before Congress to argue for universal healthcare, again wielding the language of rights. NHI, he stated, "will mean that proper medical care will be economically accessible to everyone covered by it, in the country as well as in the city, *as a right and not as a medical dole.*"[84] However, the balance of power now greatly favored NHI's opponents. First, the attention of organized labor—perhaps NHI's staunchest (and most powerful) supporters— was diverted from this cause by a number of factors. The CIO, for instance, was largely focused at the time on the expulsion of Communist affiliates.[85] Second, the "labor-capital accord" that developed during these years—exemplified by the new United Auto Workers' contract—led unions to focus more on private benefits won through collective bargaining than on the fight for universal socioeconomic rights.[86]

Additionally, sensing a real threat, the AMA soon launched a truly massive public relations fight against the WMD bill, which Poen describes in great detail. The AMA readied itself for a major campaign following Truman's election, quickly raising a "huge war chest" from its members that it used to hire the pioneering public relations firm Whitaker and Baxter, which launched what has been called "perhaps the widest-ranging and most imaginative lobbying campaign of the post-Second World War era."[87] Critically, it should be noted, this was not simply a "doctors' campaign." A burgeoning intersection of corporate forces was beginning to coalesce to impede reform. The *Journal of the American Medical Association* served as a conduit of funds between pharmaceutical companies (which advertised in its pages) and the AMA.[88] Other corporations and their interest groups entered the healthcare reform battle as well, with the AMA receiving backing from the US Chamber of Commerce, the American Enterprise Association, and corporate executives.[89] This has been called the "the formative juncture" when "healthcare providers and corporate leaders entered into an alliance against plans for social insurance . . ."[90]

Whitaker and Baxter's well-funded campaign involved the production of a great volume of literature (55 million items, according to Poen) and impressive levels of spending ($1.5 million in one year alone, around $15 million in 2015 dollars).[91] Some of the literature painted the WMD bill as little less than a battalion of invading Soviet tanks. One pamphlet produced by the AMA contained a fabricated quote from Lenin, who (it claimed) had said, "Socialized Medicine is the key-stone to the arch of the Socialist State."[92] In any event, this red-baiting campaign (together with other political dynamics) was highly effective in the court of public opinion: the 75 percent approval that NHI had in 1945 sunk to a mere 21 percent in 1949.[93]

Red-baiting was also an effective tool against the healthcare left—a notable bulwark of support for NHI within the medical community—and it accelerated during the 1940s.[94] It is worth noting that in this decade, a number of health scholars, physicians, medical students, and medical historians played influential roles in advancing the cause of universal healthcare in the US. The polymath Henry Sigerist, for instance, who had come to the US to be chair of the history of medicine at Johns Hopkins, became an increasingly prominent advocate for national health insurance (as well as admirer of the Soviet healthcare system) during the Roosevelt era, with a notable appearance on the cover of *Time* magazine in 1939.[95] In 1944, however, he was accused by the government of membership in a "Communist front," and soon left the country.[96] But the postwar years saw even greater backlash. Consider, for instance, Milton Roemer, a physician and health systems scholar who was heavily influenced by Sigerist and who did work for the federal government in the 1940s on planning for a national health insurance system.[97] Accused of political disloyalty—charges that were dropped—he nonetheless had his passport seized by the US consulate after he took a position at the World Health Organization in Geneva (he and his wife Ruth Roemer, an important public health and health rights scholar, then fled to Canada, where they played a role in the design of a universal healthcare system in the province of

Saskatchewan, before returning to the US and continuing their work in healthcare advocacy and research).[98]

Meanwhile, the left-leaning Association of Interns and Medical Students (AIMS)—which reached some 3,000 members in 1945, and which advocated against racial inequities in medicine and in favor of the WMD bill—was destroyed in a campaign of red-baiting, with some of its young members left unable to find employment.[99] One of them, Bernard Lown (now world-renowned for, among other things, the invention of direct-current defibrillation), found himself blacklisted until the late 1950s.[100] Similarly, the Physicians Forum (PF)—composed of a spectrum of progressives including New Deal liberals but also some communists—took a stand against the AMA in its support of NHI.[101] As a result, its members were hauled in front of the House Un-American Activities Committee in what one historian has described as a "purposeful" attack, "intent on decoupling medicine and social activism."[102] FBI director J. Edgar Hoover even penned an editorial in *JAMA* enjoining physicians to keep on the lookout for political subversives in their midst.[103] Even the decidedly un-radical social insurance expert and administrator Isidore Falk, who had served on the Committee on the Costs of Medical Care, Roosevelt's National Health Conference, and the Social Security Board and Social Security Administration, was also investigated by both the House and the Senate.[104] "American communism," one report from the House hearings stated, "holds this program [i.e., socialized medicine] as a cardinal point in its objectives. . . ."[105]

On the one side, in other words, was the physicians' lobby, backed by the power and purse of doctors throughout the nation, but also (as noted) by pharmaceutical companies and other business interests. On the other side was a relatively small number of policy experts, government administrators, and progressive medical groups, as well as—perhaps most importantly—the labor movement. In the middle was the government, consisting of a Democratic president who supported WMD and a conservative-dominated Congress.[106] Only labor could have substantially altered the balance of power in this equation but, as Derickson argues, it never truly exercised its full potential to do so. Although organized labor supported NHI, it essentially "deferred" to the policy elites behind the proposals; the lack of a popular movement left these intellectuals particularly vulnerable to the coming McCarthyite storm.[107] "Without question," he argues, "the social base for a large-scale movement existed . . . Although no one else did more than they did to advance this issue, the unions fell short of activating their millions of uninsured members as the basis for a popular crusade for health security."[108]

Then, as the likelihood for success on the national level faded, labor increasingly fought for privatized, decidedly non-universal health benefits, won through collective bargaining, as a way to bolster its organizational strength.[109] Indeed, the Chamber of Commerce even suggested to its members that offering private health insurance benefits to their employees would be a way to impede the passage of WMD.[110] The United Mine Workers took the first step in this direction, and were followed shortly thereafter by the steelworkers, who won the first countrywide contract that had a Blue Cross benefit.[111] The autoworkers followed soon after.

Although the unions continued to financially support the campaign for NHI, their support waned, and by the end of the 1950s, it had desiccated entirely.[112]

As a result of these historical dynamics, a "right to healthcare" did not emerge in the United States—neither during the postwar years nor after. This is not because healthcare was not *conceived* as a right. In fact, one can find various instances in which the right to health was explicitly articulated by various parties. A health commission later set up by Truman, for example, declared, "Access to the means of attainment and preservation of health is a basic human right."[113] Instead, there was simply an imbalance in power that pushed the health rights-commodity dialectic in the United States sharply rightward. Not only did healthcare not become a right, but events at this critical juncture also set the United States down a particular path of healthcare privatization. The fragmented postwar welfare state that did emerge, as labor historian Nelson Lichtenstein has argued, in turn served to divide the American workforce.[114] On the one hand was a group that had a private, "almost Western European level of social welfare protection," and on the other was a bigger, poorer, and more often black or female group, which was excluded from these benefits.[115] This dynamic towards the privatization of welfare thereby reinforced the movement towards healthcare commoditization, with the aggregate effect of taking the nation further away from a social right to healthcare.

This turn away from some sort of universal healthcare system left the United States virtually alone among high-income countries. This is not to say that other nations all followed the same path. Britain's path was somewhat unique in its sweeping scope, whereas most other nations took a more incremental approach. France, for instance, followed a progressive corporatist approach, successively widening the scope of its national health insurance system—administered by private albeit heavily regulated funds—until it eventually constituted universal coverage.[116] Canada, meanwhile, achieved a single payer universal system, albeit only at the provincial level at first. Although the Liberal postwar government was influenced by the Beveridge Report, it was the leftist Cooperative Commonwealth Federation (CCF), which took power in the province of Saskatchewan in 1944, that pushed for health insurance at the national level. Despite the initial failure to achieve federal legislation, in 1946—the same year as the passage of the National Health Service Act across the Atlantic—the CCF implemented a provincial hospital insurance plan funded through taxation. In 1962, it passed a complete health insurance program for the province. And finally, four years later, a coalition government passed a single payer health insurance bill for the nation as a whole.[117]

The program, it should be noted, came to be called Medicare—the same name as a US program passed around the same time. One of these programs created a right to health; the other, many hoped, would be a step in that direction. But, as will be explained later, this was not to be.

China and Soviet Russia: The Contradictions of Communist Healthcare

Red-baiting played an important part in the pre-emption of universal healthcare reform in the United States. National health insurance, its opponents argued, was part of a larger communist plot. But what did actual "red" healthcare look like in the most powerful communist countries of the time, the Soviet Union and China? The NHS of the (then) socialist Labour Party advanced the right to healthcare in Britain, in deed if not in word. But what we can say of the healthcare systems of the Communist bloc itself?

A word of warning, however, is first very much in order. Although this book focuses primarily on the right to *healthcare*, it has also dealt, on occasion, with the larger question of the right to *health*. Chapter 3, in particular, explored the advent of social medicine thought, and of the "social determinants" which so massively affect human health and happiness. From the larger perspective of delivering this broader "right to health," the experience of China and Soviet Russia must be considered—especially at certain moments in their histories—a mammoth failure on a mortifying scale. Any description of the Soviet healthcare *system*, for instance, should be prefaced with an acknowledgment of the Stalinist policies that were destructive to human health on a scale that is difficult to fathom. Recent work has refined the quantitative assessment of Stalin's toll: an estimated two to three million perished in the Gulags during the years of Stalin's reign, some five million starved to death from Stalinist policies that all but "ensured mass death" in the form of famine, and 682,691 people were more directly murdered, predominantly in colossal "shooting actions" undertaken by the secret police during the Great Terror.[118] Mao Zedong, on the other hand, has been called the maker of "the worst man-made human catastrophe ever," namely, the "Great Famine" that resulted from the disastrous Great Leap Forward.[119] Estimates of lives lost range from 36 to 45 million, the result largely of starvation, but also of the massive "government-instigated torture and murder of those who opposed the Communist Party's maniacal economic plans that caused the catastrophe."[120]

At this point, one might wish to simply leave the question of the "right to health" alone in these regimes. At the same time, however, one has to account for the vast improvements in health metrics made in these countries, especially China. China experienced comparatively enormous declines in infant mortality and increases in life expectancy from the 1950s to the 1980s.[121] The reality of health, and healthcare, in both Soviet Russia and China is, indeed, a complex and fraught issue, one that cannot be easily reduced to the murderousness of Stalin and Mao or their successors or predecessors. Although health gains were made, and although healthcare (like many things) underwent a decommoditization of sorts, the creation of a right to healthcare (even defined narrowly) was limited in each nation by a number of fundamental factors.

The nation that the Bolsheviks took over in October 1917 had dismal health conditions and an equally dismal health system, at least in comparison to the industrialized West.[122] Although a system of largely free rural public healthcare had been established under the Tsars in the nineteenth century, administered by units called *zemstvos*, the actual impact of this system is questionable.[123] A Health and Accident Insurance Act, somewhat analogous to the legislation in Britain and Germany, was passed in 1912, and it is argued that this law, as in Germany, was perhaps intended to deflate the energy of a displeased working class[124] (albeit evidently without much success). In any event, needs were high and resources low when the Bolsheviks took power. This period in Soviet history—the years of the "New Economic Policy," in which a mixed economy was, to some extent, encouraged—saw some ambiguous developments in healthcare. The government did not, at least initially, seek to establish a system of universal healthcare; instead, it established an insurance scheme that covered workers and their families (similar to compulsory health insurance programs in Western Europe): tellingly, however, this system excluded peasants, even though they constituted a substantial portion of the population.[125] Although the Bolshevik policy, announced shortly after the party took power, was for universal healthcare for all,[126] healthcare in early Soviet Russia was explicitly distributed on "class proletarian lines," as one scholar described, a system of "strictly differentiating the medical services of particular groups (the insured), giving priority to those in leading branches of industry and in state and collective farms."[127] Two observers (one American and one British) who visited the USSR in 1932 to study its healthcare system similarly described the "deprived persons" excluded from coverage: not only various groups from the middle and former upper classes, but also peasants, who formed the majority of the country's population.[128] This was, in other words, a distinctly non-universal system.

However, this non-universal system of social insurance was ultimately discarded in favor of a universal system in 1937, with free physician and hospital care (though with fees for drugs) for everyone.[129] Universal access coincided with a huge growth in medical personnel and facilities and, over a period of decades, striking improvements in health outcomes. From 1913 to 1973, the numbers of physicians and hospital beds soared, life expectancy more than doubled, and infant mortality fell by 90 percent.[130] Although not all of the improvements in health outcomes can be attributed to this expansion in health services, the scholar Howard Leichter makes the important point that such gains were by no means inevitable. While India and the Soviet Union had similarly poor health statistics in the early twentieth century, by the 1970s, the latter was enormously out-performing the former.[131] In light of these developments, it is not surprising that free universal care has been "historically regarded as a great sociopolitical achievement of the Soviet society."[132]

And yet, even if one admits these early achievements, there are some important qualifications to be made about the universal character of Soviet healthcare. Even though the health system was, on paper, imbued with the ideology of universalism, in practice, it continued to reflect Bolshevik political prerogatives. First, even after the turn in 1937 away from an insurance scheme-based system, a prioritization of the health of industrial workers persisted.[133] Workers had their own superior outpatient facilities and hospitals, and, by the report of one American health scholar, they were "put to the head of the line" at clinics, "ahead of housewives and oldsters."[134] They also had preferential access to the health resorts that were a part of the Soviet health system.[135] Second, although healthcare was theoretically supposed to be equally available to all, both the payment of cash and membership in the Communist Party facilitated access to superior care.[136] Lived reality—as with so much in Soviet society—diverged from the grandiose principles of its stated ideals or printed constitution.

To some extent, an analogy can be made between the Soviet approach to healthcare and its approach to economic growth more broadly, the latter of which was—as Donald Sassoon characterized it—"brutally quantitative."[137] This emphasis on quantity over quality,[138] moreover, was later accompanied by financial neglect. Even while expenditures on healthcare were rising throughout the developed world (sometimes to more than 10 percent of GDP), one observer notes that USSR health spending actually *fell*, from 6.6 percent in 1960 to a mere 4 percent in 1989, resulting in serious deficiencies and shortfalls.[139] This had real consequences. For instance, health statistics began to decline in the 1970s (the Soviets then simply ceased reporting them).[140] The comparative failure of the Soviet health system was more definitively demonstrated in a study that compared "treatable" mortality—that is to say, deaths that could potentially have been prevented through medical intervention—in Russia (and three other Soviet republics) with the United Kingdom from 1965 into the 1990s. The investigators found that whereas treatable mortality was quite similar among the nations in the 1960s, it steadily declined in the UK over subsequent decades while it remained flat in Russia. Thus, the gap in *avoidable* mortality between Russia and the UK had grown enormously larger by 1990.[141] And sadly, as will be described in the next chapter, things would only get worse with the introduction of neoliberal shock therapy in the 1990s.

A right to healthcare, clearly, is not met simply by enshrining it in the constitution. But creating a system of universal healthcare is also not enough: resource neglect, a political system that prioritizes growth over health,[142] and inequitable access on the basis of money or political status, all weaken the right to healthcare. This is to say nothing of the atrocious impact on health of the endless, systematic violations of human rights by the Soviet regime, such as the weaponization of psychiatry against political dissidents.[143]

The story in China bears some parallels to that in the USSR, but also some important divergences, with respect to both achievements and failures. As in the USSR, after Mao swept into power in 1949, his government contended with a massively underdeveloped healthcare system: for the great majority of the country, there was little in the way of modern health services available at all.[144] The following year, a National Health Congress was held in Peking, which delineated—as described by Victor Sidel and Ruth Sidel, who visited the country in the 1970s and became enthusiastic experts on Chinese healthcare—four core tenets of the new health system.[145] Key among them was an emphasis on the notion of community participation in healthcare—that "health work" should draw on the "full participation of the people themselves."[146] In a number of publications, Sidel and Sidel described the forms this could take.[147] Most notably, for perhaps the first time, medical care (albeit basic) was extended to the countryside by the so-called "barefoot doctors." These were peasants-cum-part-time-auxiliary-health-workers who, after receiving relatively basic medical training, provided healthcare to the village commune. In all, the efforts of the Mao regime made for an increase of about 100,000 doctors over a decade and a half. The communes additionally had a "cooperative medical system," which, through an insurance scheme, provided more advanced medical care. Although there were also "worker doctors" who provided care in factories, what made the Chinese system unique was that, to quote Mao's 1965 directive, it "put the stress on the rural areas."[148] As Sidel and Sidel later summarized, "China's revolution in health services brought medical care to most of the country's immense rural population—some eight hundred million people—a group that previously had largely lacked access to personnel trained in modern medical methods and to facilities equipped with modern medical technology."[149]

That China—despite the enormity of Mao's murderous depredations—experienced rapid improvements in health in these decades is not disputed. No doubt, the "barefoot doctor" was not the only factor. Literacy campaigns, mass immunizations, crackdowns on prostitution and opium use, a better diet, vector control, and advancements in public health infrastructure were all other potential contributing factors.[150] The aggregate result, however, was enormous: between the years 1952 and 1982, life expectancy nearly doubled (from 35 to 68), and infant mortality fell by more than 80 percent.[151] A 1981 paper described this as a "record of sustained and rapid progress that has seldom been matched" and attributed it in part to the "unusual emphasis on simple preventative measures ... widely distributed by auxiliary medical personnel."[152] China, the paper concluded, was a "super-achiever in mortality reduction," alongside a few other nations.[153]

And yet, the universalism of the Chinese welfare state should not be exaggerated. Critically, as the political scientist Mark Frazier notes, the Chinese Communist Party created "rigid spatial boundaries that define differential access to social welfare to this day."[154] The household registration system—or hukou—was set up by Mao during the terrible years of the famine that he helped to create, and it delineated separate rural and urban tiers of citizenship rights. Urban residents had access to higher quality welfare goods. Those in state factories, on the other hand, might also receive "superior benefits for medical care" and other services. Above them were party members and politicians, who could access the top tier of these services. Though Frazier concurs with the basic assessment of greatly improved health among the rural population, he notes that "these public goods varied widely and fell far below the benefits that urban residents received," while the "[m]obility restrictions [set up by the hukou] and administrative hierarchies created at least three tiers of citizenship and access to social policies: rural, urban, and official-dom."[155] Critically, these divisions have persevered to the present day.

Thus, in the case of both China and Soviet Russia, regimes took power that (1) murdered unfathomable numbers of people, mostly through starvation but also through more rapid methods; (2) created large new healthcare systems, albeit with different emphases (e.g., formal physicians and hospitals in the USSR, informal "barefoot doctors" based in rural areas in China); and (3) achieved major improvements in health outcomes (in the case of the USSR, at least for some time). Developments (2) and (3) could not possibly justify, explain, or exclude (1), the enormous violations of human rights committed by these regimes. Any assessment of progress towards a right to healthcare, obviously, must take into account transgressions against the right to health and life itself. However, even when examined in isolation of other rights issues, these health systems had fundamental inadequacies of their own. In the Soviet Union, underfunding and neglect combined with persistent inequities in access (whether because of one's resources or one's political affiliation). In the case of China, rigid stratification of society into three legally defined tiers created differentials in access to social services like healthcare that persist to the current day. Thus, although these regimes expanded access to a decommodified form of healthcare, with some impressive though inconsistent results, they failed in many respects to make a right to healthcare, much less health.

The Right to Health in the "International Bill of Rights"

The last chapter explored the articulation of powerful statements on the right to health, first in the 1946 World Health Organization (WHO) constitution, and then, two years later and in a somewhat more dilute form, in the Universal Declaration of Human Rights (UDHR). Though its prose may have been sweeping, the UDHR lacked any mechanism of enforcement. As noted, however, this declaration of principles was supposed to be soon followed by a legally binding "Covenant," which, together with the UDHR, would form an "International Bill of Rights." This Covenant, like the UDHR, would weave together political and socioeconomic rights into a single, unified, binding whole.

With the onset of the political tensions and conflicts of the Cold War, however, this was not to be. The international political framework of the Cold War widened the divide between these two realms of rights. Western nations became leery of the potential meaning of socioeconomic rights; in consequence, the Covenant was cut in half, with an International Covenant on Civil and Political Rights (ICCPR) on the one hand and an International Covenant on Economic, Social and Cultural Rights (ICESCR) on the other.[156] As John Tobin describes in his seminal work *The Right to Health in International Law*, the political dynamic of the Second World War—namely, the presence of the "common enemy" of fascism—was in no small part responsible for the unification of political and socioeconomic rights in the UDHR in the 1940s. The coming of the Cold War, in contrast, ruptured that harmony and signaled an end to the intention to create a unified, binding document.[157]

Such political dynamics also played out within the newly formed WHO. Global health, in fact, soon became another front of the Cold War itself. Although it boldly proclaimed the right to health in 1946, the WHO proceeded to shift its focus in a more conservative direction in the early-to-mid 1950s. It withdrew from an advocacy of health rights while increasingly embracing a technocratic vision of global health work. Meanwhile, the process of transitioning from the UDHR to the international covenants—which was necessary for human rights to have some legal force—advanced at a slow pace. Indeed, it was not until the 1970s that the covenants actually came into effect. As Moyn has sharply pointed out, human rights came to life shortly after the Second World War only to die soon thereafter.[158]

These shifts—including within the WHO—were not immediate postwar developments, and need to be explored in greater depth. The WHO's first director was the Canadian physician Brock Chisholm, a man described as "loosely identified with the British social medicine tradition."[159] Indeed, during his relatively short tenure as director-general, the WHO embraced both a right to health and a social medicine orientation towards the social determinants of health.[160] It also worked intimately with the UN Commission on Human Rights in formulating a right to health in the draft for what was initially the "International Covenant on Human Rights," and later became the International Covenant on Economic, Social and Cultural Rights (ICESCR). The WHO Secretariat argued that the right to health should (1) be defined in a "positive" sense along the lines of the WHO Constitution, (2) emphasize the social determinants of health, and, lastly, (3) include responsibilities for states to fulfill.[161] The 1952 draft of the ICESCR reflected this influence, and it included both the WHO's broad definition of health ("a state of complete physical, mental and social well-being") and an outline of "[t]he steps to be taken by the States Parties to the Covenant to achieve the full realization of this right . . ."[162]

However, this embrace was to be fleeting. In 1953, Chisholm was replaced by Marcolino Candau, who went on to direct the organization for the following two decades. As Tobin argues, this was accompanied by a shift in the WHO towards a more technocratic stance that allowed it to avoid "the politicization of its work in the bipolar world."[163] This new direction led by Candau embraced so-called "vertical" programs, or campaigns against individual illness like malaria,[164] in contrast to efforts to create and grow comprehensive national health systems. Technocracy, however, is not the same as neutrality, and some scholars argue that some of these campaigns were to an extent a reflection of US foreign policy and commercial interests. A successful campaign against malaria, for instance, might (so the theory went) help the US in its battle against communism, strengthening its ties with local governments and opening up new markets on the global stage.[165] At the same time, however, these campaigns—relying as they did on imported methods and technologies, and emphasizing implementation from above over a more cooperative approach with local elements from below—ultimately gave short shrift to the importance of community involvement. "This model of development assistance," as one review puts it, "fit neatly into US Cold War efforts to promote modernization with limited social reform."[166] It was also, in the case of malaria at least, to prove to be a major debacle.

At the same time as the WHO was focusing on these vertical programs instead of on health system development, it also distanced itself almost entirely from its earlier commitment to international health rights. Indeed, the WHO actively refused involvement in the ongoing formulation of the right to health in international legal documents.[167] In response to queries requesting WHO input on the right to health in the drafting of the ICESCR, Candau stated that the WHO had "no comments to offer concerning the right to health."[168] The WHO's "neglect for human rights development," argues health policy scholar Benjamin Mason Meier, "continued to deny the right to health a place in evolving international legal frameworks," including during debates over the UN Declaration of the Rights of the Child and the Declaration on the Elimination of Discrimination Against Women.[169] The WHO's disinterest allowed the right to health to be gradually diluted, particularly with respect to the emphasis on the social determinants of health.[170] Nonetheless, despite the vagaries of the drafting process, the final text of the ICESCR still bore some strong similarities to the WHO Constitution.[171] Article 12 ultimately read:

1. The States Parties to the present Covenant recognize the right of everyone to the enjoyment of the highest attainable standard of physical and mental health.
2. The steps to be taken by the States Parties to the present Covenant to achieve the full realization of this right shall include those necessary for:
   (a) The provision for the reduction of the stillbirth-rate and of infant mortality and for the healthy development of the child;
   (b) The improvement of all aspects of environmental and industrial hygiene;
   (c) The prevention, treatment and control of epidemic, endemic, occupational and other diseases;
   (d) The creation of conditions which would assure to all medical service and medical attention in the event of sickness.[172]

As wide as this articulation of the right to health may be, gone was the broad conceptualization of health of the WHO Constitution (a "state of complete physical, mental and social well-being") as well as the emphasis on the "legislative measures" necessary to ensure the right to health. A delineation of specific social determinants of health ("nutrition, housing, sanitation, recreation, economic and working conditions and other aspects of environmental hygiene")—which had been favored by the early WHO and had appeared in an earlier draft—likewise disappeared.[173]

Apart from this change in the orientation of the WHO, other dynamics worked against the ICESCR as well, including a rightward political shift in the United States. In 1952—amidst rising Cold War tensions and anti-communist sentiment—Republican Dwight D. Eisenhower, the first Republican to hold the office in two decades, was elected president. The following year—the same year that saw the leadership change in the WHO—the administration, turning back from Truman's policy, ended US participation in the drafting of the Covenant, and announced that it would not ratify it.[174] Describing this move as a surrender to Senator Joseph McCarthy and his ilk, Eleanor Roosevelt called it "a sorry day . . . in relation to our interest in the human rights and freedoms of people throughout the world," lamenting, "We are not willing to sign anything that binds us legally in the field of human right and freedoms."[175] Subsequent progress was slow: the covenants were not adopted until 1966 and did not receive enough votes to go into effect until ten years later. Even then, however, the ICESCR was underpowered, lacking (in distinction to the other covenants) a committee to oversee implementation until 1987, when the Committee on Economic, Social and Cultural Rights was established for this purpose.[176]

From a broader perspective, this divorce of socioeconomic and political rights came at a considerable cost: the implicit assertion that these two categories were fundamentally incompatible.[177] Additionally, the weakening of the right to health in the ICESCR should be seen not so much as a *cause* of conservatism in global health as its *effect*. Still, this conservative orientation towards health rights and global health was not to last forever. In the decades following the Second World War, nation after nation was breaking free of colonialism; new ideas were on the rise, and the health records of socialist countries were increasingly trumpeted. The 1970s saw the powerful return of health rights to the international stage, exemplified by the Declaration of Alma-Ata. But first, for a greater understanding of the developments of this era, one must turn toward Latin America and observe how some "developing" nations began to work towards a right to healthcare in this region—and what set them back.

Latin America and the Right to Healthcare

Thus far, this book has almost entirely neglected how tension along the healthcare rights-commodity dialectic was playing out in the global South where—in light of economic underdevelopment stemming from the history of imperialism—social rights were, if anything, even more "needed." However, nations in Latin America were actually pioneers in the development of socioeconomic rights, including that to healthcare. As in Western Europe, the articulation and legislation of social rights was often a response, albeit in a complicated fashion, to political pressures from below. In Latin America, however, this pressure was more likely to come from the peasantry than from the proletariat. For instance, the Mexican Revolution—a complex, bloody struggle that erupted in 1910—was, to no small extent, a peasant revolution. Mexico's revolutionary constitution of 1917 was, in fact, the first in the world to include socioeconomic rights, for instance to labor rights and conditions and social insurance.[178] However, although it included protections for occupational health and for the health of women, it contained no explicit right to healthcare.[179]

Chile was perhaps a more important pioneer with respect to healthcare. The dynamics behind the evolution of Chile's welfare state in some ways reflect those of Western Europe. In the century following its independence, Chile's large and growing mining sector gave rise to a relatively large working class, from which arose a dynamic and influential labor movement.[180] Connected with this development was the materialization of a multifaceted political left, which included anarchist groups (early in the twentieth century), a Communist party, and an anti-Stalinist Socialist Party.[181] In part in response to working-class pressure, the liberal government elected in 1918 passed legislation that created what some have described as the first public health insurance program in the hemisphere, though admittedly it was restricted to rail workers.[182] However, unrest in the 1920s led to its expansion.[183] And the 1925 Chilean constitution, unlike the Mexican one, included a specific commitment to health, if not a right to healthcare *per se*: "It is the duty of the state," reads Article 10, "to oversee the public health and hygienic well-being of the country. Each year a sufficient sum of money should be earmarked in order to maintain a national health service."[184] Laws passed in the following decade further expanded coverage, including an insurance program for white-collar workers (the *Servicio Médico Nacional de los Empleados*, or SERMENA).[185] Unlike with Great Britain, however, such health insurance measures fell short of universalism, largely neglecting some of the most vulnerable. But similar to Britain and other countries in Western Europe, the postwar years witnessed an expansion of health coverage in a more universal direction.

This expansion was fostered by a wave of democratization that swept through the region in the postwar period.[186] Until the destruction of its democracy in 1973, Chile was a pioneer in the expansion of healthcare access. Shortly after the war, the Popular Front government of Chile (together with the governments of other Latin American countries) helped to secure the inclusion of socioeconomic rights, including the right to healthcare, in the Universal Declaration of Human Rights.[187] The postwar decades, meanwhile, saw important innovations in health policy domestically. The story of healthcare in Chile is to no small extent intertwined with that of Salvador Allende, a physician and politician who, for a time, helped push the nation slowly in the direction of a right to healthcare. Born to a wealthy and politically active family, Allende had a long political career until his death in 1973. In 1933, shortly after graduating from medical school, he helped found the country's Socialist Party. Four years later, he was elected to the Chilean National Congress, and in 1939, he became the health minister under a Popular Front government.[188] Allende's commitment to health and healthcare in Chile reflected not only his background in medicine and his leftist politics, but also his embrace of social medicine thought.[189] Allende's thinking was shaped by European social medicine ideas, particularly those of Rudolf Virchow, likely a result of the influence of a German pathologist who studied with Virchow and emigrated to Chile.[190] He was also influenced by the ideas of Engels, which were described in Chapter 3.[191] In 1939, as health minister, Allende published *The Chilean Medico-Social Reality* (*La Realidad Médico-Social Chilena*). In this groundbreaking social medicine text, Allende described how the living conditions of workers gave rise to illness and how structural forces of underdevelopment, economic dependency on foreign governments, and labor exploitation created such harmful social conditions.[192] Healthcare, for Allende, was not a matter of efficiency, but of rights: "Rather than seeing improved healthcare services as a means toward a more productive labor force," Howard Waitzkin explains, "Allende valued the health of the population as an end in itself and advocated social changes that went far beyond the medical realm."[193] Such social changes would, in part, come through the agency of the working class itself, which, Allende noted, would eventually "resolve to conquer the right to well-being, health and culture."[194] The Popular Front government, he argued, would similarly work "to conquer the right to develop our culture at all levels, regardless of social classes," so as to foster "a revitalized, healthy and educated people . . ."[195] He remained steadfast in pursuing these goals. Indeed, that same year, he proposed a "National Health Service" for Chile, which eventually became law in 1952.[196]

This 1952 law has been called "the first program in the Americas to guarantee universal healthcare."[197] The law no doubt advanced the right to healthcare in the nation: by integrating many of the existing health departments, the Chilean NHS brought coverage to a majority of Chileans (70 percent, according to one figure).[198] Some also credit the NHS for Chile's superior health outcomes in coming decades.[199] However, the Chilean NHS fell short of its British name-sake in one critical way: it never achieved universal reach. Although the NHS to some extent created a "right" to healthcare in Chile by moving it towards universal coverage, a multi-tiered system continued to exist owing to the persistence of a large private health sector.[200] Additionally, the publicly funded insurance scheme for white-collar workers (SERMENA) was outside of the NHS from the beginning.[201] These tiers became entrenched with the passage of time, and by 1970, Chile had a stratified health system divided among three main levels: an NHS for workers and the poor, SERMENA for white-collar workers, and a private sector for the rich.[202] Though providing, to some extent, "universal coverage," this fragmentation would make the system vulnerable to attack in later years, which will be later discussed.

Important developments in healthcare in the region were also occurring in Cuba. The revolutionary government of Cuba has emphasized healthcare to an almost unique extent, including among socialist countries. After the socialization of the health sector in the 1960s, the National Health System (SNS) became responsible for the health of the entire population.[203] As Julie Feinsilver explains in *Healing the Masses: Cuban Health Politics at Home and Abroad*, the ideology of the Cuban health system was based on three ideas: first, the commitment that health services would be equally available to all; second, the provision of an "integral approach to healthcare"; and third, community involvement in health programs.[204] Cuba, Feinsilver, argues, uniquely combined a "First World" orientation (i.e., an emphasis on physician-level care and advanced medical technology) with "Third World" principles that emphasized community-level involvement and participation in health programs.[205] It also diverged in significant ways from the healthcare policies of both the Soviet Union and China. Unlike the Soviet Union, Cuba emphasized the health of the underserved *rural* population.[206] And unlike China, it relied on physicians, as opposed to lower-level community health workers, to serve this population.[207]

In the 1970s, the system was reorganized into neighborhood health centers called polyclinics, which delivered comprehensive primary care at the community level and included the services of internal medicine specialists, pediatricians, obstetricians, and sometimes dentists.[208] In the 1980s, the primary care, community-level focus of the health system was further bolstered by the "Family Doctor Program," in which community-based teams were responsible for everyone within circumscribed areas, and which will be further described in the next chapter. Together, such reforms achieved remarkable success. Easily surpassing those of much of the developing world, health indices in Cuba soon came to rival those of some of the richest countries.[209]

Political change in Chile also raised the possibility of a major transformation of the healthcare system. In 1970, Allende emerged victorious in a three-way presidential contest, thereby becoming what some describe as the first Marxist to come to power in an election that was both fair and democratic.[210] Allende was the candidate of the left-wing coalition "Popular Unity" (UP), and its platform described healthcare as a right of citizenship, though it stopped short of endorsing—as some had hoped—a *Servicio Único*, or a unified health service that would have, like the British NHS, Cuban SNS, or Canadian Medicare, provided care for all.[211]

Still, during the brief years of Allende's presidency, government sponsorship of healthcare reached a "zenith."[212] Allende increased spending and promoted "free healthcare as a mechanism for income redistribution," with a "long-term goal . . . [of] a unified health system with progressive financial participation of the State."[213] During the three years of UP government, immunizations rose dramatically; the number of NHS appointments increased by almost a quarter; a system of universal free emergency medical care was established; and new maternity facilities, hospitals, and clinics were built.[214] Additionally, the country embarked on a program of "decentralization" through Decreto 602, which emphasized the role of auxiliary health workers, community-level healthcare, and active participation in health programs.[215] This shift in orientation towards community health can be conceived as broadly consistent with the principles later delineated in the Declaration of Alma-Ata. Regardless, the emphasis of the government on both health and healthcare showed results. During this period, a number of health outcomes improved, including reductions in child malnutrition as well as mortality from a number of diseases.[216] However, a universal *Servicio Único* never materialized; on the contrary, progress towards a decommodified, publicly funded health service was brought to a sudden and violent end in 1973.

Cold War politics suffused the discourse of global health, human rights, and, as described earlier in the chapter in the case of the United States, health policy. In Latin America, the politics of the Cold War intersected with the "right to health" in even more dramatic ways. As the historian Greg Grandin describes, with the possible exception of the brief interlude years of Roosevelt's "Good Neighbor Policy," for the past century social-democratic governments in Latin America have often been viewed by the US government and various corporate interests as dangerous threats.[217] Throughout the 1960s and 1970s, through coup d'état after coup d'état, Washington facilitated the "counterrevolution of South America," thereby turning it into a "garrison continent."[218] Chile's unique path—eschewing Soviet authoritarianism while also embracing peaceful socialism—perhaps made it, as Grandin notes, a more threatening model for change than Cuba.[219] Indeed, shortly after Allende took power, Nixon was already requesting that the CIA look for ways to take him out.[220] Though the UP government is blamed for economic mismanagement that facilitated the coming coup,[221] an order from Nixon to "make the [Chilean] economy scream" no doubt played a critical role.[222]

On September 11, 1973, a military coup led by Augusto Pinochet, encouraged and welcomed by the Nixon administration (and followed by large-scale murder and torture), brought an end to Chile's long history of democratic government. It also brought an end to Allende's life: with military troops closing in and planes circling overhead, the physician-president took his own life.

The coup also brought to an end, also through violence, Allende's vision for a healthcare system for Chile. Reports of the human rights violations unfolding in Chile led to the formation of the American Public Health Association "Task Force on Chile," which published a report in 1977 highlighting these developments.[223] A "great many" health workers, it noted, were "among the thousands jailed, tortured, and killed," while "[p]romising health programs, representing careful developments antedating the Allende government, have been dismantled or sharply curtailed."[224] Health workers were categorized by their political reliability, 35 or more physicians were murdered, neighborhood health centers were shuttered, and community involvement in health planning was curtailed.[225] A new overall dynamic—away from health rights and towards privatization of healthcare—soon became evident. Shortly after the coup, the new health minister, a colonel in the Chilean Air Force, declared that "healthcare is not given; rather it must be obtained by the people."[226] Funding for the NHS was cut by 20 percent by the new government.[227] A leftward shift in the healthcare rights-commodity dialectic had been suddenly reversed.

To a large extent, the story of Chile ties together the political theme of this chapter—the Cold War—with that of the next one—the emergence of healthcare "neoliberalism." Under Pinochet, Chile famously served as a model for the "Chicago School" of economic thought, embracing a free market ideology that left little room for universal public programs, especially in the domain of healthcare. To this day, Chile has failed to seriously recommit to the pursuit of a truly universal healthcare system.

Yet despite the fall of Allende in 1973, this decade was, in some other respects, a hopeful one. Some poorer nations—particularly Nicaragua—attempted to move towards the provision of healthcare as a right. And in the developed world, welfare states increasingly included systems of universal healthcare. Indeed, even in the United States, this decade saw the resurrection of the campaign for national health insurance. Meanwhile, on the international stage, the optimism of the period was proclaimed in the pathbreaking Declaration of Alma-Ata.

The 1970s, in other words, were a precipice. New heights were reached, though much hope was about to be dashed.

Alma-Ata and the Advent of "Primary Care" in the Cold War

The Conference at Alma-Ata—with which this chapter began—is generally regarded as a fundamental milestone in the history of the right to health. Yet interpreting Alma-Ata as little less than an unfulfilled triumph misses the mark. The conference had many roots: the emergence of independent nations from the shadow of colonialism, growing skepticism towards medical technology, tripolar

Sino-Russo-American political rivalry, the evolution of "missionary medicine," the "discovery" of "communist" medicine (mainly that of Cuba and China), a "leftward" swing in international health governance, and more. It was not, in other words, simply a magical moment of international healthcare rights harmony. It occurred at a critical moment in world history, a postcolonial period poised between two overlapping eras: the Cold War and a resurgence of capital on the international stage that can be referred to in shorthand as the age of neoliberalism. That opposition to the principles of Alma-Ata so quickly emerged (examined in depth in the next chapter) demonstrates not that its principles were ahead of its age, but rather that its age was on the verge of ending.

But first, how and why did Alma-Ata come about? One important factor was a growing recognition of the inadequacy of the WHO's "vertical disease" approach, which had resulted from the aforementioned rightward turn within the organization. Beginning in the mid-1950s, malaria reduction—principally by way of insecticide and medication—was the priority of the WHO. Yet this program was later deemed an enormous failure, a fact that the organization could barely avoid admitting. The importance of eliminating malaria was not in question—rather, the controversy was whether this could be done without developing comprehensive health systems at the local level, particularly in rural areas. By the late 1960s, both Candau and the World Health Assembly admitted that it could not, and in 1969, the Assembly recognized that controlling malaria necessitated incorporating such measures into local health systems.[228]

However, the WHO's later embrace of what was eventually called "primary care" was by no means predetermined. Scholars emphasize a number of developments that led to this progressive turn. First were reports of success in China, which had returned to the fold of the UN in 1973. China's efforts and other community-based health initiatives seemed to provide a sort of "third way" between the bureaucratic, medicalized, centralized healthcare system of the USSR and the vertical, disease-specific programs long supported by the West.[229] Reports from the early 1970s suggested that China was accomplishing enormous progress without advanced medical technology through the aforementioned community-based "barefoot doctors," who made care accessible to all, including in rural areas.[230] This same period also saw a rise in overall skepticism about the benefits of medical technology—or indeed medicine itself—resulting in a renewed emphasis on the social determinants of health.[231]

Additionally, in 1973, a new director-general, Halfdan Mahler, of Denmark, was appointed to the WHO. Mahler's WHO partnered with UNICEF to begin to explore alternatives to the vertical model, and in 1975, the two organizations co-published a report, *Alternative Approaches to Meeting Basic Health Needs in Developing Countries*, that looked beyond the two dominant Western paradigms of high-technology healthcare and vertical programs.[232] A second publication that was to prove highly influential was *Health by the People*, edited by Kenneth Newell, an epidemiologist in charge of the new WHO division "Strengthening of Health Services."[233] It has been noted that Newell—"an active member of the UK social medicine community in the 1950s"—was likely influenced by the pioneering "community health" work of Sidney and Emily Kark in South Africa.[234] In any event, *Health by the People*, which Mahler later described as an important influence behind Alma-Ata thinking, and whose title reflected the evolving "bottom-up" ideology,[235] featured examples of successful rural health projects from a number of developing countries.

Newell's introduction to the book embraced the social medicine concept that underlying socioeconomic determinants mattered more than healthcare access itself: "[M]any of the 'causes' of common health problems derive from parts of society itself," he wrote, and so "a strict health sectoral approach is ineffective," with "other actions outside the field of health perhaps having greater health effects than strictly health interventions."[236] The book included a chapter on China, written by Sidel and Sidel, which emphasized China's success in closing the rural-urban health gap through a combination of health workers at different levels, a stress on preventive healthcare, and the fostering of cooperation between traditional and modern medicine.[237] There was also a chapter on Cuba, which argued that, in this island nation, "health is considered as one of the fundamental human rights and health services are free for everyone."[238] Another example in *Health by the People* were projects of the Christian Medical Commission, an organization that brought "medical missionaries" to developing countries.[239]

A sequence of events led from this burgeoning ethos of "primary care" to the conference at Alma-Ata in 1978.[240] Though in some ways Alma-Ata was a product of the Cold War, it also represented a transcendence of the politics of the era. For instance, the Soviet Union, which had been pushing for the WHO to reorient its attitude towards the health services of the developing world, succeeded in getting the conference held within its borders, which has been described as a "small Soviet victory in the Cold War."[241] At the same time, the "ground-up" vision of Alma-Ata that emerged—stressing decentralization, non-professional health workers, and community involvement—was to some extent a repudiation of the Soviet model.[242] And while this vision may have been, in theory at least, closer to the Chinese model, China was not even in attendance at Alma-Ata, the consequence of Sino-Soviet rivalry.[243]

Much of the groundwork had been prepared in the years ahead of the conference, and by 1978, there was a broad consensus around the idea of a primary care approach to global health.[244] The declaration began with a strong embrace of the sweeping 1946 WHO definition of health, calling the "attainment of the highest possible level of health" a "most important world-wide social goal ..." that required more than just healthcare.[245] As Condorcet had done centuries earlier, it declaimed inequality both between and within nations, and called for "economic and social development, based on a New International Economic order ..." It placed responsibility for the right to health on governments, but also emphasized that people "have the right and duty to participate individually and collectively in the planning and implementation of their healthcare." It proceeded to define and discuss "primary healthcare," which would be at the center of the health system. "Primary healthcare" would deliver care "as close as possible to where people live and work," though the definition then was more expansive than it is today.

For instance, primary care involved not only the provision of comprehensive healthcare, but also public health and health education, drawing on multiple sectors outside the healthcare system to address the social determinants of health. Transcending the politics of the Cold War, it also proposed detente and the redirection of military resources towards health.

Speaking of Alma-Ata years later, Mahler described an "almost . . . spiritual atmosphere" and a feeling of "jubilation" in its aftermath.[246] Indeed, he saw a "true revolution in thinking."[247] A journal article entitled "High Hopes at Alma-Ata," published in 1978, similarly described the "strong sense of a landmark achieved" at the end of the meeting.[248] And indeed, it seems to have inspired a whole generation of health workers. The event "gave impetus to the right-to-health movement," as Jonathan Wolff notes in his recent *The Human Right to Health*.[249] "The WHO's rallying cry of 'Health For All By the Year 2000,' first proclaimed in 1977, inspired many individuals (myself included) and movements globally," notes physician and notable health equity scholar Paula Braverman.[250] Mary Bassett, a physician who worked in Zimbabwe and who is now the Commissioner of the New York City Department of Health and Mental Hygiene, described the impact of Alma-Ata in Harare after her arrival there: "It seemed that at every meeting I attended people were talking about Alma-Ata. . . . Alma-Ata situated health advancement in its larger social context, naming national governments as the main guarantors of 'Health for All by the Year 2000'."[251]

The spirit of Alma-Ata had a powerful impact on health movements in a number of nations in the coming years. At the same time, almost as soon as it was issued, the pushback against its principles began. Although the WHO may have reoriented its vision, far more powerful international bodies—namely, the International Monetary Fund and the World Bank—differed sharply in their vision of development, health, and rights. So did, for that matter, the rich nations of the world, which controlled and funded these organizations. Back in the United States, however, the outlook for healthcare rights still seemed promising in the 1970s.

Return to the US: From Medicare to Universal Healthcare?

"The 1970s," Mahler commented in an interview about Alma-Ata many years later, "was a warm decade for social justice."[252] From the perspective of the right to health, it was no doubt a time for optimism. Developments in a number of nations suggested that the right to health was on the advance. Even in the United States, which had been left behind in the postwar movement towards universal healthcare, a window of opportunity for progress again seemed to be open. Meanwhile, some poorer countries embraced the spirit of Alma-Ata in seeking to remake their health systems, often from very poor baselines. The final sections of the chapter will turn first back to the US, and then to revolutionary Nicaragua, to see what this decade meant for the advance of the right to healthcare in one rich country and in one terribly poor one.

In the early 1950s, as the WMD campaign crumbled, reformers looked for ways to salvage something from the rubble, and came upon an idea that would later be successful: a national insurance plan that would be limited to older Americans.[253] Yet in the decade and a half that followed, there was more or less complete stagnation on the national health insurance front. This is not to say that there was no change in healthcare "access." On the contrary, there was an enormous growth in protection from the costs of illness through the rise of private insurance: the number of the insured increased more than tenfold between 1940 and 1966.[254] Having insurance, however, did not necessarily mean full financial protection for the cost of health care, and during this period organized labor fought hard for *more comprehensive* insurance coverage.[255] Additionally, this privatized welfare state fell short of a right to healthcare in other ways as well. The system discriminated along the axes of gender, race, class, age, and medical condition. For instance, private insurers had exclusions for various conditions including "normal maternity;" racial minorities and women might have to pay more in premiums; and anyone could have their coverage revoked for various reasons, including for the crime of simply growing older.[256] What's been referred to as "the deeply gendered nature of medical underwriting" essentially constituted a form of medical discrimination against women.[257] Atrocious discrimination on the basis of race—ranging from hospital segregation to "patient dumping"—were some of the enormous inequities at the heart of the American healthcare system.[258] Such inequities gave the lie to any hope that a privatized welfare state would deliver a broad "right to healthcare."

The 1960s, however, saw renewed efforts towards expanding healthcare access and reducing healthcare discrimination. In the 1960 presidential election, the Democratic platform finally included a plank on a healthcare plan for the elderly, which Truman's aides had first formulated, named "Medicare."[259] Though supported by President John F. Kennedy, Medicare nonetheless encountered strong resistance from the AMA, which began a campaign against it.[260] For a number of reasons, Kennedy was unable to advance the agenda on Medicare, despite support from a number of major constituencies.[261] Things changed, however, with the sweeping Democratic victory in the 1964 elections, which may have ensured that Medicare would be passed by Congress, albeit in an unclear form, and signed by President Johnson.[262]

What emerged—the so-called "three-layer cake" consisting of a universal hospital plan for the elderly (Medicare Part A), a voluntary physician insurance plan for the elderly (Medicare Part B), and a means-tested healthcare plan for some groups of the poor (Medicaid)—was indeed a historic advance that broadened access to healthcare for a substantial portion of the population.[263] In a 1966 address at the inauguration of the new program, Johnson affirmed (echoing, by happenstance, the language of the NHS leaflet quoted earlier) that Medicare was not "an act of charity, but . . . the insured right of a senior citizen."[264] And indeed, Medicare was even used to help roll back Jim Crow hospital segregation in the South, decreasing blatant racial healthcare inequality.[265] The Hill-Burton Act— the federal hospital building law that was all that survived of the National Health

Insurance effort of the post-Second World War period—theoretically required that federally funded hospitals be non-discriminatory, but in reality explicitly allowed for separate-but-equal facilities for blacks and whites; the result, not surprisingly, was the entrenchment of a virulent system of hospital apartheid throughout the South.[266] Although the Civil Rights Act of 1964 made such segregation theoretically illegal, in practice it accomplished little until the administration used the threat of exclusion from Medicare to require—at long last—that all hospitals that wanted to accept Medicare money (which was essentially all of them) end formal racial segregation.[267] More pernicious forms of segregation, of course, persisted—indeed, they survive to the present day.[268] Still, the successful use of Medicare to end explicit healthcare segregation was a notable "rights" victory, and demonstrates the potential power of universal federal programs.

Still—and again unlike the NHS or Canadian Medicare—not only was this expansion not universal, but it also had deficiencies that gave rise to tiered coverage. "Medicare," Beatrix Hoffman explains, "conferred a right to (partial) health coverage for seniors, but it did not confer a right to care."[269] In addition to excluding those who were not seniors, Medicare also drew on an "'insurance' approach" to health coverage that imposed cost sharing (co-payments and deductibles) and excluded certain important benefits.[270] These deficiencies encouraged many people to purchase supplementary insurance, resulting in tiers of protection, something antithetical to an equal right to medical care.[271] Medicaid, meanwhile, ultimately provided care for large numbers of Americans, but as a means-tested program for the poor, it carried with it all the deficiencies intrinsic to such programs, evident from the Poor Law medical service onward: inadequate resourcing, lower quality, and susceptibility to austerity funding. Additionally, as compared to Medicare, Medicaid had a state-based structure, allowing states to avoid participating altogether (at least for a while), to restrict eligibility to more narrow groups of the poor, to restrict benefits, and to keep reimbursement rates (and therefore physician participation rates) low.[272] Moreover, Wilbur Mills—the Ways and Means Committee chairman who played a critical role in the passage of the bill—saw Medicaid as a way to prevent the expansion of Medicare in a universal direction "by undercutting future demands to expand the social security insurance program to cover all income groups."[273]

Still, as many have noted, *some* of Medicare's supporters and architects very much conceived of the law as an initial foray towards a more fully universal program. And indeed, by the early 1970s, the prospects for national health insurance seemed to again be on the rise. A front page story in the *New York Times* in August 1971 carried this message clearly: "Subtly but unmistakably, Americans from all strata of society and all economic classes are swinging over to the idea that good healthcare, like a good education, ought to be a fundamental right of citizenship."[274] Indeed, several years earlier, a campaign for national health insurance had already begun, in part sparked by a speech from the progressive president of the United Autoworkers, Walter Reuther, to the American Public Health Association.[275]

Critically, this shift corresponded with a broader rise in social activism, in particular the Civil Rights movement. It was in the context of this new era of social movements that a number of healthcare movements grew to prominence. Though sometimes with a narrow, single-issue focus, such movements often grappled with the inadequacy of the larger healthcare system over time,[276] and they frequently employed the language of health rights. The Medical Committee for Human Rights (MCHR), for example, functioned as the medical wing of the Civil Rights Movement[277] (the name of its publication, interestingly, was *Health Rights News*).[278] Among other things, MCHR helped to secure the desegregation of healthcare facilities in the South and provided medical assistance to activists at the front lines of the Civil Rights struggle.[279] Out of the movement came a number of other campaigns aimed at broadening healthcare access in a universal direction for the nations' poor and disproportionately minority population. The "Community Health Center" (CHC) movement, for instance, has been described as an outgrowth of the MCHR.[280] According to one mission statement, CHCs were meant to realize "social, economic, and human rights in concrete ways by providing healthcare, but also by addressing the social determinants of health . . ."[281]

CHCs had their roots in the innovative health centers set up by Drs. Sidney and Emily Kark in pre-apartheid South Africa. These centers were meant to not merely provide healthcare at the community level, but also to ensure the health of a defined group of people through a multiplicity of public health interventions. The US community health center pioneer Jack Geiger visited one of these as a medical student in 1957 (they would be subsequently destroyed following the election of the Apartheid government in 1960). Geiger became a founding member of MCHR, and would visit Mississippi as a field coordinator for the organization. As the MCHR's field work came to an end, Geiger and others came to envision the creation of a CHC that would provide care to states' poor black population along the lines of what the Karks had accomplished in South Africa. Yet, as Geiger later wrote, this would be heavily premised on the notion of direct participation from the community itself, or of "making the citizens of targeted impoverished communities full participants in the planning and operation of their health services." Geiger won a grant from the Johnson administration's new Office of Economic Opportunity to create two health centers in association with Tufts Medical School—one in Mount Bayou, Mississippi, and one in Boston. The CHC at Mount Bayou not only provided healthcare, but took on major public health improvement projects with community participation. For instance, it largely brought about the end of malnutrition in the region through the creation of a five-hundred-acre cooperative farm. The CHC model was institutionalized, and spread nationwide; regulations specify that at least half of the members of the boards of these nonprofit centers have to be current patients of the CHC. CHCs today provide a crucial healthcare safety net for an estimated 20 million of the nation's poor—and disproportionately minority—population.[282]

The intersection of civil rights activism and health rights thought during this era is part of a much larger story, however.[283] The Black Panther Party, for instance, opened up healthcare clinics in urban areas, in some instances drawing on the health rights language of the international documents of the post-Second World War era.[284] Along similar lines, the National Welfare Rights Organization's "National Health Rights Committee" agitated against economic and racial discrimination in healthcare, particularly at the hospital level.[285] Asserting that "[j]ust as all people have *welfare rights*, we believe they also have *health rights*," the Health Rights Committee demanded that the American Hospital Association adopt a "patients' bill of rights" that would assure more equitable treatment, "on the basis of need rather than the basis of income."[286] This campaign would see both success and failure. "Patients' bills of rights" would indeed become commonplace in American hospitals. Yet hospitals would later drop one of the most—if not *the* most—important right: the right to healthcare itself.[287] This right was replaced by an anodyne assurance that aid would be provided with the process of paying bills.[288] Nevertheless, it seems fair to conclude that the social activists of this era expanded not only the meaning but the impact of the "right to health."

Notably, this activism corresponded with hopeful movements on the national stage. In 1970, Senator Ted Kennedy of Massachusetts first presented his "Health Security" bill, which would have created a health insurance system that—similar to the British NHS—provided "first dollar" coverage (i.e., no cost sharing) on a single payer basis for the entire country.[289] In 1971, for every one American opposed to national health insurance reform, two were in favor.[290] The bill also had major support from organized labor, which particularly supported the first dollar approach to coverage.[291] The Nixon administration responded with a far less universal proposal that would have expanded Medicaid for the poor while requiring employers to provide insurance for their workers. Nixon also embraced the newly developed "health maintenance organization" (HMO concept), which became the "centerpiece" of his healthcare agenda.[292]

It had been decades since the prospects for achieving sweeping reform had seemed this good. Though neither Kennedy nor Nixon's proposals became law, hopes were high that some sort of system of universal healthcare would be created in the years ahead, and some even envisioned a reform more radical than that of Kennedy. In the early 1970s, the congressman Ronald Dellums (D-Ca.) approached the MCHR for assistance with drafting an ambitious new healthcare bill. What emerged was Dellums Health Service Act, the "first legislation ever introduced into Congress to create a national health service." As such, it went beyond national health insurance in proposing a national health service more akin to the NHS. It furthermore envisioned "community health systems"—inspired by the aforementioned community health center (CHC)—that would provide primary care to all of those within a circumscribed area.[293]

And with the election in 1976 of a Democratic president—Jimmy Carter—and a Democratic Congress, the window of opportunity for national health reform no doubt seemed fully open to many. They were, however, wrong: a fundamental rightward shift in American, and indeed international, politics had in fact already begun. Various progressive legislative initiatives went down to defeat during the years of the Carter administration.[294] The economic strains of the decade coincided with a reassertion of business power, which was now beginning to break free from its New Deal fetters and exert itself with renewed vigor on the political stage.

In 1979, Carter released his long-awaited health insurance plan. Not only did it not meet the standard of the 1970 Kennedy plan, but it also has been described as a "rather faint echo" of the Nixon plan from earlier in the decade,[295] which "ranked with the most cautious and conservative versions of earlier health reform bills . . ."[296] Yet nothing came even of this, and the following year, Carter went down in a resounding defeat to the unapologetically conservative Ronald Reagan. Healthcare rights would only retreat further during the Reagan era.

The final years of the 1970s were pivotal elsewhere as well. In the small, poor Central American country of Nicaragua, a revolution was underway, and its success enabled a movement towards a right to healthcare. Yet this, too, collided with the rise of Reaganism and the growing hegemony of the neoliberal economic and health policy agenda.

Return to Latin America: Alma-Ata in Nicaragua

However diffusely the ideas of Alma-Ata may have spread in the late 1970s, attempts to *implement* its principles in the form of health systems were, not surprisingly, far more limited. Only a few countries successfully achieved comprehensive primary healthcare programs in the manner championed by Alma-Ata.[297] Among these was the poor Central American nation of Nicaragua, which had long suffered under a combination of authoritarianism and imperialism. The case of Nicaragua provides an important case study into how a "right to health" can be advanced, and rolled back, in an extremely poor country.

Healthcare is costly, and when provided to the poorest, it produces little in the way of profits. Thus, there should perhaps be no surprise that extractive, corrupt dictatorships frequently pay little heed to the health needs of their populations. This was certainly the case with the rule of the Somoza family over Nicaragua. The health system under their rule primarily benefited the rich and well-connected. By one estimate, a tenth of the population received some 90 percent of all healthcare services during the 1970s.[298] Health indices—such as life expectancy, child mortality, and child malnutrition—were abysmal.[299] Fundamental reform of the health sector would require—as has been the case in essentially all the nations examined in this chapter—political change. Yet unlike in Britain and Canada where such change was possible at the ballot box, in Nicaragua, the status quo was defended by secret police and the torture chamber.

It was thus only with great bloodshed that the Somoza regime was overthrown. Though it was met with enormous brutality, a left-wing insurgency led by the Sandinistas (the *Frente Sandinista de Liberación Nacional*, or FSLN) came to power in 1979 and subsequently embarked on a series of health reforms that, to no small extent, embodied some of the ideals of Alma-Ata. This is not to say that the Sandinistas were influenced by the document, but rather that both the Sandinistas and Alma-Ata drew on a common pool of healthcare ideas that were percolating throughout the 1970s. Indeed, the emphasis that the new government put on health can, in part, be traced back to its revolutionary program of 1969, which stated that it would "provide free medical assistance to the entire population . . . [and] set up clinics and hospitals throughout the national territory."[300] Additionally, the years of the civil war saw the rise of politicized community health organizations. These networks provided care in areas under Sandinista control, but also, some argue, functioned to raise political consciousness, contributing to the revolutionary movement itself.[301]

Soon after coming to power, the new government sought to expand and transform the healthcare system, efforts that were studied at the time by American nurse and health policy scholar Richard Garfield. Garfield visited the country several times, publishing a series of articles in the medical literature (and later a book) about Sandinista health reforms.[302] His accounts present a measured picture of promise and real accomplishment, followed by rollback and disappointment amidst much carnage.

Change began soon after the Sandinistas came to power: following the revolution, Garfield and a colleague describe, "the FSLN declared that health care was a right of the people and a responsibility of the government."[303] (Others have similarly noted that the right to health was a core principle of the new government's health policy.)[304] This was not simply a rhetorical step, as the Sandinistas quickly took several practical steps to transform healthcare in a universal direction: they created a Unified National Health System under a new Ministry of Health (MINSA) that was responsible for all public provision of care, energetically began building hospitals and health centers, opened the nation's second medical school, and eliminated all fees for prescription medications.[305] The government also greatly increased healthcare expenditure, with per capita government healthcare spending tripling between the pre-revolutionary period and the early 1980s.[306] Publicly funded doctor visits, public health clinics, and vaccinations all increased several-fold over this period as well.[307] Together, these reforms resulted in a major expansion of "primary care," i.e., the community-based medical care concept (so central to Alma-Ata), particularly (as in Cuba) in previously neglected rural areas.[308] The percentage of the population with access to at least some professional healthcare increased from 28 to 70 from before the revolution to 1982.[309]

Yet the changes were not only quantitative: the bottom-up, community-level emphasis that was at the core of Alma-Ata was an important aspect of the Sandinistas' health reform as well. "The insurrection of our people . . . has given us," read one 1979 statement from a city Sandinista government, "the basis for organizing a health system which responds to popular interests, and in which the *participation of the people is an indispensible* [sic] *priority at both decision-making and practical levels*" (emphasis added).[310] The revolutionary government trained massive numbers of community health workers, a system modeled in part on a similar and highly successful Sandinista system for improving literacy. These so-called primary care *brigadistas* have been likened to the Chinese "barefoot doctors"—in addition to health education, they participated in primary care campaigns, including mass vaccination and malaria treatment.[311] These campaigns were, in some cases, enormously successful. For instance, the polio vaccination campaign, led by "People's Health Councils," achieved high rates of vaccination and completely eliminated polio from Nicaragua over the course of the 1980s.[312] An enormous anti-malaria campaign likewise hinged on community involvement, with participation of around 10 percent of the populace.[313] Such successes were recognized by international bodies including the WHO and UNICEF.[314]

No doubt, of course, there were also shortcomings from a "right to health" perspective. Again, the system never had a universal reach, as a substantial private practice sector persisted, which, as elsewhere, led to a tiered system. Now, even in nations with a fully universal national health insurance or national health system, some level of private "concierge" care, mainly for the wealthy, persists, including in the UK. Richer nations, however, have been able to establish services that provide a high level of universal care (with reasonable remuneration for health workers), effectively reducing demand for private care and minimizing its size and disruptive impact on the overall system. In poorer countries, however, the persistence of private care can be more problematic, as seems to have been the case in Nicaragua. The government was reasonably concerned that it could alienate the nation's healthcare professionals, causing them to flee abroad, as had happened in Cuba.[315] However, at the same time, it lacked the resources to retain them in the public service in the manner of the British NHS. The government's tolerance of such "contradictions" alienated some in the Latin American social medicine community.[316] "[T]he goal of a single national health service," as Garfield and a colleague put it, "is tempered by the reality of resource limitations, causing continued although greatly reduced differentials in access to healthcare between those who can afford private care and the rest of the population."[317]

And yet, the early years following the revolution nonetheless saw the right to health expanding, with an increased availability of largely free care for much of the country emerging alongside a simultaneous improvement in the health of the population, in part accomplished through enormous ground-up mobilizations. Yet this dynamic of progress would soon change.

In fact, the discourse around health policy in the developing world was about to change the world over. On the one hand, the principles of Alma-Ata were, it was soon argued, unrealistic and idealistic. At the same time, IMF and World Bank-led "structural readjustment policies" resulted in reductions in public expenditures and increases in user fees for things like healthcare—demands that ran directly counter to the principle of a right to healthcare. Nicaragua, meanwhile, was soon plunged into violence. The Sandinista regime was deemed an intolerable threat by the emboldened foreign policy hawks of the newly elected Reagan administration. Although adventurism abroad had been somewhat chastened in the mid-1970s in the aftermath of the Chilean coup and the Watergate scandal, the 1980s saw the reassertion of an aggressive stance towards Central America by Washington that destroyed much of what had been accomplished in Nicaragua in the realm of health. The coming Contra war not only diverted the attentions and resources of the new government, but also directly involved and targeted healthcare facilities and workers. Healthcare, yet again, became a Cold War front.

The coming era would, more broadly, witness something of a bizarre paradox from the perspective of the right to health. On the one hand—amidst the horrendous slaughter of the soon-to-explode AIDS epidemic—the "right to health" movement would be born. On the other, a global "neoliberal" assault on public health programs—stretching from China to Chile, taking aim at both Medicare and Managua—was set to begin. The discourse of the "right to health" would rise to a new prominence on the world stage—just as actual healthcare rights were increasingly under the boot of neoliberal ideologues and actors.

Notes

1   The facts in this paragraph about the conference are drawn from Fiona Fleck, "Consensus During the Cold War: Back to Alma-Ata," *Bulletin of the World Health Organization* 86, no. 10 (2008): 746.

2   Marcos Cueto, "The Origins of Primary Health Care and Selective Primary Health Care," *American Journal of Public Health* 94, no. 11 (2004): 1867.

3   *Declaration of Alma Ata: International Conference on Primary Health Care, September 6–12, 1978,* accessed 09/11/2015, http://www.who.int/publications/almaata_declaration_en.pdf.

4   Halfdan Mahler, "Primary Health Care Comes Full Circle," *Bulletin of the World Health Organization* 86, no. 10 (2008): 748.

5   Debabar Banerji, "Reflections on the Twenty-Fifth Anniversary of the Alma-Ata Declaration," *International Journal of Health Services* 33, no. 4 (2003): 815; John J. Hall and Richard Taylor, "Health For All Beyond 2000: The Demise of the Alma-Ata Declaration and Primary Health Care in Developing Countries," *Medical Journal of Australia* 178, no. 1 (2003): 17.

6   Mahler, "Primary Health Care Comes Full Circle," 748.

7   Cuba could also be placed in this category, but is instead categorized by region with other Latin American countries.

8   Tony Judt, *Postwar: A History of Europe since 1945* (New York: Penguin Press, 2005), 66.

9   Donald Sassoon, *One Hundred Years of Socialism* (London: I.B.Tauris & Co. Ltd, 2014), 117.

10   Ibid., 118.

11   Ibid., 123–4.

12   Judt, *Postwar: A History of Europe since 1945*, 75.

13   T. H. Marshall, "Citizenship and Social Class," in *Citizenship and Social Class* (London: Pluto Press, 1992), 6.

14   M. W. Flinn, "Medical Services under the New Poor Law," in Derek Fraser (ed.), *The New Poor Law in the Nineteenth Century* (London: Macmillan, 1976), 66; Ruth G. Hodgkinson, *The Origins of the National Health Service: The Medical Services of the New Poor Law, 1834–1871* (London: The Wellcome Historical Medical Library, 1967), xv, 696.

15   Julian Tudor Hart, *The Political Economy of Health Care: Where the NHS Came From and Where It Could Lead*, 2nd ed. (Bristol: Policy Press, 2010), 173.

16   Harry Eckstein, *The English Health Service: Its Origins, Structure, and Achievements* (Cambridge, MA: Harvard University Press, 1958), 34; Nicholas Timmins, *The Five Giants: The Biography of the Welfare State*, revised & updated edition (London: HarperCollins, 2001), 105–6.

17   Timmins, *The Five Giants*, 104; Rudolf Klein, *The New Politics of the NHS*, seventh ed. (London: Radcliffe, 2013), 3; Eckstein, *The English Health Service*, 35–6.

18   Jacob S. Hacker, "The Historical Logic of National Health Insurance: Structure and Sequence in the Development of British, Canadian, and U.S. Medical Policy," *Studies in American Political Development* 12, no. 01 (1998): 90; Lesley Doyal and Imogen Pennel, *The Political Economy of Health* (Boston: South End Press, 1981), 174.

19   Eckstein, *The English Health Service*, 19.

20   Hacker, "The Historical Logic of National Health Insurance: Structure and Sequence in the Development of British, Canadian, and U.S. Medical Policy," 95.

21   Eckstein, *The English Health Service*, 115–16; Charles Webster, "Conflict and Consensus: Explaining the British Health Service," *Twentieth Century British History* 1, no. 2 (1990): 123–6.

22   Eckstein, *The English Health Service*, 117–18.

23   A point made in ibid., 102–7.

24   Ibid., 106–7.

25   *A Socialized Medical Service* (London: Socialist Medical Association, 1933), accessed September 8, 2015, http://contentdm.warwick.ac.uk/cdm/ref/collection/health/id/643, 7, also see page 4.

26   Ibid., 4.

27   Ibid.

28   Eckstein, *The English Health Service*, 108.

29   Eckstein, *The English Health Service*, 133; Derek Fraser, *The Evolution of the British Welfare State: A History of Social Policy since the Industrial Revolution*, 4th ed. (Basingstoke: Palgrave Macmillan, 2009), 245–7.

30   Fraser, *The Evolution of the British Welfare State*, 245–6.

31   Ibid., 253.

32   Inter-departmental Committee on Social Insurance and Allied Services, *Social Insurance and Allied Services: Report by Sir William Beveridge* (New York: The Macmillan Company, 1942), 5.

33   Quotes are from ibid., 10 and 14. See also pages 11 and 15.

34   Ibid., 158.

35   Fraser, *The Evolution of the British Welfare State*, 253.

36   Rodney Lowe, "The Second World War, Consensus, and the Foundation of the Welfare State," *Twentieth Century British History* 1, no. 2 (1990): 158.

37   Klein, *The New Politics of the NHS*, 8; Eckstein, *The English Health Service*, 147–8; Fraser, *The Evolution of the British Welfare State*, 262.

38   This point is made by Lowe, "The Second World War, Consensus, and the Foundation of the Welfare State," 164–5.

39   Ibid., 160.

40   Daniel M. Fox, *Health Policies, Health Politics: The British and American Experience, 1911–1965* (Princeton, NJ: Princeton University Press, 1986), 133–4.

41   Fraser, *The Evolution of the British Welfare State*, 278.

42   Charles Webster, *The National Health Service: A Political History*, new ed. (Oxford: Oxford University Press, 2002), 24.

43   Quoted in Fraser, *The Evolution of the British Welfare State*, 278.

44   T. H. Marshall, "Citizenship and Social Class," in *Citizenship and Social Class*, 34.

45   A reproduction of the full original document, from which these quotes are taken, is available at: "Introducing the National Health Service," *The Guardian*, accessed 2013, http://www.theguardian.com/society/interactive/2008/jun/16/nhs.anniversary. The leaflet has been quoted by others, including Webster, *The National Health Service: A Political History*, 24.

46   Klein, *The New Politics of the NHS*, 1.

47   Eckstein, *The English Health Service*, 2–3.

48   Ibid., 3, 44.

49   Ibid., 3, 9, 44, 45, 101.

50   "Nothing is more remarkable," Klein writes "than the shared assumption that the health service should be both free and comprehensive – and that it should be based on the principle of the collective provision of services and the pooling of financial risks through the public financing of the service." Webster disputes the interpretations of both Klein and Fox. He is not persuaded by Klein's emphasis on the "intangible operation of consensual forces," which he argues ultimately strengthens Eckstein's idea that, ultimately, the role of the Labour Party was not particularly significant. He likewise sees Fox as continuing down the path of both Eckstein and Klein. Webster, "Conflict and Consensus," 119–21, 134; Klein, *The New Politics of the NHS*, 19; Fox, *Health Policies, Health Politics*.

51   Webster, "Conflict and Consensus: Explaining the British Health Service," 135, 149.

52   Ibid., 149.

154 · Health and Death in the Cold War

53 A point made by A. W. Brian Simpson, *Human Rights and the End of Empire: Britain and the Genesis of the European Convention* (Oxford: Oxford University Press, 2004), 39.

54 Samuel Moyn, *The Last Utopia: Human Rights in History* (Cambridge, MA: Belknap Press of Harvard University Press, 2010), 64.

55 Webster, "Conflict and Consensus: Explaining the British Health Service," 149.

56 Ibid.

57 Hart, *The Political Economy of Health Care*, 4.

58 Newdick notes that the rights are statuary, not constitutional. Weait notes that the right to healthcare in the United Kingdom arises not from its ratification of the International Covenant of Economic and Social Rights (which was not brought into UK law), but instead through the operation of the NHS itself, and to some extent through its membership in the European Convention on Human Rights. Christopher Newdick, "Promoting Access and Equity in Health: Assessing the National Health Service in England," in *The Right to Health at the Public/Private Divide: A Global Comparative Study*, ed. Colleen M. Flood and Aeyal M. Gross (New York: Cambridge University Press, 2014), 112–13; Matthew Weait, "The United Kingdom: The Right to Health in the Context of a Nationalized Health Service," in *Advancing the Human Right to Health*, ed. José M. Zuniga, Stephen P. Marks, and Lawrence O. Gostin (Oxford: Oxford University Press, 2013), 209–19.

59 Weait, "The United Kingdom: The Right to Health in the Context of a Nationalized Health Service," 215.

60 Morris Fishbein, "Medicine in the Postwar World," *New England Journal of Medicine* 235, no. 21 (1946): 739.

61 Ibid., 743.

62 Monte M. Poen, *Harry S. Truman Versus the Medical Lobby: The Genesis of Medicare* (Columbia: University of Missouri Press, 1979), 32.

63 Ibid.; Philip J. Funigiello, *Chronic Politics: Health Care Security from FDR to George W. Bush* (Lawrence: University Press of Kansas, 2005), 53–4.

64 Daniel S. Hirshfield, *The Lost Reform: The Campaign for Compulsory Health Insurance in the United States from 1932 -1943* (Cambridge, MA: Harvard University Press, 1970), 163.

65 Poen, *Harry S. Truman Versus the Medical Lobby*, 33.

66 Quoted in ibid., 35.

67 Funigiello, *Chronic Politics*, 53.

68 Fox notes, however, that others in the administration were less hopeful. Poen, *Harry S. Truman Versus the Medical Lobby: The Genesis of Medicare*, 49; Fox, *Health Policies, Health Politics*, 122–3; Jill S. Quadagno, *One Nation, Uninsured: Why the U.S. Has No National Health Insurance* (New York: Oxford University Press, 2005), 26.

69 Mike Davis' so-called "barren marriage." Mike Davis, *Prisoners of the American Dream: Politics and Economy in the History of the US Working Class* (London: Verso; repr., 1991), 52.

70 Alan Derickson, "'Take Health from the List of Luxuries': Labor and the Right to Health Care, 1915–1949," *Labor History* 41, no. 2 (2000): 172.

71 Ibid., 184.

72 Quoted in ibid., 185.

73 To be clear, the first quote is that of Derickson, the second two are Derickson quoting Green. Ibid., 185.

74 His universalism, however, fell somewhat short of that of Bevan, insofar as he found an income maximum acceptable. Alan Derickson, "Health Security for All? Social Unionism and Universal Health Insurance, 1935–1958," *The Journal of American History* 80, no. 4 (1994): 1338–9.

75 Ibid., 1341; Beatrix Rebecca Hoffman, *Health Care for Some: Rights and Rationing in the United States since 1930* (Chicago: University of Chicago Press, 2012), 58; Poen, *Harry S. Truman Versus the Medical Lobby*, 64–5.

76 Quoted in Derickson, "Health Security for All? Social Unionism and Universal Health Insurance, 1935–1958," 1341.

77 Hoffman, *Health Care for Some*, 59.

78 This summary relies on the various sources that I cite throughout the section that follows.

79 The quote of Taft is taken from Poen. Derickson has a slightly different version of the quote. Poen, *Harry S. Truman Versus the Medical Lobby*, 88; Derickson, "Health Security for All? Social Unionism and Universal Health Insurance, 1935–1958," 1342.

80 Derickson, "Health Security for All? Social Unionism and Universal Health Insurance, 1935–1958," 1342.

81 Anthony J. Badger, *The New Deal: The Depression Years, 1933–40* (New York: Hill and Wang, 1995), 143; Robert H. Zieger, Timothy J. Minchin, and Gilbert J. Gall, *American Workers, American Unions: The Twentieth and Early Twenty-First Centuries*, fourth ed. (Baltimore: Johns Hopkins University Press, 2014), 152–3.

82 Poen, *Harry S. Truman Versus the Medical Lobby*, 93.

83 Funigiello, *Chronic Politics*, 70; Quadagno, *One Nation, Uninsured*, 29–30; Poen, *Harry S. Truman Versus the Medical Lobby*, 126–7, 138–9.

84 Quoted in Hoffman, *Health Care for Some*, 59.

85 Zieger, Minchin, and Gall, *American Workers, American Unions: The Twentieth and Early Twenty-First Centuries*, 177.

86 Nelson Lichtenstein, "From Corporatism to Collective Bargaining: Organized Labor and the Eclipse of Social Democracy in the Postwar Era," in *The Rise and Fall of the New Deal Order, 1930–1980*, ed. Steve Fraser and Gary Gerstle (Princeton, NJ: Princeton University Press, 1989), 122.

87 Quotes are from Funigiello, *Chronic Politics*, 78–80. I also rely on Poen, *Harry S. Truman Versus the Medical Lobby*, 144–52.

88 Colin Gordon, *Dead on Arrival: The Politics of Health Care in Twentieth-Century America* (Princeton, NJ: Princeton University Press, 2005), 216.

89 Alan Derickson, "The House of Falk: The Paranoid Style in American Health Politics," *American Journal of Public Health* 87, no. 11 (1997): 1840.

90 Ibid.

91 Poen, *Harry S. Truman Versus the Medical Lobby*, 151.

92 Quoted in: ibid., 148–9; Gordon, *Dead on Arrival*, 144. Notably, this fabricated quote was still being referenced during the Republican Presidential primary election of 2015–16, by Ben Carson. See: Jonathan Weiler, "On Ben Carson, Fake History and Obamacare," *Huffington Post*, January 23, 2014, accessed October 7, 2015, http://www.huffingtonpost.com/jonathan-weiler/on-ben-carson-fake-histor_b_4091583.html.

93 These numbers are from: Hoffman, *Health Care For Some*, 61.

94 Gordon makes note of the red-baiting tradition in health reform history: Gordon, *Dead on Arrival*, 142.

95 Elizabeth Fee, "The Pleasures and Perils of Prophetic Advocacy: Henry E. Sigerist and the Politics of Medical Reform," *American Journal of Public Health* 86, no. 11 (1996): 1637–47.

96 Ibid.

97 Emily K. Abel, Elizabeth Fee, and Theodore M. Brown, "Milton I. Roemer Advocate of Social Medicine, International Health, and National Health Insurance," *American Journal of Public Health* 98, no. 9 (2008): 1596–7.

98 Ibid.

99 John Dittmer, *The Good Doctors: The Medical Committee for Human Rights and the Struggle for Social Justice in Health Care* (New York: Bloomsbury Press, 2009), 11; Jane Pacht Brickman, "Medical McCarthyism and the Punishment of Internationalist Physicians in the United States," in *Comrades in Health: U.S. Health Internationalists, Abroad and at Home*, ed. Anne-Emanuelle Birn and Theodore M. Brown (New Brunswick: Rutgers University Press, 2013), 84, 95.

100 Brickman, "Medical McCarthyism and the Punishment of Internationalist Physicians in the United States," 90.

101 Jane Pacht Brickman, "'Medical McCarthyism': The Physicians Forum and the Cold War," *Journal of the History of Medicine and Allied Sciences* 49, no. 3 (1994): 390; Jane Pacht Brickman, "Minority Politics in the House of Medicine: The Physicians Forum and the New York County Medical Society, 1938–1965," *Journal of Public Health Policy* 20, no. 3 (1999): 282–309.

102 Jane Pacht Brickman, "'Medical Mccarthyism': The Physicians Forum and the Cold War," 395.

103 Brickman, "Medical McCarthyism and the Punishment of Internationalist Physicians in the United States," 89–90.

104 Derickson, "The House of Falk: The Paranoid Style in American Health Politics," 1836–43.

105 Quoted in ibid., 1839.

106 Hacker, "The Historical Logic of National Health Insurance: Structure and Sequence in the Development of British, Canadian, and U.S. Medical Policy," 116.

107 Derickson, "The House of Falk: The Paranoid Style in American Health Politics," 1840.

108 Ibid.

109 Quadagno, *One Nation, Uninsured*, 49; Gordon, *Dead on Arrival*, 67.

110 Gordon, *Dead on Arrival*, 62.

111 Derickson, "Health Security for All? Social Unionism and Universal Health Insurance, 1935–1958," 1349.

112 Ibid., 1354–6.

113 Quoted in Theodore R. Marmor and James Morone, "The Health Programs of the Kennedy-Johnson Years: An Overview," in *Toward New Human Rights: The Social Policies of the Kennedy and Johnson Administrations* (Austin: Lyndon B. Johnson School of Public Affairs, University of Texas at Austin, 1977), 162.

114 Lichtenstein, "From Corporatism to Collective Bargaining: Organized Labor and the Eclipse of Social Democracy in the Postwar Era," 144.

115 Ibid.

116 Victor G. Rodwin, "The Health Care System under French National Health Insurance: Lessons for Health Reform in the United States," *American Journal of Public Health* 93, no. 1 (2003): 31–7.

117 The discussion of health reform in Canada in this paragraph relies on Hacker, "The Historical Logic of National Health Insurance: Structure and Sequence in the Development of British, Canadian, and U.S. Medical Policy," 99–106.

118 Timothy Synder, "Hitler Vs. Stalin: Who Killed More?," *The New York Review of Books*, March 10, 2011, accessed October 8, 2015, http://www.nybooks.com/articles/archives/2011/mar/10/hitler-vs-stalin-who-killed-more.

119 Roderick MacFarquhar, "The Worst Man-Made Catastrophe, Ever," *The New York Review of Books*, February 10, 2011, accessed October 8, 2015, http://www.nybooks.com/articles/archives/2011/feb/10/worst-man-made-catastrophe-ever. The quoted text is from the headline of the article.

120 Ian Johnson, "China: Worse Than You Ever Imagined," *The New York Review of Books*, November 12, 2012, accessed October 8, 2015, http://www.nybooks.com/articles/archives/2012/nov/22/china-worse-you-ever-imagined.

121 William C. Hsiao, "Correcting Past Policy Mistakes," *Daedalus* 143, no. 2 (2014), 55; Judith Banister and Samuel H. Preston, "Mortality in China," *Population and Development Review* 7, no. 1 (1981): 98–110.

122 Howard M. Leichter, *A Comparative Approach to Policy Analysis: Health Care Policy in Four Nations* (Cambridge: Cambridge University Press, 1979), 202–5.

123 Christopher Lawrence, "Continuity in Crisis: Medicine, 1914–1945," in *The Western Medical Tradition: 1800 to 2000* (New York: Cambridge University Press, 2006), 353; Leichter, *A Comparative Approach to Policy Analysis*, 206–7; R. V. Korotkikh, "The Social and Ethical Implications of Universal Access to Health Care in Russia," *Kennedy Institute of Ethics Journal* 3, no. 4 (1993), 411–12.

124 Leichter, *A Comparative Approach to Policy Analysis*, 208.

125 Ibid., 213–14.

126 Lawrence, "Continuity in Crisis: Medicine, 1914–1945," 355; Korotkikh, "The Social and Ethical Implications of Universal Access to Health Care in Russia," 412.

127 Gordon Hyde, *The Soviet Health Service: A Historical and Comparative Study* (London: Lawrence & Wishart, 1974), 100.

128 These points, and the quote from *Red Medicine: Socialized Health in Soviet Russia*, is from Brickman, "Medical McCarthyism and the Punishment of Internationalist Physicians in the United States," 45, 50.

129 Leichter, *A Comparative Approach to Policy Analysis*, 214; Hyde, *The Soviet Health Service*, 125–7.

130 These statistics are from Leichter, *A Comparative Approach to Policy Analysis*, Table 7.2, 227.

131 Ibid., 228.

132 Korotkikh, "The Social and Ethical Implications of Universal Access to Health Care in Russia," 411.

133 Hyde, *The Soviet Health Service*, 23; Leichter, *A Comparative Approach to Policy Analysis*, 214–15.

134 Leichter here is quoting Milton Roemer. Leichter, *A Comparative Approach to Policy Analysis*, 214–15. Quote on 215.

135 Ibid., 221.

136 Ibid., 232.

137 Donald Sassoon, *One Hundred Years of Socialism*, 194.

138 Kate Schecter, "Soviet Socialized Medicine and the Right to Health Care in a Changing Soviet Union," *Human Rights Quarterly* 14, no. 2 (1992): 206–15.

139 Korotkikh, "The Social and Ethical Implications of Universal Access to Health Care in Russia," 412.

140 Julie Margot Feinsilver, *Healing the Masses: Cuban Health Politics at Home and Abroad* (Berkeley: University of California Press, 1993), endnote 28, pp. 243–4.

141 Evegueni M. Andreev et al., "The Evolving Pattern of Avoidable Mortality in Russia," *International Journal of Epidemiology* 32, no. 3 (2003): 437–46.

142 Schecter argues that Soviet government emphasized "economic growth" over "human welfare" from "Lenin through Brezhnev," and that this emphasis is reflected in its healthcare system. Schecter, "Soviet Socialized Medicine and the Right to Health Care in a Changing Soviet Union," 209.

143 Leichter, *A Comparative Approach to Policy Analysis*, 232–3.

144 Victor W. Sidel, "Medical Care in the People's Republic of China," *Archives of Internal Medicine* 135, no. 7 (1975), 916; Victor W. Sidel, "The Barefoot Doctors of the People's Republic of China," *New England Journal of Medicine* 286, no. 24 (1972), 1293.

145 Sidel, "Medical Care in the People's Republic of China", 918.

146 Ibid.

147 The following brief description of this system draws mainly on two of these publications from the 1970s. Sidel, "The Barefoot Doctors of the People's Republic of China"; Sidel, "Medical Care in the People's Republic of China."

148 Quoted in Sidel, "The Barefoot Doctors of the People's Republic of China," 1294.

149 Victor W. Sidel and Ruth Sidel, "Barefoot in China, the Bronx, and Beyond," in *Comrades in Health: U.S. Health Internationalists, Abroad and at Home*, ed. Anne-Emanuelle Birn and Theodore M. Brown (New Brunswick: Rutgers University Press, 2013), 123.

150 Hsiao, "Correcting Past Policy Mistakes": 55; Therese Hesketh and Wei Xing Zhu, "Health in China. From Mao to Market Reform," *British Medical Journal* 314, no. 7093 (1997), 1544.

151 William C. Hsiao, "Correcting Past Policy Mistakes," 55.

152 Banister and Preston, "Mortality in China," 107–8.

153 Ibid., 108.

154 Mark W. Frazier, "State Schemes or Safety Net? China's Push for Universal Coverage," *Daedalus* 143, no. 2 (2014), 69–80.

155 The information and the quotes throughout this paragraph are drawn from ibid., 71–2.

156 Yamin describes this separation, increasingly "entrenched during the Cold War," as a "misleading one." Alicia Ely Yamin, "Will We Take Suffering Seriously? Reflections on What Applying a Human Rights Framework to Health Means and Why We Should Care," *Health and Human Rights* 10, no. 1 (2008), 52. On this split, see also: Brigit C.A. Toebes, *The Right to Health as a Human Right in International Law* (Antwerpen: Instersentia/Hart, 1999), 40–1; Daniel Tarantola, "A Perspective on the History of Health and Human Rights: From the Cold War to the Gold War," *Journal of Public Health Policy* 29, no. 1 (2008), 43.

157 John Tobin, *The Right to Health in International Law* (Oxford: Oxford University Press, 2012), 31.

158 Moyn, *The Last Utopia*.

159 Theodore M. Brown, Marcos Cueto, and Elizabeth Fee, "The World Health Organization and the Transition from 'International' to 'Global' Public Health," *American Journal of Public Health* 96, no. 1 (2006), 64.

160 In the remainder of this paragraph, I draw on the work of Benjamin Mason Meier, "The World Health Organization, the Evolution of Human Rights, and the Failure to Achieve Health for All," in *Global Health and Human Rights: Legal and Philosophical Perspectives*, ed. John Harrington and Maria Stuttaford (London; New York: Routledge, 2010), 168–71.

161 Ibid., 169.

162 Quoted in ibid., 171.

163 Tobin, *The Right to Health in International Law*, 32. Others make similar points, for instance Helena Nygren-Krug, "The Right to Health: From Concept to Practice," in *Advancing the Human Right to Health*, 40.

164 Discussed in Brown, Cueto, and Fee, "The World Health Organization and the Transition from 'International' to 'Global' Public Health," 65; Meier, "The World Health Organization, the Evolution of Human Rights, and the Failure to Achieve Health for All," 172.

165 This and the point in the following sentence rely on Brown, Cueto, and Fee, "The World Health Organization and the Transition from 'International' to 'Global' Public Health," 65.

166 Ibid.

167 Meier, "The World Health Organization, the Evolution of Human Rights, and the Failure to Achieve Health for All," 172–5.

168 Quoted in ibid., 173.

169 Ibid., 174.

170 Ibid., 173–5.

171 This point is emphasized by Toebes, who traces the drafting history of Article 12 in depth. Toebes, *The Right to Health as a Human Right in International Law*, 52.

172 United Nations, "International Covenant on Economic, Social and Cultural Rights" (1966), accessed multiple times, available as of January 11, 2016, at: http://www.ohchr.org/en/professionalinterest/pages/cescr.aspx.

173 Quoted in Meier, "The World Health Organization, the Evolution of Human Rights, and the Failure to Achieve Health For All," 170–1. For the details of the drafting history, see Toebes, *The Right to Health as a Human Right in International Law*, 40–52.

174 Mary Ann Glendon, *A World Made New: Eleanor Roosevelt and the Universal Declaration of Human Rights* (New York: Random House, 2001), 205–7; M. Glen Johnson, "The Contributions of Eleanor and Franklin Roosevelt to the Development of International Protection for Human Rights," *Human Rights Quarterly* 9, no. 1 (1987): 46.

175 Quoted in Johnson, "The Contributions of Eleanor and Franklin Roosevelt to the Development of International Protection for Human Rights," 46–7.

176 Dianne Otto, "Linking Health and Human Rights: A Critical Legal Perspective," *Health and Human Rights* 1, no. 3 (1995), 276.

177 Glendon, *A World Made New*, 202.

178 Though it was shortly followed by Germany and the Soviet Union in the following two years. Toebes, *The Right to Health as a Human Right in International Law*, 79; Wright-Carozza, "From Conquest to Constitutions: Retrieving a Latin American Tradition of the Idea of Human Rights," *Human Rights Quarterly* 25, no. 2 (2003): 304.

179 Wright-Carozza, "From Conquest to Constitutions: Retrieving a Latin American Tradition of the Idea of Human Rights," 304; Tobin, *The Right to Health in International Law*, 22.

180 Stephen Reichard, "Ideology Drives Health Care Reforms in Chile," *Journal of Public Health Policy* 17, no. 1 (1996): 82–3.

181 Richard Muir and Alan Angell, "Commentary: Salvador Allende: His Role in Chilean Politics," *International Journal of Epidemiology* 34, no. 4 (2005): 737; Edwin Williamson, *The Penguin History of Latin America* (London; New York: Penguin Books, 1992), 486–9.

182 Joseph L. Scarpaci, "Restructuring Health Care Financing in Chile," *Social Science and Medicine* 21, no. 4 (1985): 417; Reichard, "Ideology Drives Health Care Reforms in Chile," 83.

183 Reichard, "Ideology Drives Health Care Reforms in Chile," 83; Francisco Mardones-Restat and Antonio Carlos de Azevedo, "The Essential Health Reform in Chile; a Reflection on the 1952 Process," *Salud Publica de México* 48, no. 6 (2006), 505.

184 Quoted in Toebes, *The Right to Health as a Human Right in International Law*, footnote 80, p. 90.

185 Scarpaci, "Restructuring Health Care Financing in Chile": 417; Mardones-Restat and de Azevedo, "The Essential Health Reform in Chile; a Reflection on the 1952 Process", 506.

186 Greg Grandin, *Empire's Workshop: Latin America, the United States, and the Rise of the New Imperialism* (New York: Metropolitan Books, 2006), 40–1.

187 Johannes Morsink, *The Universal Declaration of Human Rights: Origins, Drafting, and Intent*, (Philadelphia: University of Pennsylvania Press, 1999), 130–1; Mary Ann Glendon, "The Forgotten Crucible: The Latin American Influence on the Universal Human Rights Idea," *Harvard Human Rights Journal* 16 (Spring 2003): 35–7.

188 The facts about Allende thus far in this paragraph are drawn from: Sara K. Tedeschi, Theodore M. Brown, and Elizabeth Fee, "Salvador Allende: Physician, Socialist, Populist, and President," *American Journal of Public Health* 93, no. 12 (2003), 2014–15.

189 Howard Waitzkin, "Commentary: Salvador Allende and the Birth of Latin American Social Medicine," *International Journal of Epidemiology* 34, no. 4 (2005): 739–41.

190 Ibid., 739.

191 Howard Waitzkin, *Medicine and Public Health at the End of Empire* (Boulder, CO: Paradigm Publishers, 2011), 16.

192 Waitzkin, "Commentary: Salvador Allende and the Birth of Latin American Social Medicine," 740.

193 Ibid.

194 Salvador Allende, "Chile's Medical-Social Reality," in *Salvador Allende Reader: Chile's Voice of Democracy*, ed. James D. Cockcroft (Melbourne: Ocean Press, 2000), 38.

195 Ibid., 36.

196 Mardones-Restat and de Azevedo, "The Essential Health Reform in Chile; a Reflection on the 1952 Process," 506.

197 Tedeschi, Brown, and Fee, "Salvador Allende: Physician, Socialist, Populist, and President," 2015.

198 John W. Sloan, *Public Policy in Latin America: A Comparative Survey* (Pittsburgh, PA: University of Pittsburgh Press, 1984), 117.

199 Mardones-Restat and de Azevedo, "The Essential Health Reform in Chile; a Reflection on the 1952 Process," 508.

200 Howard Waitzkin, *Medicine and Public Health at the End of Empire*, 44–5.

201 Sloan, *Public Policy in Latin America: A Comparative Survey*, 117.

202 There was also a military service. Anamaria Viveros-Long, "Changes in Health Financing: The Chilean Experience," *Social Sciences and Medicine* 22, no. 3 (1986), 381.

203 Feinsilver, *Healing the Masses*, 33; Felipe Eduardo Sixto, "An Evaluation of Four Decades of Cuban Healthcare," *Association For the Study of the Cuban Economy*, accessed September 10, 2015, http://www.ascecuba.org/c/wp-content/uploads/2014/09/v12-sixto.pdf, 326.

204 Feinsilver, *Healing the Masses: Cuban Health Politics at Home and Abroad*, 28.

205 Ibid., 62.

206 Sixto, "An Evaluation of Four Decades of Cuban Healthcare," 326.

207 Feinsilver, *Healing the Masses*, 30, 103.

208 C. W. Keck and G. A. Reed, "The Curious Case of Cuba," *American Journal of Public Health* 102, no. 8 (2012): e14; Feinsilver, *Healing the Masses: Cuban Health Politics at Home and Abroad*, 36–7; Sixto, "An Evaluation of Four Decades of Cuban Healthcare," 326; Steve Brouwer, *Revolutionary Doctors: How Venezuela and Cuba Are Changing the World's Conception of Health Care* (New York: Monthly Review Press, 2011), 59.

209 Sixto, "An Evaluation of Four Decades of Cuban Healthcare," 340; Keck and Reed, "The Curious Case of Cuba," e13–e22.

210 James D. Cockcroft, Introduction to *Salvador Allende Reader: Chile's Voice of Democracy* (Melbourne: Ocean Press, 2000), 1.

211   Waitzkin, *Medicine and Public Health at the End of Empire*, 46.

212   Scarpaci, "Restructuring Health Care Financing in Chile," 417.

213   The quotes are from: Viveros-Long, "Changes in Health Financing: The Chilean Experience," 381. See also: Howard Waitzkin and Hilary Modell, "Medicine, Socialism, and Totalitarianism: Lessons from Chile," *New England Journal of Medicine* 291, no. 4 (1974), 171–7.

214   Waitzkin, *Medicine and Public Health at the End of Empire*, 48–9; "History of the Health Care System in Chile," *American Journal of Public Health* 67, no. 1 (1977), 35.

215   Waitzkin, *Medicine and Public Health at the End of Empire*, 49–51; Waitzkin and Modell, "Medicine, Socialism, and Totalitarianism: Lessons from Chile," 173.

216   "History of the Health Care System in Chile," 35.

217   Grandin, *Empire's Workshop: Latin America, the United States, and the Rise of the New Imperialism*, 13–51.

218   Ibid., 49.

219   Ibid., 59–60.

220   Odd Arne Westad, *The Global Cold War: Third World Interventions and the Making of Our Times* (Cambridge; New York: Cambridge University Press, 2010; repr., 7th), 201.

221   Ibid.

222   Quoted in Vijay Prashad, *The Darker Nations: A People's History of the Third World*, A New Press People's History (New York: New Press, 2007), 147.

223   Paul B. Cornely et al., "Report of the APHA Task Force on Chile," *American Journal of Public Health* 67, no. 1 (1977): 71–3.

224   Ibid.: 72.

225   Waitzkin and Modell, "Medicine, Socialism, and Totalitarianism: Lessons from Chile," 175; Waitzkin, *Medicine and Public Health at the End of Empire*, 51–2.

226   Quoted in Reichard, "Ideology Drives Health Care Reforms in Chile," 88.

227   "History of the Health Care System in Chile," 35.

228   This paragraph draws on Brown, Cueto, and Fee, "The World Health Organization and the Transition from 'International' to 'Global' Public Health," 65–70; Elizabeth Fee, Marcos Cueto, and Theodore M. Brown, "WHO at 60: Snapshots from Its First Six Decades," *The American Journal of Public Health* 98, no. 4 (2008): 630–1; Socrates Litsios, "The Christian Medical Commission and the Development of the World Health Organization's Primary Health Care Approach," *The American Journal of Public Health* 94, no. 11 (2004), 1885; Lesley Magnussen, John Ehiri, and Pauline Jolly, "Comprehensive Versus Selective Primary Health Care: Lessons for Global Health Policy," *Health Affairs* 23, no. 3 (2004), 167.

229   The importance of China is emphasized by: Magnussen, Ehiri, and Jolly, "Comprehensive Versus Selective Primary Health Care: Lessons for Global Health Policy," 168; M. Cueto, "The Origins of Primary Health Care and Selective Primary Health Care," *American Journal of Public Health* 94, no. 11 (2004): 1865; Brown, Cueto, and Fee, "The World Health Organization and the Transition from 'International' to 'Global' Public Health," 66.

230   For instance, Sidel, "The Barefoot Doctors of the People's Republic of China."

231   Cueto, "The Origins of Primary Health Care and Selective Primary Health Care," 1864–5.

232   Ibid., 1866.

233   Litsios, "The Christian Medical Commission and the Development of the World Health Organization's Primary Health Care Approach," 1886–7.

234   Ibid., 1890.

235   Mahler, "Primary Health Care Comes Full Circle," 747.

236   Kenneth W. Newell, Introduction to *Health by the People*, ed. Kenneth W. Newell (Geneva: World Health Organization, 1975), accessed October 4, 2015, http://apps.who.int/iris/bitstream/10665/40514/1/9241560428_eng.pdf, x_xi.

237   Victor W. Sidel and Ruth Sidel, "The Health Care Delivery System of the People's Republic of China," *Health by the People*, 11–12.

238   Arnaldo F. Tejeiro Fernandez, "The National Health System in Cuba," *Health by the People*, 15.

239   Its journal *Contact* may also have been the first to use the term "Primary Healthcare," Cueto notes. Cueto, "The Origins of Primary Health Care and Selective Primary Health Care," 1865;

Litsios, "The Christian Medical Commission and the Development of the World Health Organization's Primary Health Care Approach," 1891.

240   On this topic, see: Cueto, "The Origins of Primary Health Care and Selective Primary Health Care," 1864–74; Socrates Litsios, "The Long and Difficult Road to Alma-Ata: A Personal Reflection," *International Journal of the Health Services* 32, no. 4 (2002): 709–32; Litsios, "The Christian Medical Commission and the Development of the World Health Organization's Primary Health Care Approach," 1884–93.

241   Cueto, "The Origins of Primary Health Care and Selective Primary Health Care," 1867.

242   Litsios, "The Long and Difficult Road to Alma-Ata: A Personal Reflection," 718.

243   Cueto, "The Origins of Primary Health Care and Selective Primary Health Care," 1867.

244   Ibid., 1867.

245   *Declaration of Alma-Ata.*

246   Mahler, "Primary Health Care Comes Full Circle: An interview with Dr Halfdan Mahler," 747–8.

247   Ibid.

248   "High Hopes at Alma-Ata," *Lancet* 2, no. 8091 (1978), 66.

249   Jonathan Wolff, *The Human Right to Health* (New York: W.W. Norton & Company, 2012), 9.

250   Paula Braverman, "Find the Best People and Support Them," *Comrades in Health*, 180.

251   Mary Travis Bassett, "From Harlem to Harare," *Comrades in Health*, 207.

252   Mahler, "Primary Health Care Comes Full Circle: An interview with Dr. Halfdan Mahler," 748.

253   The plan was devised by Wilbur Cohen and I. S. Falk, and approved by Oscar Ewing. Funigiello, *Chronic Politics*, 89–90; Wilbur Cohen, "From Medicare to National Health Insurance," *Toward New Human Rights: The Social Policies of the Kennedy and Johnson Administrations*, ed. David C. Warner (Austin: Lyndon B. Johnson School of Public Affairs, University of Texas at Austin, 1977), 145; Theodore R. Marmor, *The Politics of Medicare* (New York: A. de Gruyter, 2000), 9.

254   Quadagno, *One Nation, Uninsured*, 49.

255   Hoffman, *Health Care for Some*, 92, 102.

256   Ibid., 97–9.

257   Gordon, *Dead on Arrival.* 80–1.

258   Hoffman, *Health Care for Some*, 88–9.

259   Quadagno, *One Nation, Uninsured*, 62.

260   Hoffman, *Health Care For Some*, 121.

261   Ibid., 119–22.

262   Marmor, *The Politics of Medicare*, 45.

263   Regarding the so-called "three-layer cake" term, see Funigiello, *Chronic Politics*, 145; Quadagno, *One Nation, Uninsured*, 73.

264   Quoted in Funigiello, *Chronic Politics*, 164.

265   Quadagno, *One Nation, Uninsured*, 87–91.

266   Ibid., 77–80.

267   Hoffman, *Health Care For Some*, 126; Funigiello, *Chronic Politics*, 161; Quadagno, *One Nation, Uninsured*, 86–92; P. Preston Reynolds, "The Federal Government's Use of Title VI and Medicare to Racially Integrate Hospitals in the United States, 1963 through 1967," *American Journal of Public Health* 87, no. 11 (1997): 1850–8.

268   See, for instance: J. Greene, J. Blustein, B. C. Weitzman, "Race, Segregation, and Physicians' Participation in Medicaid," *The Milbank Quarterly* 84, no. 2 (2006): 239–72.

269   Hoffman, *Health Care For Some*, 132.

270   Marmor, *The Politics of Medicare*, 59.

271   Ibid., 154.

272   Paul Starr, *Remedy and Reaction: The Peculiar American Struggle over Health Care Reform*, Revised edition. ed. (New Haven: Yale University Press, 2013), 47.

273   Marmor, *The Politics of Medicare*, 60.

274   Quoted in Hoffman, *Health Care For Some*, 163.

275   Quadagno, *One Nation, Uninsured*, 110.

276   A point made by Beatrix Hoffman, "Health Care Reform and Social Movements in the United States," *American Journal of Public Health* 93, no. 1 (2003), 79.

277   Dittmer, *The Good Doctors.*

278   Ibid., 208–9.

279   Ibid.

280   Dittmer deems it the "most significant and enduring achievement in the field of healthcare to come out of the civil rights years." Ibid., 229.

281   A mission statement quoted in ibid., 230–1.

282   The entirety of this paragraph draws from Geiger's own account of CHCs: H. Jack Geiger, "Contesting Racism and Innovating Community Health Centers," *Comrades in Health*, 101–8, quote on page 112.

283   Hoffman, "Health Care Reform and Social Movements in the United States," 80.

284   Hoffman, *Health Care For Some*, 153.

285   Beatrix Hoffman, "'Don't Scream Alone': The Health Care Activism of Poor Americans in the 1970s," in *Patients as Policy Actors* (New Brunswick, NJ: Rutgers University Press, 2011), 132–47.

286   Quoted in ibid., 138.

287   Ibid., 142–4.

288   Ibid.

289   Starr, *Remedy and Reaction*, 53; Funigiello, *Chronic Politics*, 173.

290   Gordon, *Dead on Arrival: The Politics of Health Care in Twentieth-Century America*, 33.

291   Hoffman, *Health Care For Some*, 164.

292   Funigiello, *Chronic Politics*, 175; Quadagno, *One Nation, Uninsured*, 116.

293   The history of the Dellums bill and the quotes in this paragraph all draw from Len S. Rodberg, "Anatomy of a National Health Program. Reconsidering the Dellums Bill after 10 Years," *Health PAC Bulletin* 17, no. 6 (1987): 12–16, quote on 12. Notably, Rodberg was involved in the drafting of the bill.

294   Judith Stein, *Pivotal Decade: How the United States Traded Factories for Finance in the Seventies* (New Haven, CT: Yale University Press, 2010), 204.

295   Starr, *Remedy and Reaction*, 61.

296   Funigiello, *Chronic Politics*, 191.

297   Magnussen et al., for instance, list Cuba, Mozambique, Nicaragua as three examples of success stories in the 1980s, although they mention that progress in the latter two was "short-lived," which seems a fair assessment. Others list Nicaragua among those nations that moved in the direction of the Alma-Ata vision of comprehensive primary care, including Lawn et al., Magnussen, Ehiri, and Jolly, "Comprehensive Versus Selective Primary Health Care: Lessons for Global Health Policy," 169–70; J. E. Lawn et al., "Alma-Ata 30 Years On: Revolutionary, Relevant, and Time to Revitalise," *Lancet* 372, no. 9642 (2008): Table I and p. 922.

298   This fact and the points of the preceding two sentences are drawn from Richard Garfield and Glen Williams, *Health Care in Nicaragua: Primary Care under Changing Regimes* (New York: Oxford University Press, 1992), 12.

299   Richard M. Garfield and Eugenio Taboada, "Health Services Reforms in Revolutionary Nicaragua," *American Journal of Public Health* 74, no. 10 (1984), 1138; David C. Halperin and Richard Garfield, "Developments in Health Care in Nicaragua," *New England Journal of Medicine* 307, no. 6 (1982), 389.

300   Garfield and Williams make the point that the FSLN's healthcare agenda preceded Alma-Ata, and cite the "Historic Program of the FSLN." "The Historic Program of the FSLN," in *Sandinistas Speak*, ed. T. Borge (Pathfinder Press, 1982), last accessed January 12, 2016, http://www.pathfinderpress.com/core/media/media.nl?id=15173&c=ACCT136348&h=db7095d92bf092a22b4e, p. 20; Garfield and Williams, *Health Care in Nicaragua*, 233–4.

301   David Werner, Foreword to *Health Care in Nicaragua: Primary Care under Changing Regimes*, by Richard Garfield and Glen Williams (New York: Oxford University Press, 1992), vi–vii; Garfield and Williams, *Health Care in Nicaragua*, 18.

302   His publications are cited throughout this section.

303   Garfield and Williams, *Health Care in Nicaragua*, 239.

304   John M. Donahue, "Planning for Primary Health Care in Nicaragua: A Study in Revolutionary Process," *Social Science & Medicine* 23, no. 2 (1986), 151.

305   Garfield and Williams, *Health Care in Nicaragua*, 19–28.

306   Ibid., 87.

307   Douglas Lefton, "Nicaragua: Health Care under the Sandinistas," *Canadian Medical Association Journal* 130, no. 6 (1984), 782.

308   Patti Lane, "Economic Hardship Has Put Nicaragua's Health Care System on the Sick List," *Canadian Medical Association Journal* 152, no. 4 (1995), 580.

309   Garfield and Williams, *Health Care in Nicaragua*, 32.

310   Quoted in Tom Frieden and Richard Garfield, "Popular Participation in Health in Nicaragua," *Health Policy and Planning* 2, no. 2 (1987), 162.

311   Ibid., 162–70.

312   Garfield and Williams, *Health Care in Nicaragua*, 51.

313   Richard M. Garfield and Sten H. Vermund, "Health Education and Community Participation in Mass Drug Administration for Malaria in Nicaragua," *Social Science and Medicine* 22, no. 8 (1986), 876.

314   Donahue, "Planning for Primary Health Care in Nicaragua: A Study in Revolutionary Process," 153.

315   Howard Waitzkin et al., "Social Medicine Then and Now: Lessons from Latin America," *American Journal of Public Health* 91, no. 10 (2001), 1596.

316   Ibid., 1596.

317   Garfield and Taboada, "Health Services Reforms in Revolutionary Nicaragua," 1141.

7
The Right to Health in the Age of Neoliberalism

"The cause of the outbreak is unknown," the *New York Times* reported in 1981, "and there is as yet no evidence of contagion." In retrospect, these were portentous words. The article briefly described the sudden and unexplained emergence of Kaposi's Sarcoma—an unusual form of cancer that arises from the cells that line blood vessels—in some forty-one gay men who mainly lived in New York City and San Francisco.[1] These were the first days of what was soon an international epidemic, the consequences of which were more catastrophic than anyone could have possibly imagined.[2] HIV/AIDS has since claimed, according to the World Health Organization, around 35 million lives around the world. And despite decades of advancements in therapy, some 1.1 million people are still dying each year from complications related to the disease.[3]

The emergence of HIV/AIDS coincided with another development—also deadly, and also in its earliest stages. A rightward political shift—often described under the rubric of "neoliberalism"—was unfolding globally. First rising to prominence in the 1970s, the ideology of neoliberalism—articulated by economists, supported by think tanks, funded by corporate dollars, and embraced (and coldheartedly enacted) by politicians across the political spectrum—was ascendant just as the HIV epidemic began its deadly expansion. The rise of neoliberalism—and attendant shifts towards privatization, public austerity, and free-market ideology—had multifold consequences in the realm of health, beginning with the rollback of the ideals of Alma-Ata and their replacement with the icy market logic of institutions like the World Bank. Together, these developments were tantamount to a crucial historic turn in the healthcare rights-commodity dialectic: within the emerging framework, healthcare was first and foremost contextualized as a commodity—and an increasingly global and lucrative one at that.

And yet—perhaps paradoxically—both of these developments contributed to the emergence of a new "human right to health" discourse and movement. In the 1990s and 2000s, the "right to health" became an increasingly prominent concern in both academic and activist circles. It also appeared in new international legal instruments and national constitutions. Indeed, it was only in this recent era that the "human right to health" became an important theoretical and organizational concern.

This chapter will trace—in broad outline—the meaning and contradictions of the "right to healthcare" in the neoliberal age. It will begin with a brief discussion of the political context, that is, the emergence of what can be termed the "neoliberal healthcare agenda." It will then explore the turn away from Alma-Ata, the changing orientation of the World Health Organization, and the World Bank-promoted retreat from the public provision of healthcare in the developing world. Next, it will explore the "why" and the "how" of the "right to health" movement, looking at some of its key moments, both in activism and in international and national law. It will also discuss the meaning of these developments for many of the case nations discussed in the last chapter—Chile, Nicaragua, Cuba, China, the United Kingdom, and the United States—as well as some new ones, including South Africa, Brazil, Colombia, and India. It will conclude by turning to some recent developments, including the passage of the Affordable Care Act in the United States and the onset of austerity of Europe.

The modern concept of the right to health was first articulated in the postwar era, but it gained currency and power only in our own. Still, even though this has been something of a golden era for the "right to health" as a *discourse*, it has been a far more mixed period for this right in *practice*. Yet the unsteady, unstable politics of our day are wavering even as this chapter is being written: where things will stand when it is published remains unclear.

Exit Alma-Ata, Enter the World Bank

The historic healthcare conference at Alma-Ata—explored in the last chapter—was representative of an early crest for the "right to health" movement in the developing world. Yet it was a moment that most probably did not first see as a peak. Yet it is now clear that the conference marked the turning of a tide: almost immediately in its wake, the rollback of its expansive notion of health rights began. This rollback coincided with the onset of a brutal era of neoliberalism. With it came the emergence of a distinct neoliberal healthcare agenda, which has had enormous ramifications for global health, continuing into our own age.

The sources of this political shift must first be briefly discussed. In the US, some describe the political change of this era as the culmination of a decades-long effort by businessmen to turn back the gains of the New Deal.[4] Other historians attribute it to structural changes in the global economy in the 1970s that led financial interests to gain dominance over manufacturing ones.[5] Others emphasize the sudden and historic influx of corporate dollars into lobbying and political campaigns as a key factor in "America's slow, steady slide toward economic oligarchy . . ."[6] In contrast to these more materialist interpretations, Daniel Stedman Jones, in his important study of the rise of neoliberalism, emphasizes the neoliberal victory in the war of *ideas* (albeit one that was made possible by the changing economic circumstances of the 1970s).[7]

Like all wars, this one was not won in a single battle. Jones discerns three main "phases" of neoliberalism.[8] The initial phase, which he describes as beginning in the interwar period and extending into the postwar era, saw the formation of an intellectual coalition of Austrian and German economists, most prominently Ludwig von Mises and Friedrich Hayek. His second phase extends from the 1950s to 1980, and it was during this period that a popularized version of neoliberal thought congealed as a powerful political program. "These US-based neoliberals," as he puts it, "formed the intellectual nodes at the heart of a transatlantic network of think tanks, businessmen, journalists, and politicians, who spread an increasingly honed political message of the superiority of free markets."[9] The third phase begins with the election of Margaret Thatcher in the United Kingdom and Ronald Reagan in the United States, and saw historic successes of the neoliberal program, at both the state and the international level. In these years, neoliberalism was advanced by key international institutions, including the International Monetary Fund (IMF), the World Bank (WB), and the World Trade Organization (WTO),[10] and this was to have a profound effect on the practical "right to health" in the developing world. One can perceive these developments coldly and rationally, but in truth, they caused much death and dismay and appropriately caused much revulsion.

In short, the ideology of the WB rapidly displaced that of Alma-Ata. Indeed, almost immediately after the passage of the Alma-Ata Declaration, some policymakers began arguing that it had gone too far. In a highly influential paper in the *New England Journal of Medicine* in 1979, two physicians argued that although the "goal set at Alma Ata is above reproach . . . its very scope makes it unattainable because of the cost and numbers of trained personnel required."[11] The authors instead argued for a form of "selective primary care directed at preventing or treating the few diseases" with the greatest impact. Lassa fever, for instance, carried a high mortality rate, but was only treatable by serum injection—and so was not a good target. Similarly, parasitic infection with the nematode Ascaris, though it caused widespread infection and disability, could only be controlled through prolonged courses of therapy, and so was also not worth the cost and effort. The authors were not even convinced that it was worthwhile to treat childhood pneumonia with antibiotics, even though this had become standard practice in high-income countries, and even though they themselves cited its life-saving effects in India! Overall, they favored a more cost-effective "selective approach" focusing on "a circumscribed number of diseases . . . in a clearly defined population," which for them meant children three years old and younger and women of childbearing age. This was a prescription for death.

Indeed, this vision is as stark a contrast to the broad vision enunciated in the WHO Constitution—and reconceptualized at Alma-Ata—as can be imagined, though it rapidly achieved a hegemonic position in global health discourse. That same year, the Rockefeller Foundation sponsored a conference in Italy organized around the *New England Journal* paper.[12] The conference was supported by the World Bank, influenced by US groups and ideas, and attended by the president of the World Bank as well as James Grant from UNICEF (who came away very influenced by what he had heard).[13] Grant—who became the executive director of UNICEF in 1980—thereafter embraced the principles of so-called "selective primary care," which in coming years was essentially reduced to four basic interventions (growth monitoring, oral rehydration, breastfeeding, and immunization—or the so-called "GOBI" interventions) for certain population groups *in lieu* of the comprehensive vision of universal primary healthcare promised at Alma-Ata.[14] "This narrow selection of specific conditions for these population groups," scholars later noted, "was designed to improve health statistics, but it abandoned Alma Ata's focus on social equity and health systems development."[15] Some have characterized this turn in even harsher terms, calling it a "massive assault on the intellect of public health workers," with people reduced to the "hapless recipients of prefabricated, market-driven, technocentric, and scientifically very questionable programs imposed by international agencies."[16] Others have similarly interpreted this turn as a regression to the "vertical programs" of an earlier era, with the community-centric ethos of Alma-Ata basically abandoned.[17]

Not all were in agreement with this shift in priorities away from a more rights-based framework, particularly within the WHO, which was increasingly at loggerheads with UNICEF in the debate over comprehensive versus selective primary healthcare in the coming years.[18] However, the WHO was increasingly marginalized during the 1980s, as a result of the emergence of stridently pro-market bodies like the WB and the action of conservative national governments, especially that of the United States. In the US, in part in response to pharmaceutical industry pressure, the Reagan administration promptly ceased all payments to the WHO's regular budget.[19] (Notably, the administration had already been in conflict with the WHO earlier in the decade over its anti-tobacco program and its efforts to regulate breast milk substitutes.)[20] As a result, by the early nineties, the WHO was "almost completely sidelined" in matters of global health policy.[21] So-called "extrabudgetary" funding from high-income nations and powerful groups like the World Bank for individual "vertical" health programs did provide much-needed funds for the WHO, but at the same time, this method of funding effectively subordinated the WHO to the prerogatives of these nations and international bodies.[22]

And just as the WHO was being sidelined, the WB began its rise as a commanding global health policy actor. It is difficult to not be impressed by its ability to first adopt a new vision of health, and then to shift the international discourse in its direction. By the early 1980s, it adopted a number of key neoliberal assumptions about healthcare, including an emphasis on cost sharing ("user fees"), privatization of care provision, private insurance, and health system austerity. There was nothing inevitable about this: it reflected the "capture" of the WB by neoliberal actors and ideas. Indeed, in its 1980 World Development Report, the WB had actually voiced *opposition* to user fees for basic goods like healthcare and endorsed the idea of healthcare as a human right.[23] This soon changed amidst the influx of new free market economists from the US and UK, and the WB began to embrace the emerging "conservative counter-narrative . . ."[24]

Then, over the course of the 1980s, the WB played an increasingly important role in funding healthcare projects in the developing world, which allowed it to impose its vision of commodified healthcare.[25] Some have noted a key "turning point" in 1981, with the publication of the WB report *Accelerated Development in Sub-Saharan Africa*, which emphasized private insurance, liberalization of the trade in pharmaceuticals, and user fees for health services.[26] "[G]overnments should seek ways to generate revenues from at least some beneficiaries of publicly provided health services . . ." it notes, continuing, "Methods such as industrial insurance schemes and user fees for public services may be unpopular, but may be the only alternative to systems which are too poor to provide many services at all."[27] The imposition of user fees was even more strongly articulated in two key later documents, *Paying for Health Services in Developing Countries: An Overview* (1985) and *Financing Healthcare: An Agenda for Reform* (1988).[28] The latter document laid out a vision of health system reform based on four key propositions: (1) the imposition of user fees for many health services (2) support for private insurance (3) an increased role for private (both for-profit and not-for-profit) organizations, and (4) "decentralization."[29] The promotion of user fees was probably the WB's most successful (and most deadly) program. The rationale behind it deserves a closer look.

The WB's proposal for user fees was clothed in the language of neoliberal economics, and was based on the argument that such fees would, paradoxically, *increase* healthcare access. Why would charging desperately poor people for healthcare help these folks, one might reasonably ask? Well first, as the document describes, fees would raise revenue for the government. And second, "higher charges could improve access of the poor to health services." For though for some it might appear that "free healthcare would make it easier for the poor to 'afford' services," in truth "appearances are deceptive." Free healthcare, according to the report, represented a subsidy to the rich; charging fees would thus generate revenue in order to "extend appropriate services to the underserved." And third, user fees would improve the efficiency of the overall healthcare system: fees deter frivolous use of healthcare, and "[c]onsumers will be more sensible in their demand for services."[30] This last point underscores a key principle of neoliberal healthcare ideology that has accrued great popularity in our own era: individuals need to have "skin in the game" so that they use healthcare wisely as diligent "customers." The emphasis on user fees, in other words, is based not only on practical considerations, but also on a distinct neoliberal ideological conceptualization of healthcare. The document notes that unlike vaccinations (which benefit society at large), "curative" care is essentially a consumer good that benefits only the particular individual who elects to purchase it: "[A]ll the benefits of a mended broken bone," it notes, "are captured by the patient." That is obviously incorrect (there is a benefit to society, even economically, in not having its population walking around on crutches), but it is nonetheless a wonderfully lucid distillation of neoliberal healthcare thought.

Admittedly, the document does also favor a form of "compulsory" health insurance so as to spread risk, but not a universal public system. "Only effective competition will guarantee that administrative costs will be minimized and a variety of options offered," it (incorrectly[31]) notes, and so "[w]henever possible, governments should thus avoid crowding out private insurers."[32] And although its emphasis on decentralization might seem laudable from the perspective of community-based healthcare, in reality, the WB's vision for decentralization entailed a retreat from solidarity and redistribution by shifting costs onto local governments, with individuals "transformed from citizens with a right to health into individually paying customers . . ."[33]

The neoliberal vision of the WB was further solidified by its 1993 World Development Report, *Investing in Health.* Health policy scholar John Lister has described the report as perhaps the WB's "most influential policy document" with respect to health policy, as it essentially "proposed the consolidation of a two-tier global health system . . ."[34] The document makes the case for the economic benefits of health system reform, and envisions a publicly-funded "nationally defined package of essential clinical services [that] would leave the remaining clinical services to be financed privately or by social insurance . . ."[35] The publicly-funded "minimum package of essential clinical services," however, would be restricted to cost-effective and mostly preventive measures, such as "sick-child care, family planning, prenatal and delivery care, and treatment for tuberculosis and STDs," and would generally exclude "expensive drug therapies for HIV" or cancer treatment "other than pain relief."[36] As others have noted, this two-tier health system approach represented a stark rejection of the ethical philosophy of healthcare rights. Rather than ensure equitable access to all, the state guarantees a form of Poor Law medicine for the poor (see Chapters 1 and 3), while the better-off buy healthcare to the extent that they can afford it, as consumers.[37]

Unfortunately, these documents were not mere academic think pieces. The WB had the economic muscle (and the political desire) to implement its ideas, in particular through its power over international lending. For example, the WB's recommendations on healthcare were translated into health policy through the "structural adjustment programs" of the 1990s,[38] which allowed lenders to impose conditions on debtor nations in exchange for the receipt of funds. As a backdrop, the global economic crisis of the 1970s had contributed to unsustainable debt in many low-income countries.[39] The IMF and the WB responded with bailouts attached to various "conditionalities" (such as reductions in public spending, liberalization of capital flows, privatization, and deregulation) that were to prove enormously detrimental both for countries' economies and the health of their citizens.[40] "These changes," it is noted, "greatly transformed the health sectors of dozens of developing countries as deep budget cuts, staff layoffs, and user fees were applied throughout the 1980s and 1990s; this had tragic consequences for millions of people who were too poor to afford the user fees."[41] In 1985, for instance, Ghana was required to cut public spending, which led to a steep increase in user fees for a wide range of medical services; reportedly, women would be detained after childbirth until they had paid their hospital bills.[42] Nigeria similarly acceded to a structural adjustment program in 1986, with terrible results: public expenditures decreased and user fees were implemented and raised.[43] Whereas the nation had something of a universal public system into the early years of the 1980s, in Nigeria more recently, approximately 70 percent of healthcare spending is "out of pocket."[44]

We will probably never know how many lives, precisely, were cut short as a result of the imposition of the neoliberal healthcare agenda on the African continent. Still, some general approximations can be made. One study, for example, used a simulation model to quantify the impact of these fees on the survival of children younger than five in twenty African nations.[45] The investigators estimated how user fees affected the use of common healthcare interventions for these children, and then estimated how the reduced use of these interventions affected survival. By their estimate, removing user fees might have led to approximately 233,000 fewer deaths annually. Even relying on their more conservative approximation, this would translate into millions of fewer deaths over two decades.[46]

Some argue, rather reasonably, that the structural adjustment policies of the WB or IMF should be seen as an explicit violation of the human right to health.[47] World Bank-imposed reductions in health spending constituted a violation of "the concept of progressive realization" of health as it is described in the ICESCR, and its policies "play a role in the inability of these countries to comply with their core obligations to realize the right to health."[48] And unfortunately, these developments unfolded in parallel with the deadly global explosion of HIV/AIDS, and indeed may have exacerbated the impact of the epidemic. STD clinics in Kenya, for example, began charging fees at this very time, deterring use.[49] Fortunately, as the evidence of harm mounted, activist campaigns succeeded in forcing the recalcitrant WB to (partially) retreat from its stance on fees.[50] Yet the WB's 2004 move to a "no blanket policy" stance on user fees was not accompanied by an embrace of free care for the poor, nor by an attempt to reverse fees where they had already been implemented.[51] Nor could it—nor can it—undo the grave harm that was already inflicted.

Healthcare and Neoliberalism: A Return to Chile, Nicaragua, China, Russia, and Cuba

The neoliberal healthcare agenda affected nations in different ways, and was often shaped by the political dynamics of the late Cold War. The last chapter discussed health system reforms in Chile, Nicaragua, China, Soviet Russia, and Cuba with respect to what they accomplished from the perspective of "health rights," and how they failed. It is worth briefly returning to these five nations, with an eye to how the dynamics of neoliberal health policy played out in each case.

As described in the last chapter, Chile had a relatively long history of state involvement in healthcare, which expanded in a promisingly more universal direction under the presidency of Salvador Allende. Yet, in the brief period following his overthrow and death, many of these reforms were rolled back. And subsequently, a neoliberal healthcare agenda was unflinchingly implemented during the years of the dictatorship of Augusto Pinochet. This is, of course, not surprising: Pinochet's Chile was famous for its role as a "laboratory" for the neoliberal economic ideas associated with Milton Friedman and the University of Chicago. This was prominently manifested in the arena of healthcare—indeed, along many of the same lines outlined by the WB—including reduced public expenditures, privatization, the promotion of private health insurance, an increase in user fees, and decentralization.

For example, from 1981 onward, individuals covered by the public social security system FONASA could instead elect to receive private health insurance through a new system called ISAPREs (Instituciones de Salud Previsional), a change described by some as "one of the most ambitious reform programs in the area of social services" that was carried out by Pinochet's regime.[52] The result was a deterioration in equitable access to healthcare, however. The ISAPREs tended to take on a population that was disproportionately young, healthy, wealthy, and male (indeed, some plans entirely excluded women of childbearing age).[53] Those from the middle class, in contrast, were more likely to be covered by the FONASA, which imposed high cost sharing (about half of the cost of both inpatient and outpatient care), while the poor were treated by the National Health Service System (SNSS, the previous NHS).[54] In 1977, fees were introduced for users of the SNSS, and in 1986, a new law required that SNSS users provide income information from their employer so as to set the level of cost sharing.[55]

Other aspects of the neoliberal healthcare agenda were also implemented under Pinochet. An agreement signed with the IMF in 1984, for instance, constrained public health spending.[56] And while public spending fell, private spending increased, a change endorsed by the 1987 WB report *Financing Health Services in Developing Countries*, as discussed earlier.[57] Following the Pinochet era, the new democratic government increased public spending on health, although the fragmentation and inequity that had been imposed by the neoliberal reforms of the Pinochet era remained.[58] In short, the combination of a military coup and neoliberal reform produced a sharp shift in the rights-commodity healthcare dialectic in Chile, one that contributed to the emergence of a less equitable health system.

There are clear parallels between the situation in Chile and that in Nicaragua. The last chapter explored the expansion of public healthcare under the Sandinista government, some elements of which could be interpreted as consistent with the principles of Alma-Ata. Yet whatever gains were made in that period were rapidly rolled back in the face of the brutal Contra war—supported and funded by an aggressive Reagan administration—which was accompanied by a policy of economic strangulation. The Contras firepower was aimed not merely at government troops, but at easier targets like health facilities. "Stop your medical work," threatened a note posted by Contra troops at one health clinic, "or we will burn the clinic and you with it."[59] It was not an idle threat. Tragically, over the course of the war, hospitals, health clinics, and schools were targeted by the Contras and destroyed; health workers and volunteer *brigadistas* were captured, tortured, and murdered; and various public health projects were aborted.[60] At the same time, the increasingly adverse fiscal state of the country led to a financial squeeze of the health sector.[61]

A more robust neoliberal healthcare turn, however, awaited 1990, when—facing both unceasing military and economic war—the Nicaraguan people voted the Sandinistas out of power, and Violeta Chamorro as the new president.[62] The changes instituted by the Chamorro government did much to recommodify healthcare in Nicaragua in the 1990s along the various policy lines endorsed by the World Bank. First, there was austerity: in response to rising foreign debt and pressure from the IMF and WB, the government drastically reduced spending.[63] Between 1990 and 1995, for instance, there was a 40 percent reduction in public health spending.[64] Second, there was an increase in user fees: although small fees had been instituted by the Sandinistas in the mid-1980s in a time of financial stress, the Chamorro government created a new system of fees, including ones for primary care, which had previously been exempted.[65] Third was decentralization, another one of the four policies advocated by the WB in 1987. While decentralization, at face value, might seem logical—i.e., a shift of control of health resources to the community level, where needs can be more accurately assessed—in reality, the "main outcome" of decentralization in Nicaragua, scholars argue, was "a dismantling of the principles and structures of universality, accessibility, and primary care that were developed under the Sandinistas."[66] Fourth was privatization: as public provision fell, private provision—and private insurance—rose.[67] "[P]rivate practice came back with a vengeance," while, at the same time, the deterioration of public provision resulted in declining preventive visits for things like nutritional care.[68] The cumulative effect of these developments was a clear shift in the rights-commodity dialectic: those who could afford superior private care bought it, while those who could not were left with an inferior, deteriorating public system.[69]

Thus, in the case of both Chile and Nicaragua, US intervention sadly contributed to right-wing political change, which led to the embrace and imposition of neoliberal economic reforms that, in turn, resulted in dramatic shifts within the rights-commodity dialectic of these nations. "Foreign" pressure, however, was by no means a necessary precondition for nations to take steps in this direction. China is a good example. As discussed in the last chapter, an expansion of public healthcare did occur under Mao, particularly in rural areas, which may have contributed to the impressive improvement of life expectancy in China over this era. However, even putting aside the terrible health consequences stemming from the monstrous human rights record of the regime, the system had a multitude of weaknesses from the perspective of health equity and health rights. Change, therefore, was needed, though two very different paths existed: one towards more universal and comprehensive coverage, and the other towards greater inequity and commodification. There might have been, in other words, either a leftward or a rightward shift in the rights-commodity dialectic.

It was to be the latter. Criticism of this turn does not merely come from left-wing sources. In a 2005 *New England Journal of Medicine* article entitled "Privatization and its Discontents—the Evolving Chinese Healthcare System," mainstream US health policy scholars David Blumenthal and William Hsiao wrote: "Ironically, the citizens of the United States, a bastion of capitalism, now enjoy far more protection against the cost of illness than the citizens of China, a nominally socialist nation."[70] The health sector was not excluded, it turned out, from the market-oriented reforms of Deng Xiaoping, and the public system rapidly withered as a result. Beginning in the 1980s, the Chinese healthcare system began to undergo a transformation roughly analogous to the sorts of neoliberal changes experienced by other nations: (1) a fall in healthcare spending by the central government (2) effective decentralization of healthcare funding to provincial and local governments, resulting in funding deficits that had to be covered by increased out-of-pocket payments by patients (3) the end of the cooperative medical system, which had previously provided free care in rural areas, and its replacement by fee-for-service care (4) "financial independence" for hospitals, which increasingly relied on user fees from patients, and (5) the emergence of new modes of payment, including private insurance.[71] The new out-of-pocket payments worsened the economic position of poor families,[72] the decentralization of funding increased inequities in healthcare between urban and rural areas, and the end of the communes "rip[ped] apart the healthcare safety net for most of rural China."[73] Barefoot doctors lost their jobs and began instead supplying expensive healthcare services, despite their lack of qualifications, for cash.[74] A supercharged commercial ethos suffused the health-care system, resulting in falling quality, declining respect for doctors, rising corruption, and high prices.[75] As a result, as Hsiao has noted, "[i]n China's privatized, market-based healthcare system, the wealth of consumers is a critical determinant of both their access to services and the quality of services they receive."[76]

The neoliberal healthcare agenda pursued with a vengeance in China in the 1980s and 1990s facilitated an impressive rightward shift in the rights-commodity healthcare dialectic. More recent reforms, some achieved and some proposed, could conceivably broaden China's health system in a more universal direction.[77] Yet even with coverage widening under new insurance schemes, serious inequities and shortcomings remain. The government seems determined to continue to nurture the growth of a for-profit hospital sector,[78] for instance, while the new coverage schemes still result in high levels of cost sharing (i.e., user fees).[79] Additionally, the use of medical savings accounts in these insurance schemes—in which members make contributions to dedicated accounts to be used for healthcare—is funda-mentally inequitable.[80] Time will tell how "universal" China's new universal health reforms will, in practice, actually prove to be.

Next is post-Soviet Russia. As described in the last chapter, although the Soviet health system represented an advance in access to healthcare, its health system increasingly failed the nations' citizens as it was deprived of resources. Indeed, as noted, although deaths amenable to medical intervention were fairly similar in the UK and Russia in the 1960s, in subsequent decades they steadily fell in the former but remained largely unchanged in the latter, contributing to a widening gap in life expectancy between the two nations.[81] However, with the end of Communism, the situation in Russia only further deteriorated, as neoliberal "shock therapy" policies—in part designed by economists like Jeffrey Sachs—wrought economic and human disaster on a gargantuan scale. For some post-Communist countries—especially Russia—shock therapy meant the mass privatization of large industries, which in turn led to skyrocketing unemployment, increased psychosocial stress, a rise in unhealthy behaviors like alcohol use, increased suicides, and a historic fall in life expectancy.[82] Two researchers who have studied the health impact of the transition from Communism describe how some 10 million Russian men essentially "disappeared" in the 1990s, constituting the worst demographic disaster in any country on the globe in the post-Second World War era that wasn't in the middle of a conflict or a famine.[83] The deterioration, however, was not only in health, but in healthcare, with reduced healthcare access as the health system faced austerity, privatization, and an increase in user fees.[84] Although the contribution of changes in healthcare access to changes in life expectancy is unclear, one study did show that mortality amenable to medical intervention shot up sharply in the 1990s in post-Soviet Russia.[85]

Finally, a country that resisted this neoliberal turn was Cuba. The island nation created a system of universal healthcare in the 1960s and 1970s that has undoubtedly contributed to its superior health outcomes. Of course, this system was (and is) imperfect. Some contend, for instance, that the polyclinic system suffered from a lack of care continuity and an insufficient emphasis on preventive care.[86] These inadequacies helped lead to the major health system reform Cuba undertook in the 1980s, referred to as the "Family Doctor Program." [87] This new program can be seen as an embrace of the community-oriented health rights focus of Alma-Ata, albeit oriented around doctors, not lower-level health workers.[88] Indeed Cuba "remained devoted to the Alma-Ata vision and added new features to its own healthcare system every decade to make that vision become a reality"— even after the onset of enormous economic strain following the collapse of the Soviet Union.[89] As part of the Family Doctor Program, neighborhood-based teams of doctors and nurses have taken on responsibility for the care of all of the individuals within their circumscribed geographical area.[90] Everyone receives one or more annual visits (depending on medical needs), while those requiring specialist care can be directed to polyclinics for higher-level care.[91] These teams typically have to live in the very neighborhoods they care for, and are responsible for both direct clinical care and population health.[92]

Whatever one thinks of other aspects of the Cuban regime, it is difficult not to acknowledge its important advances in healthcare: it has achieved universal coverage, highly impressive health metrics, and marked success in reducing health inequalities, while also sending enormous numbers of clinicians abroad for humanitarian missions.[93] In 2009, for instance, Cuba had twice as many doctors per capita as the United States, in addition to some 20,000 serving on international missions abroad in poor nations.[94] Notwithstanding real flaws,[95] it seems fair to conclude that a right to quality healthcare was created in Cuba to a degree unique among low-income countries.[96] Moreover, this right was maintained into the neoliberal era, despite highly adverse economic conditions, even as it retreated in so many other nations. The nation's achievements in health have been well recognized, even by those critical of the government in other respects. Following the death of Fidel Castro in November 2016, for instance, David Blumenthal of the *Commonwealth Fund* asserted that "[w]hen it comes to healthcare, Cuba is a success story with few parallels . . . Cuba has demonstrated that a poor country can dramatically improve the health of its population through long-term, consistent investments in primary care and public health."[97]

Notably, the evolution of this right in Cuba largely preceded the rise to prominence of the "right to health" as an ethos and a movement, similar to the case of the British NHS. However, in nations where creating a "right to health" through legislation was precluded by the domestic political context, the "right to health" movement had a significant impact in the coming decades, as examined in subsequent sections.

HIV/AIDS and the Human Right to Health Movement

Although the human right—including the human right to health—emerged in international law in the wake of the Second World War, it was decades before the "right to health" would became an important discourse and paradigm. Indeed, in the early postwar decades, as Moyn has argued, human rights (across the board) went into a hibernation of sorts, embraced by neither the anticolonial movement nor the great powers.[98] Moyn argues that it was the very death of alternative political visions—including a more democratic socialism in both the East (after the Prague Spring) and the West (after the Chilean coup against Allende)—that laid the groundwork for the re-emergence of the human rights discourse in the late 1970s.[99] Yet, within this new human rights discourse, social and economic rights had a much smaller role than they had in the rights discourse of the 1940s, at least initially.[100] And while the Declaration of Alma-Ata might be seen as an exception to this, it is generally true that the human right to health did not become a distinct and prominent discourse and movement until the 1990s.[101]

Why did it emerge only in the 1990s? Scholars Colleen Flood and Aeyal Gross outline seven developments that contributed to the resurgence of concern with the right to health: (1) the political impact of the end of the Cold War (2) rising concern over social and economic rights in low-income and postcolonial countries (3) the emergence of the HIV epidemic (4) the inclusion of health rights in many new constitutions, especially in Latin America and Africa (5) the impact of the neoliberal economic agenda, like structural adjustment (6) the galvanizing role of free trade agreements, which often restricted access to medications (including for HIV/AIDS), and (7) market-based health system reforms, including in high-income nations.[102] The remainder of this chapter will explore each factor not already covered in varying degrees of detail, starting with the emergence of HIV/AIDS.

The rise of the HIV/AIDS epidemic is rightly seen as a crucial trigger of the health rights movement. Jonathan Wolff, for instance, documents the connections between the two, noting that "HIV/AIDS gave the human right to health movement an impetus and a clear focus." HIV/AIDS human rights activism proceeded in two distinct waves: in the first, the primary rights concern was that of *discrimination*, and in the second, it was the right to HIV *treatment*.[103]

As one history of the movement describes, early activism around HIV/AIDS played a critically important role in shaping both discourse and policy in the early years of the epidemic.[104] An early wave of activists—gay men predominantly from

New York and San Francisco who were themselves living with HIV/AIDS—organized against the stigmatization and marginalization of those with AIDS which amounted to "social death" for these individuals that preceded their physical death.[105] The activists came together in Colorado in 1983 and promulgated the influential "Denver Principles," a "Statement From the Advisory Committee of People with AIDS" that reads as a manifesto against the discrimination, exclusion, marginalization, and neglect of those living with AIDS.[106] The document included recommendations for better care and awareness from healthcare professionals; support for the "struggle" against discrimination in the workplace, in housing, and in the community; political action by those living with AIDS; and, more generally, the protection of the "rights of people with AIDS."[107] Notable among these rights is the right to "receive quality medical treatment ... without discrimination of any form, including sexual orientation, gender, diagnosis, economic status or race." Joe Wright argues that the principles of this early activism had a critical influence on later AIDS activism, including on the US advocacy group ACT UP and the Treatment Action Campaign (TAC) in South Africa. He argues that later, "[T]he global legacy of the People With AIDS agenda was to persistently reduce seemingly complex policy debates to their simple essence: should people living with HIV die of a treatable disease to support other competing priorities? Because activists helped simplify and then answer the myriad forms of that question, millions of people lived who otherwise would have died."[108]

By the 1990s, "human rights" had become an important organizing framework in global health circles as well. Jonathan Mann, while directing the WHO's Global Program on AIDS, came to a novel articulation of the relationship between "human rights" and the HIV/AIDS epidemic.[109] Following a request for assistance from the government of Uganda to deal with its worsening epidemic, the WHO formed a new body, the Global Program on AIDS (GPA), headed by Mann, in 1987.[110] Mann was responsible for the formation of a human rights office within GPA, and his advocacy of a nondiscriminatory approach towards people living with HIV/AIDS helped lead to an important 1988 resolution by the World Health Assembly as well as the first WHO Global AIDS Strategy, both of which condemned discrimination against those living with HIV/AIDS.[111] Mann was also responsible for the WHO's Global Strategy on AIDS, a document that explicitly argued against discrimination and for access to healthcare for those living with the disease.[112]

In the early years of the epidemic, nations relied on traditional (often discriminatory) public health tools to deal with the epidemic: quarantines, mandatory testing, restrictions on travel, and so forth.[113] These measures, for instance, were employed against HIV-positive Haitian refugees in a particularly reprehensible fashion in the early 1990s by the US government.[114] Mann turned this traditional thinking on its head. He argued that respect for the civil and political rights of those living with HIV/AIDS would actually help control the epidemic, whereas a punitive approach would merely drive those with the disease—who were often already marginalized and excluded—underground.[115] This argument is sometimes referred to as the "AIDS Paradox," which is essentially the idea that the "most effective way of preventing the spread of the virus responsible for AIDS is by protecting the human rights of those most at risk."[116]

Mann perceived a changing tide at the WHO, however, with the departure of Halfdan Mahler in 1988 (who, as described in the last chapter, had overseen the formulation of the Declaration of Alma-Ata) and his replacement by Hiroshi Nakajima, who at one point suggested that there might be a tradeoff between the rights of those with AIDS and those of members of society at large.[117] Still, Mann's health rights advocacy continued after he left the WHO in 1992: in subsequent years, he was involved in the founding of the François-Xavier Bagnoud Center for Health and Human Rights at the Harvard School of Public Health, and he became the editor of a new journal, *Health and Human Rights*, in 1994.[118]

It is worth noting, however, that even at this stage, an equal right to *healthcare* was not necessarily the central concern of such activists, policymakers, and scholars. In the first issue of *Health and Human Rights*, for instance, Mann had proposed a "three-part framework" on the intersection between health and human rights.[119] The first of his health–human rights relationships stresses how public health measures and policies can have human rights ramifications; the second emphasizes how human rights violations themselves affect health, and the third proposes that the "promotion and protection of human rights and promotion and protection of health are fundamentally linked."[120] Less is said, however, about an intrinsic human right to *equal medical care*. Broadly speaking, Mann explains, "individual and population vulnerability to disease, disability and premature death is linked to the status of respect for human rights and dignity."[121] An enormous range of concerns thus fell under the umbrella of "health and human rights," and the right to healthcare itself was only one concern among them. NGOs took this doctrine in a variety of directions in coming years. The organization Physicians for Human Rights, formed in the mid-1980s, for instance, conducted on-the-ground studies of the ways in which traditional violations of human rights impacted health.[122] Others, in the tradition of nineteenth-century social medicine, focused on the "societal roots of health problems,"[123] like the intersection of the "environmental health dimension" with the right to health.[124] Advocacy of a universal right to *healthcare*, in contrast, was to some extent a delayed development.

The embrace of a right to healthcare was perhaps fostered by technological change. The 1990s saw the development of increasingly effective treatments ("antiretroviral therapy," or ART) that turned HIV/AIDS into a treatable condition. "ART brought a human injustice into focus—those who could not afford treatment had no less right to live," notes one history of the epidemic, "than people who could afford treatment."[125] And indeed, by 1998, Mann was arguing that the lack of access to HIV treatment was itself a form of discrimination,[126] essentially affirming a human right to healthcare. More broadly, however, there was no consensus among power-brokers that life-saving ART could—or should—be made universally available to the poor in low-income nations, even though these nations were facing the greatest burden of disease. Indeed, even the WHO and UNAIDS (the organization that took over HIV/AIDS policy from GPA) contended that ART was not cost-effective.[127] Yet these organizations failed in their narrow view of political economy. The *only* the reason why ART was not cost-effective was because the pharmaceutical industry priced these drugs out of reach of the budgets of the health systems of poor nations, an artifact of patent monopolies. The new neoliberal economic order, in turn, had helped to ensure that this remained the rule of law throughout the globe. Antiretroviral drugs were, it was argued, a commodity, made available not on the basis of needs (i.e., infection by HIV), but by economic means.

Thankfully, it is here where activists—articulating an explicit doctrine of the right to health—fought back. In part, they relied on developments in the realm of law. At this historic juncture, a "right to health" was increasingly diffusing into both international law and national constitutions.

The Right to Health in Law: International and Domestic

The international political order underwent a profound—and largely unpredicted —transformation with startling rapidity in 1991. The Soviet Union collapsed, the Cold War came to a close, and a new era began. The end of the Cold War, some argue, "mark[ed] the most significant paradigm shift in the history of the right to health," for it helped to usher in a new emphasis on social and economic rights within the human rights hierarchy.[128] In 1993, the Vienna Declaration, the result of the World Conference on Human Rights, posited the "interdependence and interrelatedness of all human rights," suggesting that "economic, social and cultural rights are to be treated with the same emphasis as and on an equal footing with civil and political rights."[129] This document references the right to health in several places, such as the "rights of everyone to a standard of living adequate for their health and well-being, including food and medical care, housing and the necessary social services."[130]

Subsequent years also saw efforts to "mainstream" the human right to health within the WHO, as well as the elucidation of the meaning of the human right to health in international law at the UN.[131] Until the 1990s, the actual "right to health" obligations for states under international law (as outlined in Article 12 of the ICESCR, for instance) were largely unclear.[132] The Committee on Economic, Social and Cultural Rights, formed in 1985 for the purpose of overseeing the ICESCR, moved to clarify the meaning of Article 12 with its 2000 "General Comment 14," a milestone document for the right to health in international law that bears the obvious influence of the Declaration of Alma-Ata.[133] This document frankly acknowledges the distance between the goal of the right to health and the lived reality for much of the globe.[134] It recognizes the (commonsensical) notion that the right to health is "not to be understood as a right to be healthy," but that it is instead a combination of "freedoms" from certain harms as well as "entitle-ments" to a "system of health protection which provides equality of oppor-tunity for people to enjoy the highest attainable level of health," which includes both healthcare and access to the "underlying determinants of health . . ."[135] It outlines the AAAQ schema of the meaning of the right to health for states parties, which must ensure the "availability" of "health-care facilities, goods and services"; their "accessibility" on a nondiscriminatory basis; their cultural and ethical "acceptability" to all groups and individuals; and the scientific and medical "quality" of health services.[136]

Perhaps most importantly, the General Comment clarified the meaning of the "progressive realization" of economic and social rights. Article 2 of the ICESCR had stated that each state party was to "take steps . . . with a view to achieving progressively the full realization of the rights recognized in the present Covenant . . ."[137] Yet this clause, as many note, arguably opened the door to limitless delays in actually expanding healthcare access. General Comment 14, in contrast, clarified that this provision does not give states the right to endlessly put off the implementation of healthcare rights, but instead requires that they "move as expeditiously and effectively as possible towards the full realization of article 12" and avoid taking any "retrogressive" steps.[138] It also drew on a previously described framework in which states had three levels of rights obligations: "to respect, protect, and fulfill."[139] Finally, and most importantly, General Comment 14 suggests that there are certain "core obligations" that states must ensure outside the confines of "progressive realization," among which include access to healthcare on a "non-discriminatory basis," "essential drugs," and the "equitable distribution of all health facilities, goods, and services."[140] "[A] State party cannot," it notes, "under any circumstances whatsoever, justify its non-compliance with the core obligations . . ."[141] This delineation of a set of "core obligations" that cannot be delayed under the principle of "progressive realization" was a major leap beyond Article 12 of the ICESCR.[142]

The UN Commission on Human Rights also embraced economic and social rights in the post-Cold War era. Whereas prior to the World Conference on Human Rights in Vienna, the body had mainly focused on civil and political rights, in the 1990s and 2000s, it began to focus increasingly on socioeconomic rights.[143] At the urging of Brazil and other developing nations, and over the votes of the US and Australia, the UN Commission on Human Rights established a "Special Rapporteur on the Right to Health" in 2002.[144] The first Special Rapporteur, Paul Hunt, saw his role as heavily shaped by the principles of General Comment 14, and later described three primary goals of his work: amplifying the human rights discourse on the international stage, clarifying the meaning of the right, and investigating how it might be operationalized.[145] The work to define the realization of the right to health led to a study, published in the *Lancet*, that sought to define the extent to which nations around the world were progressing towards a right to health. However, the study, which concluded that "those with responsibilities for health systems are giving inadequate attention to the right-to-health analysis," seemed more concerned with right to health metrics, the legal recognition of a right to health, and disaggregated data collection than with the very foundation of the right to healthcare—universal healthcare without financial barriers.[146]

But how important and meaningful was the advance of the human right to health in international law, from its earliest days in the WHO Constitution and the UDHR, to its clarification in the ICESCR (and various other UN treaties), to its more egalitarian articulation in Alma-Ata, and to its detailed delineation in General Comment 14? On one level, as scholar John Tobin plainly notes in his landmark study on the right to health, "the fact that there is a right to health in international law is now beyond dispute."[147] But how much does it *actually* matter in light of the relative weakness of international law? The international "right to health" does not prescribe (much less mandate) that a certain percentage of a state's resources go towards health, but instead requires only that a state take on the task of progressively providing a right to health, in light of its own resources and limitations.[148] Although these declarations and treaties have shaped the international discourse around health rights, their ability to compel nations to create systems of universal healthcare is limited. As Flood and Gross note, the advance of the right to health in international law may be "inspiring and influential," but at the same time, it collides directly with the basic reality of state sovereignty.[149] That is not to say that it has had no impact in the domestic sphere: as they note, domestic courts sometimes turn to international treaties in their deliberations, which can thereby function as "an important normative force."[150] Still, in the final analysis, the creation of a right to health necessitates the creation of health systems by national governments, something no supranational body or treaty can do.

Notably, however, alongside the congealing and strengthening of the right to health in international law were parallel developments in domestic law. Many states in this era created new constitutions that incorporated socioeconomic rights, including that of healthcare. Indeed, by 2011, more than half of all UN member states had a right to medical services, either as a guarantee or an aspiration, in their constitutions.[151] The incorporation of health rights into state constitutions increased rapidly in the final decades of the twentieth century: whereas only a third of constitutions adopted before 1970 had one or more health right protection, 60 percent of constitutions adopted in the 1970s did, followed by 75 percent in the 1980s, 94 percent of those in the 1990s, and 97 percent of those in the 2000s.[152]

Perhaps the most famous inclusion of socioeconomic rights within a new national constitution took place in South Africa. After decades of struggle, apartheid rule was finally brought to an end in the early 1990s. The end of apartheid, the release of Nelson Mandela from decades of imprisonment, the holding of free elections, and the election of the African National Congress (ANC) to the government proceeded rapidly, albeit during years of continued political strife. Following the 1994 elections, the legislature set out to draft a new constitution.[153] Though not all were in agreement with the inclusion of socioeconomic rights in this document—some thought they would allow the courts to impinge on the prerogatives of the legislature—they ultimately achieved a prominent place in the Bill of Rights of the new constitution, which went into effect in 1997.[154] Section 27 of the South African Bill of Rights declares a universal right to "healthcare services, including reproductive healthcare," "sufficient food and water," "social security," and "emergency medical treatment." The section notably includes a provision that echoes the progressive realization principle of the ICESCR: "The state must take reasonable legislative and other measures, within its available resources, to achieve the progressive realization of each of these rights."[155] Along similar lines, Section 28 notes that all children have a right to "basic nutrition, shelter, basic healthcare services and social services . . ." Although this was to some extent a strong articulation of a right to healthcare, some have described the language of Section 27 as a "markedly narrower formulation" than the "highest attainable standard" found in international law, insofar as the latter imposed a requirement for a broader swath of public health measures.[156] Yet others stress that the positive right provided by Section 27 speaks to the core principles of availability, accessibility, acceptability, and quality (AAAQ) outlined in General Comment 14, and that it effectively compels the government to realize the right to health through the provision of health services on the basis of need.[157]

But what was to be the actual impact of the new positive rights found in the constitutions being written or modified in this era? On the one hand, a right to healthcare need not, as in the case of the UK or Canada, be based on a constitutional right to healthcare. Moreover, it is clear that the adoption of a constitutional right to healthcare does not suddenly catalyze the formation of a universal, equitable system of healthcare. The impact of constitutional rights to healthcare is complex, differing from nation to nation. However, more and more, they are being used to litigate the right to health services in nations throughout the globe. And in South Africa, the constitutional right to health was used to create a right of access to life-saving HIV medications. Yet even as the notion of a right to medicines emerged through this and other struggles, a paradoxical and contrary process of medicine commodification was simultaneously occurring.

Medicines and the Rights–Commodity Dialectic: The Case of South Africa

The combination of the global neoliberal turn and the ravages of the HIV/AIDS epidemic cast into sharp relief the meaning of the healthcare rights-commodity dialectic for medicines. As seen earlier in the chapter, the IMF and the WHO, undergirded by the economic strength of wealthy nations, used their power to advance the privatization and commodification of health services. When it came to drugs, however, the more important transnational body was the World Trade Organization (WTO). The WTO, the pharmaceutical industry, and governments of high-income nations sought to ensure that drugs remained a patent-protected commodity throughout the globe, which had deadly consequences in the case of HIV/AIDS. At the same time, activists throughout the world pushed back against the WTO's hegemonic position, using the framework of the human right to health.

In 1995, the responsibilities of the General Agreement on Tariffs and Trades (GATT), which had been designed after the Second World War to facilitate trade negotiations between nations, was assumed by the newly formed WTO.[158] While some have emphasized how the WTO worked to accelerate the evolution of a privatized, international healthcare industry,[159] its role in the protection of pharmaceutical patents was more impactful. As Smith et al. emphasize, the combination of the globalization of the international pharmaceutical market and the lack of patent protection for drugs in the developing world led high-income nations to push for the adoption of the TRIPS agreement (Trade-Related Aspects of Intellectual Property Rights) at the WTO. TRIPS greatly strengthened patent protection for pharmaceuticals on the global stage, giving at least twenty years of protection for drugs (although low-income nations were given extra time to comply).[160] This brought about a "giant shift in the global market for medicines," with noncompliance punishable by trade sanctions.[161] There were also some protections, however. The agreement contained "flexibilities" (later confirmed by the so-called Doha Declaration) that allowed states to undertake such measures as "compulsory licensing" (i.e., they could give a national drug producer permission to produce the patented drug) and "parallel import" (i.e., they could import the drug from a nation that did not respect the patent) when required for public health reasons.[162] Yet nations' efforts actually to utilize these flexibilities have been curtailed by the power of high-income nations, together with that of the pharmaceutical industry itself.[163]

As a result of these dynamics, by the end of the twentieth century, HIV/AIDS drugs—which at that point were highly effective at controlling the virus and saving lives—were deemed too expensive for poor countries, including by the WHO and UNAIDS.[164] That the new HIV/AIDS drugs might be provided to the poor of Africa was deemed entirely infeasible, and that drug prices might be lowered was seen as an intolerable infringement on drug patents and global trade pacts.[165] But many of those poor people—allied with activists around the globe—saw things rather differently.

As Lisa Forman narrates, in the late 1990s, both the US government and a number of pharmaceutical companies sought to use legal challenges and trade threats to prevent the government of South Africa from using a law (the "Medicines Act") that would allow it to produce and obtain medications cheaply. "A dramatic global battle for AIDS medicines ensued," she writes, "coalescing around moral arguments and human rights claims for medicines and mass actions by social networks of health and human rights activists."[166] In the United States, for instance, activists targeted Vice President Al Gore, whose presidential campaign had benefited from the largesse of the pharmaceutical lobby and who had (according to the State Department) undertaken an "assiduous, concerted campaign" to convince South African President Thabo Mbeki to modify this new pharmaceutical law to protect the industry.[167] Activists from ACT-UP and the group AIDS Drugs for Africa followed Gore around the campaign trail, chanting such things as "Gore's greed kills."[168] As a result of such pressures, the US eventually backed away from its trade threats, although the pharmaceutical industry then responded by directly challenging the law in South African courts.[169]

The pharmaceutical companies' suit was met by a major mobilization of civil society groups in South Africa, including the Treatment Action Campaign (TAC), which had been founded a few years earlier by Zackie Achmat, a long-time left-wing political activist as well as a gay man living with AIDS.[170] To an extent, the TAC drew on ideas from American AIDS activists (such as "treatment literacy") and formed connections with such groups as Gay Men's Health Crisis and ACT-UP, which came to South Africa in 1999.[171] From the beginning, TAC activists saw their mission in terms of the language of rights—"the right of access to treatment"—to be won predominantly through grassroots activism, but also through legal action.[172] The TAC worked with organizations both domestically and internationally to mount an enormous public campaign just as the pharmaceutical companies' case against the Medicines Act was starting.[173] They succeeded in shaming the pharmaceutical industry on the world stage to a sufficient degree that it ultimately withdrew its case against the law, perhaps realizing that it had more to lose in the court of public opinion than it had to gain financially from a successful suit.[174]

Notably, the TAC introduced the language of the "human right to health" into this struggle. As Forman notes, until the TAC joined the government's case, human rights were little invoked by either party. However, the TAC injected human rights arguments into the case, contending that the human right to health in the South African constitution gave the government the authority to pass the Medicines Act, and that this right should supersede the property rights of corporations.[175] The combination of the TAC's activism in the streets and the mobilization of international allies abroad was probably just as important as what transpired in the courtroom.[176] The impact of this campaign was enormous: the defeat of the pharmaceutical industry led to a sort of "norm cascade," helping to lead not only to the Doha Declaration—which theoretically strengthened the TRIPS flexibilities that gave nations the ability to produce or purchase inexpensive drugs—but also to an increase in international financial commitments for fighting the epidemic as well as further reductions in drug prices for poor nations.[177]

Yet the TAC earned its international fame in a battle not against the pharmaceutical industry, but against the South African government itself. This struggle led to what is perhaps the most famous "right to healthcare" legal case, *Minister of Health and Others v. Treatment Action Campaign and Others*. Although South Africa's post-apartheid constitution guaranteed a range of socioeconomic rights, including healthcare, how the courts would apply these provisions was unclear. Indeed, the "first major case" dealing with a socioeconomic right— *Soobramoney v. Minister of Health* (1997)—left some doubt about the actual meaning of these rights, to the disappointment of some rights activists.[178] Mr. Soobramoney was an unemployed man with chronic kidney disease who required hemodialysis to survive, which he was unable to afford at a private hospital.[179] The public health system, however, only had a limited number of dialysis machines, and so it only offered dialysis to those with chronic kidney disease who were eligible for a kidney transplantation (and he was not).[180] The Constitutional Court found that this hospital's system for allocating dialysis was not in fact in violation of Section 27, which as noted affirmed the right to healthcare. It argued that, where resources are limited, rationing decisions must be made. In this particular case, it found the hospitals' guidelines to be a "rational response to scarce resources which maximized the number of people who could access dialysis."[181]

Essentially, the court was relying on the "progressive realization" clause of Section 27, which is consistent with a similar provision in the ICESCR.[182] No doubt, this may seem rather reasonable: all health systems must make allocation decisions that are invariably constrained by resource availability. If a low-income nation elects not to develop a lung transplantation program, and instead allocates its healthcare resources to programs that yield greater overall societal benefit, is this an implicit violation of the right to health? Few would contend so. On the other hand, some have criticized the *Soobramoney* ruling from a rights perspective. The ruling, they argue, gave excessive leeway to the executive branch, did little positively to define the meaning of socioeconomic rights, and failed to at least consider international treaties (like ICESCR) as the Constitution directs it to do.[183] Moreover, because the Court narrowed its gaze to the "available resources" clause of Section 27, and not as much to the "progressive realization" clause, it avoided the question of whether the government was indeed actually working towards the progressive expansion of access.[184]

In contrast, the 2000 *Grootboom* case (*Government of the Republic of South Africa and Others v. Grootboom and Others*) initiated a new era of socioeconomic rights litigation, albeit with respect to housing, not healthcare. The plaintiffs in the case had been evicted by the state from private land without any provision for housing or other basic necessities.[185] However, although this decision was celebrated as a milestone in the litigation of socioeconomic rights (the Court decided in favor of the plaintiffs), it was actually narrow in scope and, as a result, may have limited the impact of future socioeconomic rights litigation. While the Court found that, under a "reasonableness standard," the State had failed to fulfill its obligations under Section 26 of the Constitution, it also argued against the notion that there were "minimum core" obligations to provide a particular set of housing services, as General Comment 14 had argued in the case of healthcare.[186] In any event, the ultimate outcome for the plaintiff, Irene Grootboom, demonstrates the shortcomings of rights litigation: she died "homeless and penniless" eight years after the decision.[187]

However, it was the case *Minister of Health and Others v. Treatment Action Campaign and Others* that turned the tide for health rights. As described earlier, the TAC had initially focused its activism on the pharmaceutical industry, succeeding, for instance, in getting companies to drop their suit against the Medicines Act. Yet its efforts to expand access to HIV treatment soon brought it into conflict with the ANC government itself, which was reluctant to make these now affordable—and sometimes free—medications widely available. A major barrier was President Thabo Mbeki's unfortunate embrace of discredited science about HIV, and his championing of an "African" solution to the epidemic (for instance, he backed an unsafe and ineffective South African-produced drug).[188] The *TAC* case hinged on the government's failure to make nevirapine—to which it had free access—available to pregnant women with HIV, for whom it had been proven highly efficacious in stopping vertical transmission.

Beginning in 1999, TAC pressed the government for its reasons for not making nevirapine widely available. In 2000, the government announced that it would make the drug available at only two sites in each of the nations' nine provinces. When again pushed by TAC for its reasons for pursuing such a limited strategy of dispensing a free medication, the government proceeded to question the efficacy of the drug and to cite the cost of the health infrastructure needed to provide it.

TAC then sued the government, contending first that the denial of nevirapine to pregnant women was constitutionally unreasonable, and second that the government was constitutionally mandated to establish a comprehensive program to block vertical transmission. The suit thus drew on both Section 27 (i.e., the right to healthcare) and Section 28 (i.e., the rights of children) of the Bill of Rights. The Constitutional Court decided, in contrast to the *Soobramoney* case, that the government had indeed failed to demonstrate reasonableness in its policy. Its concerns about the safety of the drug, for instance, were belied by its use in a limited number of public sites and by its common use in the private health sector. The Court required that the government make the drug available in the public health system and set up a comprehensive program to deal with the problem of vertical transmission.[189]

However, as in the *Grootboom* case, the Court again failed to embrace the idea of the "minimum core" of services to which all members of society had a right, as some have noted. It stated, for instance, that it would be "impossible to give everyone access even to a 'core' service immediately," and that one could only expect that the government progressively realize socioeconomic rights.[190] Thus, "the judgement can be seen," Forman argues, "to illustrate the Court's effort to guard a strong judicial role in enforcing the right to health, while at the same time signaling its self-restraint to government."[191] The case is nonetheless clearly a milestone in the litigation of the right to health. Clearly, the popular mobilization that preceded, accompanied, and followed the case was at least as important as the case itself, if not even more so. Indeed, continued political pressure and legal challenges from TAC and others pushed the South African government to establish what has been described as "the fastest growing ARV treatment programme in the world."[192] The benefits—in terms of lives saved and suffering averted—have been incalculable.

These South African campaigns, considered together, constitute a heroic turning point in the "right to health" grassroots movement. However, it is also important to acknowledge the limitations of the "right to health" in South Africa. Even today, its healthcare system remains riven by entrenched inequalities. As in so many other nations, South Africa has in essence two healthcare systems: a private health sector for the well-off, and a public sector for the majority of the country, which is mostly poor and of color.[193] Indeed, although the private sector provides care to 16 percent of the nation and the public sector to 84 percent,[194] the private sector employs a majority of the nation's doctors (up to 79 percent in 2007, from 40 percent in 1980).[195] Thus, although a pioneer in the health rights movement in one respect, South Africa has failed to create a basic right to equitable healthcare. Efforts are currently underway to help breach this private–public gap with a proposed and highly ambitious National Health Insurance program.[196] This reform could potentially create a more universal health system in South Africa, although much remains uncertain.[197] Some skeptics urge caution regarding the impact of this program on health, noting that medical care alone will not address the critically important underlying social factors—namely, poverty and inequality—that have actually been exacerbated by ANC neoliberalism.[198] Nonetheless, if actually implemented, National Health Insurance would no doubt be a step towards a right to healthcare in South Africa.

This complex dynamic—between the right to health in law and the actual equity of the provision of care by health systems—has parallels in nations throughout the world. Although the *TAC* case is the most famous example, healthcare rights are increasingly being litigated worldwide, especially in Latin America. The meaning and implications of this new era of social rights litigation for the cause of healthcare equality nevertheless remains ambiguous. The cases of Brazil, Colombia, India, and Canada are particularly instructive in this regard, for they speak to the complex manner in which political change, health system universality, rights litigation, and neoliberalism intersect—and often clash.

Rights, Litigation, and Privatization: Brazil, Colombia, India, and Canada

Postwar health systems succeeded in many cases in creating effective rights to healthcare, even though these achievements were not pursued or understood in a "human rights" framework. In contrast, in more recent years, health reform has increasingly been advanced with the language of human rights. This section will briefly explore the experiences of four nations—Brazil, Colombia, India, and Canada—in which the litigation of rights—whether an explicit human right to healthcare in the case of Brazil or Colombia or a right to "life" in the case of Canada and India—has been wielded in the name of "access" to health services for individuals and groups. However, the meaning of this litigation has differed from nation to nation, with varying consequences for the effective "right to health" in each case. For instance, while individuals have increasingly used rights arguments in the courts in Brazil and Colombia to obtain access to particular procedures or (especially) expensive pharmaceuticals, in Canada the "right to life" has been used to pry open the public healthcare sector to private competition.[199] Indeed, in Canada, "rights" litigation has the potential to lead to the *deterioration* of equitable access to healthcare. Rights litigation must be understood in the political context of the neoliberal healthcare agenda in each nation—an agenda that has favored the role of private insurance, user fees, and the privatization of delivery over the universal public provision of healthcare.

In Brazil, a discourse of human rights has had a particularly prominent impact on healthcare. As in many Latin American states, Brazil suffered under a right-wing authoritarian government for decades following a 1964 military coup d'état. As with the case of Chile, this political milieu was conducive to the growth of the private health industry.[200] During the 1970s, a health reform movement—opposed to the dictatorship and allied with democracy activists, trade unions, and other progressive political elements—began to formulate a more progressive public alternative.[201] Following the dissolution of the dictatorship, this movement and its allies played a critical role in the prominent inclusion of health rights in Brazil's 1988 constitution, despite resistance from the private healthcare industry.[202]

Article 6 of the Brazilian constitution sets forth that "[e]ducation, health, work, leisure, security, social security, protection of motherhood and childhood, and assistance to the destitute, are social rights," and Article 196 states that "[h]ealth is a right of all and a duty of the State . . ."[203] Perhaps more remarkably, the Brazilian constitution demands a "unified public health system" (the SUS, or *Sistema Único de Saúde*) to provide universal healthcare for the nation.[204] Thus, in Brazil, the creation of a public health system was tied to an explicit constitutional articulation of a right to health. That right was to become the foundation not only of health system reform, but also of an enormous quantity of health rights litigation in coming years.

Yet the impact of each development—the creation of the SUS and the rise of healthcare rights litigation—is more multifarious with respect to the "right to healthcare" in Brazil than one might first assume. The SUS was no doubt a soaring achievement with respect to healthcare access, and its "Family Health Strategy," in which multidisciplinary teams of healthcare workers take responsibility for the care of everyone within geographically circumscribed areas, has justly earned much praise.[205] However, the establishment of the SUS occurred alongside an implicit acceptance of certain overarching neoliberal health reform principles, namely, the promotion, protection, and indeed subsidization of a large private health sector for the well-off. As a result, although the SUS offers free care to a majority of the country and has resulted in a huge expansion of coverage and care, healthcare inequality has persisted as a result of the reliance of the middle and upper classes on a separate tier of private health insurance.[206] To a large extent, the SUS continues to function as a "poor person's program," providing a lower tier of coverage for the majority of the nation, while those who are better off are able to afford and access a (sometimes) higher quality of care in the private sector. "Dysfunctional public hospitals," notes one scholar, "largely contrast with very functional and efficient private hospitals and healthcare clinics that are only accessible to a quarter of the Brazilian population – those who can afford these services."[207] As a result, despite the progress that has been achieved so far, healthcare inequality is still pervasive in Brazil.[208]

A major part of this problem—and a particularly common issue among two-tier systems—is the chronic relative underfunding of the SUS.[209] Although the private sector is only used by a quarter of the population, it takes in about half of the nation's total healthcare spending.[210] This better-off minority relies on a growing private health insurance industry that is subsidized by the government through tax deductions.[211] This is an overall pattern seen in nation after nation throughout the globe: a powerful private health sector invariably impedes the realization of an equal right to healthcare, with lower tiers of coverage for lower social classes of the population. Thus, although articulating a doctrine of the human right to health—and although no doubt achieving a truly historic expansion of access for enormous numbers of people through the SUS—Brazil has not yet achieved a universal system that provides equitable care across class boundaries.

How about the impact of healthcare rights litigation in Brazil? Here, too, there are some ambiguities with respect to the right to healthcare. The prominence of health rights in the Brazilian constitution has facilitated an enormous increase in litigation for particular healthcare goods and services.[212] Somewhat similar to the case of South Africa, this litigation accelerated after people living with HIV/AIDS turned to the courts to obtain access to newly emerging treatments. In 2000, a milestone Supreme Court decision in their favor helped pave the way for a major increase in the number of individual suits for other treatments and therapies.[213] One scholar, however, has argued that this turn to the courts could actually have detrimental consequences from the perspective of health equity, in that the relatively small minority that is able to afford a private lawyer to petition for expensive, uncovered therapies may actually be draining public resources that might be better used in other ways.[214] It remains unclear whether this characterization of health rights litigation is entirely fair, or universally applicable across the country. One study, for instance, found that in the state of Rio Grande do Sul, more than half of those who filed "health-related lawsuits" from 2002 to 2009 earned less than the minimum wage.[215] Even so, these are instances of individual, not systemic, repairs. For instance, the authors note that "judicialization is now a part of the medical lexicon" as physicians encourage patients to litigate to obtain access to prescribed medications. This has effectively created a "parallel infrastructure" in which public and private actors interact to "enact one-by-one rescue missions," even while broader "systemic challenges . . . remain under-explored."[216]

From the perspective of the healthcare rights-commodity dialectic, Brazilian developments may therefore be seen as contradictory. On the one hand, Brazil has succeeded in creating something of a right for the nation's poor in the establishment of the SUS, including its widely lauded "Family Medicine Strategy." Additionally, "right to healthcare" litigation has provided a mechanism for individuals to achieve access to particular services or drugs on a case-by-case basis. On the other hand, an embrace of certain aspects of neoliberal healthcare ideology—in particular, the nurturing of a large private insurance and health delivery sector—has resulted in the inequities intrinsic to two-tier systems.

Similar dynamics have been playing out in other nations, such as neighboring Colombia. Colombia's 1991 constitution, like that of Brazil, included a guarantee to health services, and in so doing helped create a framework wherein individuals could launch "tutela claims," a type of lawsuit that is resolved quickly and need not involve lawyers, to ensure protection of their right to health services from both the public and private sector.[217] An important step forward in this regard was a 1992 Constitutional Court ruling that extrapolated a right to healthcare from the constitution's right to life, making it justiciable (though later, the Court came to see the right to health as justiciable on its own grounds).[218] A flood of litigation for health services—including drugs, operations, and devices—followed, such that an estimated one out of three hundred Colombians filed a tutela claim for a health service or good in 2008.[219] As in Brazil, the implications of these dynamics are not entirely clear. To some extent, they have allowed individuals to gain access to drugs to which they would otherwise be denied, albeit in a fashion that is highly beneficial to the pharmaceutical industry and that could potentially drain resources from other important public health priorities. Part of the reason for this, as Lamprea notes, is that the rise in tutela claims was accompanied by a deregulation of pharmaceutical prices. As a result, he states, "right to health" claims often result in individuals' obtaining access to "high-end" drugs at exorbitant prices, with the costs borne by the public sector. This has led to both financial strain within the health system and a larger "pharmaceuticalization" of healthcare in Colombia: even as drug expenditures rose, some metrics of public health—including vaccination rates and cervical cancer rates—worsened.[220] At the same time, on other occasions, health rights litigation in Colombia has led to more systemic change. In one key case (T760/08), the Constitutional Court decided to bundle a number of individual tutelas into a single suit, and called for a major reform of the health system itself, which it argued had failed to adequately provide access to health services, effectively denying individuals the right to health.[221]

Part of the equity problem, therefore, lies less with the manner of litigation than with the structural neoliberal characteristics of the health system itself, which is the result of the history of health reform in Colombia. In 1993, Colombia embarked on a major health system reform that proponents argued would take the nation towards universal healthcare through a managed competition model.[222] This reform was based in no small part on the 1993 World Bank report discussed earlier, particularly its emphasis on private insurance.[223] The "managed competition" model is itself more directly modeled on the ideas of Alain Enthoven, a scholar who first studied military strategy for the Pentagon before turning to health policy.[224] The idea of managed competition—namely, that all individuals purchase health insurance plans from competing private insurers—has influenced healthcare reform efforts throughout the globe, including in the Netherlands, the United Kingdom, and the United States.[225] Yet while managed competition is often described as a potent method for reaching the end goal of universal coverage, in practice, it typically allows for the persistence of inequities in coverage and access. In Colombia, for instance, some have rendered a very negative judgment on the overall impact of its "neoliberal health reform":

[I]n Colombia, the country that has followed very closely the WB [World Bank] reform blueprints, in spite of a very substantial increase in healthcare expenditures, a large percentage of the population continues to be uncovered, the poor continue to have difficulties in accessing services because of high co-payments, there are no measurable efficiency and medical care quality improvements, public healthcare has deteriorated, and health equity has suffered.[226]

In lieu of a single one-tier public system, in which equitable access to health services is provided as a matter of right, a system reliant on private insurers—whether in Colombia or elsewhere—often perpetuates a "tiered" health system in which unequal access is inevitable and cost-related barriers to care persevere.

A nation with even starker tiers and health inequities is India, which has also seen some important health rights litigation in recent years. After gaining independence, India did not pursue a broad national health service of the sort called for by the Bhore Committee, and instead aggressively embarked upon disease-specific vertical programs.[227] Although India had some significant successes,[228] continued underinvestment decade after decade has left it with a markedly inadequate public health infrastructure. In some respects, India today has worse health measures—notwithstanding its superior per capita income—than either Bangladesh or Nepal, and it has the worst health among the BRIC nations.[229] India contends with enormous health inequalities between states, a low rate of insurance coverage, high out-of-pocket exposure to healthcare costs, and growing inequalities in health financing.[230] Indeed, healthcare expenses force millions of Indians into poverty annually.[231] Healthcare is starkly divided between two poles: an expensive for-profit private sector used by both wealthy Indians and medical tourists from abroad, and an underfinanced and grossly inadequate public sector for the nation's poor.[232] The political muscle of the private healthcare sector, together with the pharmaceutical industry, helps perpetuate this status quo.[233]

This is, then, the health system context for the rise of health rights litigation in India. Notably, unlike in Brazil (or, to some extent, Colombia), there is no right to health in India's constitution. However, the Supreme Court in India has extrapolated a right to health from the "right to life" in the constitution.[234] For instance, the case *Paschim Banga Khet Mazdoor Samity v. State of West Bengal* involved a man who, after falling off a train and severely injuring his head, was turned away for emergency care by seven different hospitals, which all claimed they lacked adequate facilities to care for him. The Court found that the State's failure to establish a system of emergency treatment constituted a violation of the right to life, and obligated the state to create a system in which patients could be stabilized and then transferred to an appropriate facility.[235] The right to health derived from the constitutional right to life, but also from international treaties like the UDHR, which was at the center of a number of other cases.[236] However, the collective impact of these suits is controversial. While litigation on the individual level runs the risk of distributing health resources in a disproportionate fashion, "public interest litigation" that addresses broader systemic issues, like access to HIV treatment, has indeed "advanced the right to health of all people, by extending the relief given by courts to everyone. . . ."[237] Others, however, cast doubt on the impact of health rights cases, noting that "even if the Supreme Court or High Courts set a precedent of health as a right, the orders are rarely respected in daily practice."[238] While it seems fair to conclude that the courts can do some good, litigation can clearly not compensate for an utterly inadequate public healthcare system (to say nothing of issues pertaining to the social determinants of health).

Nor is it clear that anything is set to radically change from the health system perspective. In the past decade or so, a number of government initiatives has expanded coverage, such as the 2005 National Rural Health Mission (NRHM).[239] Yet even here, the prerogatives of the private health sector have taken precedence. As one scholar writes, the National Rural Health Mission has been "merely tinkering with the system . . . because while the government on the one hand talks about NRHM, on the other it is letting the corporate sector, including multinational corporations, have an unregulated and open environment to boost the private health sector and profit from it."[240] And following the 2014 election of the right-wing Hindu nationalist Bharatiya Janata Party, the prospects for significant reform may have actually worsened. Despite headlines that grandly described Prime Minister Narendra Modi's healthcare plan as a "universal healthcare rollout,"[241] his government has actually cut central public health spending (as a proportion of GDP), while his "New Health Policy," despite much acclaim, has again emphasized the role of private sector financing.[242] A real right to healthcare in India would require a system of universal healthcare, like the national health service first proposed by the Bhore Committee in 1946. This, however, appears nowhere on the horizon.

Canada, in contrast to the three nations just discussed, has long had a single-payer, single-tier healthcare system. But the litigation it has experienced has, paradoxically, pushed the rights-commodity dialectic *rightward*. Mobilization on both the provincial and the federal level in Canada culminated in the passage of the Canada Health Act (CHA) in 1984, which required that provincial health insurance plans meet certain basic criteria in order to receive federal funding, including both "universality" and "accessibility."[243] Accessibility excluded the use of user fees that would impede healthcare use. And this provision had teeth: the national government is supposed to hold back one dollar in funding for each dollar collected in user fees by the province.[244] However, because the CHA only stipulated the coverage of physician and hospital services, out-of-pocket spending on healthcare—for things like pharmaceuticals and long-term care—remains substantial.[245] Although private insurance is available for these uncovered services, for publicly covered services, provinces have long enacted restrictions on private health insurance in order to prevent the emergence of a two-tier system, a natural consequence of a powerful private health sector.[246] It is these sorts of restrictions that are now under attack.

Whereas in Brazil and Colombia, human rights litigation has essentially been pursued for the purpose of obtaining more care (whether from the private or public sector), human rights litigation in Canada has taken a much different turn: the right to life, it has been argued, confers a right to receive, and provide, *private* healthcare.[247] In the 2005 *Chaoulli v. Quebec* decision, the Supreme Court decided in favor of the plaintiffs, finding that Quebec's ban on private insurance constituted a violation of the right to life and to security (as found in Quebec's *Charter of Rights and Freedoms*) in that it forced these individuals to endure the waiting times for care of the public system.[248] In Colombia and India, the right to life was interpreted by the courts as a right to healthcare; in Quebec, in contrast, the right to life was translated into a right to private health *insurance*, giving those who could afford it preferential access to healthcare over those relying on the public system. Gross summarizes this development best: "[T]he idea of access was interpreted [in *Chaoulli*] in a way that actually reinforces the relationship between wealth and healthcare, opening the door to a system where the determining factor will not be need but rather the ability to pay for private health insurance."[249] As Gross emphasizes, some saw the *Chaoulli* decision as the death knell of the Canadian public health system: a "parallel" private health sector would emerge, the middle- and upper-class patients would leave the public system, and the public system would then degenerate into a lower-tier program for the poor. In reality, however, the actual effects of *Chaoulli* have thus far been limited, in part because the decision wound up only applying to Quebec.[250] Still, some observers have described an overall cultural shift towards healthcare privatization in the province of Quebec over the last ten years, proceeding along both legal and illegal lines.[251]

Yet perhaps even more worrying is the fact that *Chaoulli* may be just the first round in a larger campaign to roll back the right to equitable healthcare in Canada. The next greatest legal threat to the right to healthcare in Canada is the suit launched by Dr. Brian Day, a surgeon who operates for-profit surgical clinics (the trial is underway at the time of writing). Day, following the precedent of *Chaoulli*, is arguing that restrictions on private practice are violating the right to life and security (as protected by the Canadian *Charter of Rights and Freedoms*) of patients who are forced to go on waiting lists for procedures. He argues that physicians should be able to "extra-bill," i.e., to charge patients a premium on top of the payment rendered by the public system, in exchange for preferential treatment. Such extra payments might either be out-of-pocket or come via private insurance plans. Additionally, Day's lawyers are arguing that physicians should be able to work simultaneously in both the private and public health sectors, which is currently restricted under British Columbia law.[252] Were they to win—and if this model becomes the law of the land throughout Canada—it could very well result in the death of equitable access to healthcare.[253] In this case, health "rights" litigation may actually have the effect of rolling back the right to health in Canada.

In assessing the impact of health rights litigation across nations, scholars generally recognize both its potential and its shortcomings. Gloppen, for instance, notes that litigation can be used to increase government accountability to the right to health, but acknowledges the possible downsides, such as increasing healthcare inequality as a result of inequitable access to courts. Additionally, though strengthening the right to health on the individual level, litigation might subvert "long-term planning and rational priority setting," thereby weakening the "collective right to health."[254] Flood and Gross emphasize that health rights litigation plays a very different role depending on the nature of the health system. They note that, perhaps ironically, nations with strong public healthcare systems— like the United Kingdom or Sweden—lack constitutional or justiciable "rights" to healthcare; in contrast, states with mixed public and private financing are more likely to have a constitutional right to healthcare as well as more health rights litigation. Still, in many of these nations, they assert that successes in the arena of health rights litigation may be "overshadowed" by the enormous inequity in the public/private healthcare divide. And while they acknowledge the potential for health rights litigation to be regressive (such as in the case of Canada, or when it predominantly serves the interests of the pharmaceutical industry), they also see in it the potential for greater equity. Though acknowledging that courts cannot take the place of good health policy, they argue that courts could have a role in "holding governments to a standard of rationality and reasonability and ensuring that governmental decision making adheres to human rights standards," while at the same recognizing that health rights need to be "advanced directly in the political sphere."[255] They also assert that courts should focus more on larger systemic issues—say, onerous co-payments or the denial of care to groups of people like migrants—than on case-by-case grievances, as the latter might end up increasing government expenditure on extremely expensive therapies for individuals at the expense of other more important priorities.[256]

At the same time, as Yamin has fairly argued, one should not too sharply separate political mobilization from "court-centric strategies." Whether in South Africa or Latin America, political movements for health rights can precede, prompt, push forward, and expand upon court cases.[257] As Meier and Yamin have argued in the case of HIV/AIDS policy, a move away from a rights focus may effectively translate into an embrace of "cost-effectiveness" arguments and an acceptance of limited resources, instead of an effort to transcend them.[258] Moreover, Cabrera and Ayala contend that health rights litigation is essentially one way of contending with state failure to assure the right to healthcare through a universal health system. The political context, they assert, determines whether such litigation is progressive or regressive from the perspective of the right to health. But though case-by-case litigation can both help individuals and effect policy change, health system reform is ultimately a more potent road to healthcare equity.[259]

There are merits to each of these arguments. No doubt the achievement of any social right—or for that matter any political goal—requires efforts in multiple domains and dimensions, and might include a combination of legal strategies, electoral campaigns, grassroots movements, and so forth. Such efforts can be mutually reinforcing. Yet it is also clear that the neoliberal healthcare agenda—pushed forward by international healthcare capital—is an equally potent force in pushing the healthcare rights-commodity rightward in nation after nation. Indeed, there may be victories for health rights causes in the courts at the very same time as a nation's health system is further privatized. The essential equity implied by the presence of a "right" is undermined by two-tier or multi-tier systems in which healthcare access depends on means, not needs.

Yet this is also precisely what happens in nations where the right to health has no legal status. The final section of this chapter will turn back mostly to the United States and the United Kingdom—the first of which entered this period without a social right to health, the other with one—to examine the impact of the neoliberal healthcare agenda on the healthcare rights-commodity dialectic in these nations in more recent years.

The Healthcare Rights–Commodity Dialectic in a Time of Austerity and Reaction

In the United States, over the course of the 1970s (as described in the last chapter), the Democratic Party retreated from its previous support for a public, one-tier national health insurance system. Early in the decade, Massachusetts senator

Ted Kennedy had proposed a single-payer program, which would have provided most care free at the point of use for everyone, roughly analogous to what the Canadian system or the NHS had accomplished (the Dellums bill would have gone significantly further, as noted). Yet by the end of the decade, President Jimmy Carter had abandoned such a vision, and the proposals of subsequent Democratic presidents inexorably moved closer to that of Nixon than to that of Kennedy. Though many associate the onset of the neoliberal era with the election of Reagan in 1980, the 1970s were in many senses a "pivotal decade" when it came to the historic neoliberal shift in American political economy.[260] This was certainly the case with respect to healthcare: the healthcare "center" shifted, as Republicans abandoned Nixonian health policy and Democrats abandoned healthcare universalism.[261]

Many of the goals of the neoliberal healthcare agenda examined elsewhere in this chapter were being pursued in the US during these years as well. These included (1) the embrace of "cost sharing," or user fees, as a necessary tool for health system efficiency (or an abandonment of the idea of care free at time of use), (2) the promotion of a corporatized managed care organization (MCO)/ health maintenance organization (HMO) industry and "managed competition" as a health reform model, and (3) the progressive corporate consolidation of the healthcare delivery sector.[262] These goals were promoted in the US—in many instances—using the same language and arguments seen elsewhere. For instance, the embrace of cost sharing as an important reform tool—whether through co-payments, deductibles, or co-insurance—echoes the WB's promotion of "user fees" in Africa, with proponents using some of the same arguments. Free healthcare was deemed to carry a "moral hazard": individuals would use more healthcare than they needed, resulting in unnecessary use and a "welfare loss" for the nation as a whole.[263] Indeed, according to proponents of cost sharing, what was needed was *more* cost sharing, not less—and certainly not none at all.

Neoliberal economists advanced these ideas through economic analysis and punditry from the 1970s onward. The economist Martin Feldstein, for instance, in a 1973 article in the *Journal of Political Economy* argued that "American families are in general overinsured against health expenses," and that it would be "reasonable to conclude that an increase in the average co-insurance rate [the percentage of the cost of a health service paid out-of-pocket] would increase welfare and that the net gain would probably be quite substantial."[264] Similarly, perhaps the single most important neoliberal economist, Friedrich Hayek, had briefly made a more philosophical case against a "free health service" in his *Constitution of Liberty* some decades earlier. Hayek argued that the notion that healthcare needs were somehow "objectively ascertainable" was a fallacy: individuals might benefit from healthcare in different ways, so they should therefore choose for themselves whether to spend money on more healthcare or on other "material advantages."[265] Healthcare, in these sorts of analyses, was reducible to a consumer good. Make it free and demand would soar, impoverishing everyone in the process.

The second development was the emergence of the HMO. Although there were progressive examples of managed care arrangements earlier in the century, the modern HMO was explicitly proposed as an alternative to national health insurance during Nixon's presidency.[266] It was conceptualized as an important step in a much larger transition towards a corporatized healthcare universe: HMO-godfather Paul Elwood saw the introduction of a "free-market economy" into the health industry as having "some of the classical aspects of the industrial revolution": "conversion to larger units of production, technological innovation, division of labor, substitution of capital for labor, vigorous competition, and profitability as the mandatory condition of survival."[267] Although HMOs got off to a slow start, they rapidly grew as a result of the efforts of the Reagan administration, increasingly consolidating into large for-profit corporate entities (and, indeed, spreading internationally).[268] Moreover, HMOs became the center of a new model of healthcare reform, as Alain Enthoven's "managed competition," which envisaged a regulated marketplace of competing HMOs, emerged as a popular alternative to universal healthcare systems for many policymakers and politicians. Aspects of these proposals drifted into the mainstream of health policy discourse, strongly coloring President Bill Clinton's health reform proposal in the 1990s—and, to some extent—President Barack Obama's Patient Protection and Affordable Care Act (ACA).[269] Internationally, meanwhile, the ideas of managed competition would be drawn on by health policy actors in Colombia, the United Kingdom, the Netherlands, and elsewhere.[270]

The third development was the progressive corporate consolidation of the healthcare sector itself. "The 'health industry' used to mean just doctors and drug companies," maintained a 1969 editorial entitled "The Medical Industrial Complex" in the progressive health policy journal *Health-PAC*. "Now it's doctors, drugs, hospital supplies, electronic equipment, computers, health insurance, construction, real estate, and profit-making chains of hospitals and nursing homes."[271] In more recent years, consolidation has extended in new directions, with hospitals fusing into ever-larger "health systems." In some cases, these health systems have then looked to merge with insurers, while insurers have sought to merge with other insurers. In contrast, the physician lobby—once a powerhouse largely responsible for the destruction of Truman's national health insurance campaign—has been largely relegated (in a relative sense) to the sidelines.

In part as a result of these varied dynamics—and hand-in-hand with the broader right-wing political turn of these decades—efforts to achieve a system of universal healthcare were unsuccessful during the neoliberal era. Indeed, following the establishment of Medicare and Medicaid, there was no major health system transformation until 2010, when President Barack Obama signed the ACA. Although this law expanded coverage to millions, continued adherence to key neoliberal health principles has meant that the law did not create a right to healthcare for the nation.

Before delving further into the implications of the ACA for health rights, some parallels with contemporaneous developments unfolding in the UK are worth noting. The UK entered the neoliberal period with something of a legal right to healthcare; with the election of Margaret Thatcher in 1979, many hoped that this could be undone. "Just as socialism had grasped its opportunity in 1945," historian

Charles Webster notes, "so in 1979 it was the chance for Thatcherism to reconstruct a [healthcare] system still permeated by Bevanist assumptions."[272] Right-wing ideologues—buoyed by the changing political *milieu*—had a number of goals in these years: the re-establishment of a system of private insurance, the shrinking of the NHS into a lower-tier service for the poor, the privatization of the healthcare delivery sector, and the raising of user fees for care at time of use, among other things.[273] These were, of course, the very same principles of the neoliberal healthcare agenda seen again and again in nation after nation. However, in the UK, such goals were well beyond what the public would have accepted. As a result, what was actually pursued during the Thatcher years was instead a slow strategy of piecemeal changes, which together nonetheless amounted to a "continuous revolution . . ."[274]

A detailed accounting of this process—and those that followed during the years of the Labour government elected in 1997—is beyond the scope of this chapter. However, among the most significant changes of this era were (1) the 1991 implementation of an "internal market" (partially informed by the work of Enthoven) that helped open the door to corporate healthcare providers; (2) the infiltration of corporate capital and culture throughout the NHS, including an increasing role of for-profit companies in the provision of care; (3) an increasingly business-modeled approach towards hospital policy, planning, and management; (4) the progressive privatization of long-term care, often with adverse consequences for those relying on these services; and (5) the implementation, under Labour, of the Private Finance Initiative approach to hospital building, the wastefulness of which led to later reductions in hospital budgets and hospital beds.[275] Such changes—along with increases in user fees (there was a more than 500 percent increase in co-payments for prescription drugs during the years of the Thatcher administration[276])—no doubt amounted to a novel degree of healthcare recommodification in the UK. As policy scholar and physician Allyson Pollock describes, these changes resulted in the production of new inequities and a decline in the principle of universality: "Healthcare moved increasingly . . . away from being a right, back towards a commodity – as it had been before 1948."[277]

To an extent, there is some evidence for parallel recommodification of healthcare elsewhere in Europe during this period as well, though by no means evenly or diffusely. One study of eight European nations found that while the public share of healthcare financing increased during the 1970s, it fell from 1990 to 2002.[278] Additionally, the study suggested a transition towards for-profit healthcare delivery in some of the nations studied.[279] In more recent years, some nations have clearly embraced a neoliberal healthcare agenda. For instance, in the Netherlands, a 2006 law reformed the nation's social health insurance system along the lines of Enthoven's "managed competition" strategy, with competing for-profit insurers vying for the business of citizens; critics have charged that that these reforms have led to a deterioration of health system performance and equity.[280] Even Sweden—that archetype of the social democratic welfare state—saw some privatization of care delivery in this period.[281]

Yet in the past five years, even greater health system changes have occurred—in very different ways—on both sides of the Atlantic. The increasingly financialized capitalist system entered an acute crisis in the year 2008, unleashing economic recessions in nations throughout the globe: unemployment soared, public revenues dropped, severe austerity policies were enacted, and many governments fell. In the UK, the Conservative-led government elected in 2010 implemented a program of harsh austerity, which included a historic stagnation in funding for the NHS that continues to this day. NHS spending growth, theoretically protected, was nonetheless constrained to a fraction of its historical rate, an effective cut in light of population growth.[282] These historical reductions in funding have resulted in rising waiting times for care,[283] plans for sharp reductions in hospital beds and facilities,[284] and a squeeze of the workforce that precipitated a strike of "junior doctors" (akin to residents in the American system).[285] Moreover, in 2012, Prime Minister David Cameron's government passed its Health and Social Care Act, which some contend is setting the NHS down the road of not only privatization, but also eventual dismemberment. Indeed, according to its critics, the very promise of universal, comprehensive, free care may be under threat as a result of the changes instituted by the law.[286] "The effect [of the law]," write Pollock and lawyer David Price, "is to transform the [English] NHS from a nationally mandated public service required of the government into a service based on commercial contracting. . ."[287]

The logic of austerity has similarly been used to weaken the public health systems of nations throughout Europe, including Greece, Spain, Ireland, and Portugal.[288] The health systems of these nations changed along what one might call the four axes of the neoliberal healthcare agenda: a decline in the universal reach of the public healthcare system, increases in user fees, privatization of delivery, and reductions in public spending.[289] Although these changes have been incremental and have affected nations to varying degrees, together they have amounted to an unambiguous shift in the healthcare rights-commodity dialectic in Europe, marked by reductions in equitable access and an overall retreat from the principles of universalism that emerged with great promise in the decades after the Second World War.

The United States, therefore, may seem to be the exception: in recent years, it has actually seen a historic *expansion* of healthcare coverage with the Affordable Care Act. Before the ACA, the last significant effort towards major system-wide healthcare reform had occurred during the early years of the Clinton administration, and the political damage inflicted by the defeat of this effort was perceived as a cautionary tale for Democrats for years to come. But as the conservative years of the George W. Bush administration came to a close—and with the ranks of the uninsured actually rising in the first decade of the new millennium—many hoped that major change might again be on the horizon, and that a right to healthcare could be finally realized.

It's therefore of little surprise that healthcare reform figured prominently in the 2008 Presidential race—first in the Democratic primary, then in the general election. In the second debate, for instance, journalist Tom Brokaw asked Barack Obama and John McCain a simple question: "Is healthcare in America a privilege, a right, or a responsibility?" [290] McCain's answer was somewhat nebulous: healthcare is a responsibility in that we should "have available and affordable healthcare to every American citizen," though he noted he was a "little nervous" about the prospect of mandates. Obama's response, in contrast, was far clearer:

> Well, I think it should be a right for every American. In a country as wealthy as ours, for us to have people who are going bankrupt because they can't pay their medical bills – for my mother to die of cancer at the age of 53 and have to spend the last months of her life in the hospital room arguing with insurance companies because they're saying that this may be a pre-existing condition and they don't have to pay for her treatment, there's something fundamentally wrong about that.

But despite this strong rhetorical embrace of healthcare rights, what Obama (and other leading Democrats primary contenders) had in mind fell far short of a real "right" to healthcare—a fact that would shape the form of the legislation that ultimately came about. Similarly, key legislators like Montana senator Max Baucus, the chairman of the Senate Finance Committee, were dead set against a more ambitious single-tier national health program from the beginning.[291] No doubt such politicians were in part acquiescing to the powerful "medical-industrial complex" that had attained a position of great influence: the pharmaceutical industry, the insurance industry, and even the medical device industry now wielded significant political and economic power. Over the course of the making of the ACA, deals were made between the administration and/or Baucus and these powerful industries.[292] These compromises ultimately limited the scope and impact of reform.

Thus, what emerged from this process was less what Ted Kennedy first proposed in the early 1970s, and was more akin to the counterplan proposed by Nixon shortly thereafter, combined with other policy ideas drawn from later (mostly Republican) healthcare proposals.[293] Among its key provisions were an individual mandate requiring all to have healthcare or pay a fine; an employer mandate requiring employers above a certain size to provide coverage or pay a fine; insurance reforms outlawing exclusions or discriminations based on pre-existing conditions and requiring coverage of children up to age 26 on family plans; a major expansion of Medicaid, the program signed by Johnson that provided healthcare to some categories of the poor; and a program of subsidies for the purchase of private insurance on "exchanges" for those who are not covered by their insurer or the government.[294] As a result of these provisions, uninsurance rates have dropped substantially, although full universal coverage was neither reached nor was in sight at the end of Obama's presidency. Indeed, some 29 million remained uninsured in 2015.[295] Moreover, because ideas about the importance of "skin in the game"—the notion of "moral hazard" described earlier—were built into the law, deductibles and co-payments on the ACA marketplaces can be quite high, while potential cost sharing exposure has continued to grow for employer-based plans.[296] An estimated 31 million non-elderly adults remain underinsured, with out-of-pocket costs continuing to prevent many from actually obtaining the care they require.[297]

These and other limitations, however, are intrinsic to the structure of the reform itself. Today, in the United States, healthcare remains highly commoditized, though it is available to a substantially greater percentage of the population as a result of the ACA's subsidization of private health insurers as well as its expansion of Medicaid. In contrast, there is something of a "right" to healthcare for those age 65 and over via Medicare, though even that public program has important limitations, including high cost sharing. And profound healthcare inequalities no doubt remain.[298] "In terms of both racial and income inequalities," as Yamin and Carmalt note, "the Affordable Care Act fails to treat health and healthcare as a basic right, as opposed to a market commodity, and as a consequence, perpetuates the current structural failure to address the underlying causes of inequalities in the system."[299]

Meanwhile, at the same time, as Thomas Piketty's book *Capital in the Twentieth First Century* helped bring to center stage, economic inequality has been rising with a vengeance: with the rate of interest accruing to the owners of capital exceeding the overall growth rate of the economy, this will likely remain the status quo barring fundamental change.[300] And perhaps unsurprisingly, alongside rising economic inequality have been rising health inequalities by economic status, beginning perhaps around the time that the neoliberal era began, and continuing into the twenty-first century.[301] Likewise, racial health inequalities—the toxic legacy of slavery and subsequent oppression—remain all too real, flowing both from ongoing institutional racism and from a fragmented healthcare system.[302] And disturbing reports of *worsening* population health—driven by a host of factors—began emerging in 2015 and 2016.[303] Indeed, in June 2016, a stunning development was reported: for the first time in over ten years, overall mortality rates were actually *on the rise* for the country as a whole.[304]

It is true, however, that there has also been opposition to the neoliberal healthcare agenda, both in the US and internationally. For instance, there has been substantial resistance against healthcare austerity in Europe. In the UK, leftist MP Jeremy Corbyn, who was elected leader of the Labour Party in 2015, promised to reverse the privatization of the NHS.[305] In Spain, healthcare workers and allies have mobilized against the privatization of hospitals and against the exclusion of undocumented immigrants from the health system.[306] More broadly, around the globe, activists, healthcare workers, patients, and politicians continue to engage in struggles for the right to healthcare, whether they draw on the language of rights or not.

At the same time, a broad and perhaps epochal political shift may have begun in recent years. In the wake of the 2008 economic crisis, the global Occupy movement initiated a major turn in the political discourse against rising economic inequality. More recently, in the US, the unexpected and insurgent success of the campaign of Bernie Sanders, the democratic socialist senator of Vermont, in the Democratic presidential primary put healthcare rights back into the center of the discussion in late 2015 and early 2016. Sanders strongly supported a "single-payer" national health insurance program that would provide universal comprehensive coverage without user fees—a reform that would discard the key neoliberal healthcare principles that prevailed in recent decades, and instead move the nation towards a rights-based healthcare system. As a result, early 2016 saw a heated resurgence in the debate over universal healthcare reform.[307] Around this time, a group of more than 2,000 physicians signed onto a revised single-payer proposal[308]—drafted by a group that included this author—that was endorsed by the organization *Physicians for a National Health Program* together with the largest nurse's union in the nation. Sanders lost the primary, but polling evidence suggests that he had the winning argument on healthcare: a May 2016 poll found that some 58 percent of the nation supported a federally funded healthcare reform analogous to single payer.[309]

However, while Sanders' success provided reason for optimism for those seeking to advance the cause of healthcare rights in early 2016, subsequent events gave reason for pessimism. The election of Donald Trump to the Presidency in November 2016 will likely result in even greater healthcare commoditization in the US, at least in the short term. Trump's precise plans were not entirely clear during the campaign. His website called for the repeal of the ACA and some other changes that would "bring much-needed free market reforms to the healthcare industry,"[310] while at the same time he claimed that he was opposed to cuts in Medicaid and Medicare and would go on to promise "insurance for everyone."[311] Yet what mattered was less Trump's agenda than the long-standing Republican vision.[312] And indeed, in May 2017 House Republicans managed to pass the "American Health Care Act," a bill that would erode protection for those with pre-existing conditions, slash federal funding for Medicaid, and convert the ACA's insurance subsidies into a more regressive tax-credit (among much else). It was estimated that this bill would strip insurance coverage—far too often already inadequate—from some 24 million people, while increasing financial barriers to care for many more.[313] The assault of GOP-care, if it comes to fruition, could ruthlessly end the lives of tens of thousands,[314] and compound suffering for many more. It would also likely further the corporatization of healthcare, making healthcare access even more contingent on economic status.

At the time of this writing, the fate of this widely disliked and vicious piece of legislation—dubbed "Trumpcare" by many—is unclear. Either way, however, it is clear that the struggle for healthcare rights must go on. Indeed, perhaps there is some reason for hope: with Obamacare the reform of the past, and GOP-Care the unpopular (and likely deadly) "reform" of the present, a progressive front may at long last converge on, fight for, and achieve that long-eluded goal: the creation of a right to healthcare in the form of a universal public system. Such a shift in the healthcare rights-commodity dialectic will only occur, as this book has traced historically, through political struggle.

Yet at the time this sentence was written—with the passage of Trumpcare a real possibility, if by no means an inevitability—the outcome of that struggle seems anything but certain.

Notes

1   Lawrence Altman, "Rare Cancer Seen in 41 Homosexuals," *New York Times*, July 3, 1981, accessed April 14, 2016, http://www.nytimes.com/1981/07/03/us/rare-cancer-seen-in-41-homosexuals.html.

2   Recent research, however, has shown that the virus probably possibly first arrived in NYC around the year 1970, disproving the notion that so-called "Patient Zero" was the index patient who brought HIV to the US. Jon Cohen, "'Patient Zero' No More," *Science* 351, no. 6277 (2016), 1013.

3   HIV/AIDS numbers here are from: World Health Organization, "Global Health Observatory (GHO) Data: HIV/AIDS," accessed January 12, 2017, http://www.who.int/gho/hiv/en/. The 1.5 million deaths are for 2015.

4   Kim Phillips-Fein, *Invisible Hands: The Making of the Conservative Movement from the New Deal to Reagan* (New York: W. W. Norton & Company, 2009).

5   Judith Stein, *Pivotal Decade: How the United States Traded Factories for Finance in the Seventies* (New Haven, CT: Yale University Press, 2010).

6   Jacob S. Hacker and Paul Pierson, *Winner-Take-All Politics: How Washington Made the Rich Richer—and Turned Its Back on the Middle Class* (New York: Simon & Schuster, 2010), 6.

7   Daniel Stedman Jones, *Masters of the Universe: Hayek, Friedman, and the Birth of Neoliberal Politics* (Princeton: Princeton University Press, 2012).

8   The three phases are summarized on these pages: ibid., 6–8.

9   Ibid., 4–5.

10   Ibid., 8.

11   Julia A. Walsh and Kenneth S. Warren, "Selective Primary Health Care," *New England Journal of Medicine* 301, no. 18 (1979), 967–74.

12   Marcos Cueto, "The Origins of Primary Health Care and Selective Primary Health Care," *American Journal of Public Health* 94, no. 11 (2004), 1868.

13   Theodore M. Brown, Marcos Cueto, and Elizabeth Fee, "The World Health Organization and the Transition from 'International' to 'Global' Public Health," *American Journal of Public Health* 96, no. 1 (2006), 67.

14   Cueto, "The Origins of Primary Health Care and Selective Primary Health Care," 1869; Brown, Cueto, and Fee, "The World Health Organization and the Transition from 'International' to 'Global' Public Health," 67.

15   Lesley Magnussen, John Ehiri, and Pauline Jolly, "Comprehensive Versus Selective Primary Health Care: Lessons for Global Health Policy," *Health Affairs* 23, no. 3 (2004),169.

16   Debabar Banerji, "Reflections on the Twenty-Fifth Anniversary of the Alma-Ata Declaration," *International Journal of the Health Services* 33, no. 4 (2003), 816.

17   John J. Hall and Richard Taylor, "Health for All Beyond 2000: The Demise of the Alma-Ata Declaration and Primary Health Care in Developing Countries," *Medical Journal of Australia* 178, no. 1 (2003), 17–20.

18   Brown, Cueto, and Fee, "The World Health Organization and the Transition from 'International' to 'Global' Public Health," 67–8.

19   Ibid., 67.

20   John Lister, *Health Policy Reform: Global Health Versus Private Profit* (Faringdon: Libri Publishing, 2013), 5, 54.

21   Ibid., 5.

22   Brown, Cueto, and Fee, "The World Health Organization and the Transition from 'International' to 'Global' Public Health," 68.

23   Rick Rowden, "The Ghosts of User Fees Past: Exploring Accountability for Victims of a 30-Year Economic Policy Mistake," *Health and Human Rights* 15, no. 1 (2013), 176.

24   Ibid.

25   Lister, *Health Policy Reform*, 5.

26   Rowden, "The Ghosts of User Fees Past," 176.

27 The Africa Strategy Review Group, "Accelerated Development in Sub-Saharan Africa: An Agenda for Action" (Washington, DC: The World Bank, 1981), accessed March 23, 2016, http://www-wds.worldbank.org/external/default/WDSContentServer/WDSP/IB/2000/04/13/000178830_98101911444774/Rendered/PDF/multi_page.pdf, 88. I was led to this citation by Rowden, "The Ghosts of User Fees Past."

28 Lister, *Health Policy Reform*, 82; Rowden, "The Ghosts of User Fees Past: Exploring Accountability for Victims of a 30-Year Economic Policy Mistake," 176–7.

29 World Bank, *Financing Health Services in Developing Countries: An Agenda for Reform* (Washington, DC: World Bank, 1988), accessed September 10, 2015, http://documents.worldbank.org/curated/en/1989/07/440431/financing-health-services-developing-countries-agenda-reform, 3–7.

30 All quotes from this paragraph thus far are from ibid., 26.

31 Public single payer systems, there is no doubt, have much lower administrative costs than multi-payer systems like the US. See, for instance: Steffie Woolhandler, Terry Campbell, and David U. Himmelstein, "Costs of Health Care Administration in the United States and Canada," *New England Journal of Medicine* 349, no. 8 (2003), 768–75.

32 World Bank, *Financing Health Services in Developing Countries: An Agenda for Reform*, 34, 38.

33 Rowden, "The Ghosts of User Fees Past: Exploring Accountability for Victims of a 30-Year Economic Policy Mistake," 178.

34 Lister, *Health Policy Reform*, 82. The document is also discussed in: Virginia A. Leary, "The Right to Health in International Human Rights Law," *Health and Human Rights* 1, no. 1 (1994), 52; Hall and Taylor, "Health for All Beyond 2000: The Demise of the Alma-Ata Declaration and Primary Health Care in Developing Countries," 19; A. C. Laurell and O. L. Arellano, "Market Commodities and Poor Relief: The World Bank Proposal for Health," *International Journal of the Health Services* 26, no. 1 (1996), 1–18.

35 World Bank, *World Development Report 1993: Investing in Health* (New York: Oxford University Press, 1993), accessed October 2, 2015, https://openknowledge.worldbank.org/handle/10986/5976, Box 1, p 6.

36 Ibid., 7, 10.

37 Laurell and Arellano, "Market Commodities and Poor Relief: The World Bank Proposal for Health," 1–18.

38 Ronald Labonté and David Stuckler, "The Rise of Neoliberalism: How Bad Economics Imperils Health and What to Do About It," *Journal of Epidemiology and Community Health* 70 no. 3 (2015), 312–18.

39 Ibid.

40 Ibid.; Dorothy Logie and Michael Rowson, "Poverty and Health: Debt Relief Could Help Achieve Human Rights Objectives," *Health and Human Rights*, 3 No. 2 (1998), 82–97; C. Holden, "Privatization and Trade in Health Services: A Review of the Evidence," *International Journal of Health Services* 35, no. 4 (2005), 675–89.

41 Rowden, "The Ghosts of User Fees Past: Exploring Accountability for Victims of a 30-Year Economic Policy Mistake," 178.

42 Raymond A. Atuguba, "The Right to Health in Ghana: Healthcare, Human Rights, and Politics," in *Advancing the Human Right to Health*, ed. José M. Zuniga, Stephen P. Marks, and Lawrence O. Gostin (Oxford: Oxford University Press, 2013), 103–4.

43 Remigius N. Nwabueze, "The Legal Protection and Enforcement of Health Rights in Nigeria," in *The Right to Health at the Public/Private Divide: A Global Comparative Study*, ed. Colleen M. Flood and Aeyal M. Gross (New York: Cambridge University Press, 2014), 375–6.

44 Ibid., 376.

45 Chris James et al., "Impact on Child Mortality of Removing User Fees: Simulation Model," *British Medical Journal* 331, no. 7519 (2005), 747–9.

46 This point was made by Rob Yates. Rob Yates, "Universal Health Care and the Removal of User Fees," *The Lancet* 373, no. 9680: 2078–81. I owe this citation and that of the *BMJ* study by Chris James et al. to Rowden, "The Ghosts of User Fees Past: Exploring Accountability for Victims of a 30-Year Economic Policy Mistake."

47 Rachel Hammonds and Gorik Ooms, "World Bank Policies and the Obligation of Its Members to Respect, Protect and Fulfill the Right to Health," *Health and Human Rights* 8, no. 1 (2004), 26–60.

48 Ibid., 45.

49 Rowden, "The Ghosts of User Fees Past: Exploring Accountability for Victims of a 30-Year Economic Policy Mistake," 177.

50 Lister, *Health Policy Reform*, 8.

51 Ibid., 8, 13.

52 Arturo Vargas Bustamante and Claudio A. Méndez, "Health Care Privatization in Latin America: Comparing Divergent Privatization Approaches in Chile, Colombia, and Mexico," *Journal of Health Politics, Policy and Law* 39, no. 4 (2014), 851.

53 Núria Homedes and Antonio Ugalde, "Why Neoliberal Health Reforms Have Failed in Latin America," *Health Policy* 71, no. 1 (2005), 88; Joseph L. Scarpaci, "Restructuring Health Care Financing in Chile," *Social Science and Medicine* 21, no. 4 (1985), 424; Stephen Reichard, "Ideology Drives Health Care Reforms in Chile," *Journal of Public Health Policy* 17, no. 1 (1996), 88; Jean-Pierre Unger et al., "Chile's Neoliberal Health Reform: An Assessment and a Critique," *PLoS Med* 5, no. 4 (2008): 0543–4.

54 Scarpaci, "Restructuring Health Care Financing in Chile," table 2, p. 419.

55 Reichard, "Ideology Drives Health Care Reforms in Chile," 90.

56 Scarpaci, "Restructuring Health Care Financing in Chile," 423. On declining public health spending, see also: Anamaria Viveros-Long, "Changes in Health Financing: The Chilean Experience," *Social Sciences and Medicine* 22, no. 3 (1986), 382–4.

57 World Bank, *Financing Health Services in Developing Countries: An Agenda for Reform*, 41.

58 Thomas C. Tsai and John Ji, "Neoliberalism and Its Discontents: Impact of Health Reforms in Chile," *Harvard International Review* 31, no. 2 (2009), 33–4; Thomas J. Bossert and Thomas Leisewitz, "Innovation and Change in the Chilean Health System," *New England Journal of Medicine* 374, no. 1 (2016), 1–5.

59 Quoted in Richard Garfield and Glen Williams, *Health Care in Nicaragua: Primary Care under Changing Regimes* (New York: Oxford University Press, 1992), 67.

60 Richard M. Garfield and Eugenio Taboada, "Health Services Reforms in Revolutionary Nicaragua," *American Journal of Public Health* 74, no. 10 (1984), 1143–4; Lefton, "Nicaragua: Health Care under the Sandinistas," 784; Tom Frieden and Richard Garfield, "Popular Participation in Health in Nicaragua," *Health Policy and Planning* 2, no. 2 (1987), 162–70 Garfield and Williams, *Health Care in Nicaragua*, 67–86.

61 Lane notes that public health spending by the government began to decline in the late 1980s, and that Sandinistas began to "experiment with private wards in public hospitals." Patti Lane, "Economic Hardship Has Put Nicaragua's Health Care System on the Sick List," *Canadian Medical Association Journal* 152, no. 4 (1995), 582.

62 Richard Garfield, Nicola Low, and Julio Caldera, "Desocializing Health Care in a Developing Country," *Journal of the American Medical Association* 270, no. 8 (1993), 989–93.

63 Lane, "Economic Hardship Has Put Nicaragua's Health Care System on the Sick List,": 581; Anne-Emanuelle Birn, Sarah Zimmerman, and Richard Garfield, "To Decentralize or Not to Decentralize, Is That the Question? Nicaraguan Health Policy under Structural Adjustment in the 1990s," *International Journal of Health Services* 30, no. 1 (2000), 115.

64 Lane, "Economic Hardship Has Put Nicaragua's Health Care System on the Sick List," 581.

65 Birn, Zimmerman, and Garfield, "To Decentralize or Not to Decentralize, Is That the Question? Nicaraguan Health Policy under Structural Adjustment in the 1990s," 118–19.

66 Ibid., 112.

67 Ibid., 120.

68 Garfield and Williams, *Health Care in Nicaragua*, 165, 227, quote on 165.

69 Garfield and Williams emphasize that privatization resulted in a "fundamental inequality in the health system." Ibid., 164.

70 David Blumenthal and William Hsiao, "Privatization and Its Discontents—the Evolving Chinese Health Care System," *New England Journal of Medicine* 353, no. 11 (2005), 1165.

71 Therese Hesketh and Wei Xing Zhu, "Health in China: The Healthcare Market," *British Medical Journal* 314, no. 7094 (1997), 1616–18.

72 Ibid.

73 Blumenthal and Hsiao, "Privatization and Its Discontents: the Evolving Chinese Health Care System," 1167.

74 Ibid.

75 William C. Hsiao, "Correcting Past Policy Mistakes," *Daedalus* 143, no. 2 (2014), 56–7.

76 Ibid.

77 These reforms are discussed in: Philip D. Chen and Di Wu, "China's Evolution in Progressively Realizing the Right to Health," in *Advancing the Human Right to Health*, 159–71; David Blumenthal and William Hsiao, "Lessons from the East – China's Rapidly Evolving Health Care System," *New England Journal of Medicine* 372, no. 14 (2015), 1283; Winnie Yip et al., "Early Appraisal of China's Huge and Complex Health-Care Reforms," *Lancet* 379, no. 9818 (2012), 833–42; Winnie Yip and William Hsiao, "Harnessing the Privatisation of China's Fragmented Health-Care Delivery," *Lancet* 384, no. 9945 (2014), 805–18.

78 Yip and Hsiao, "Harnessing the Privatisation of China's Fragmented Health-Care Delivery," 807.

79 Winnie Yip et al., "Early Appraisal of China's Huge and Complex Health-Care Reforms," *Lancet* 379, no. 9818 (2012), 838.

80 Christina S. Ho, "Health Rights at the Juncture between State and Market: The People's Republic of China," in *The Right to Health at the Public/Private Divide: A Global Comparative Study*, 284–5.

81 Evegueni M. Andreev et al., "The Evolving Pattern of Avoidable Mortality in Russia," *International Journal of Epidemiology* 32, no. 3 (2003), 437–46.

82 Lawrence King, Patrick Hamm, and David Stuckler, "Rapid Large-Scale Privatization and Death Rates in Ex-Communist Countries: An Analysis of Stress-Related and Health System Mechanisms," *International Journal of Health Services* 39, no. 3 (2009), 461–89.

83 David Stuckler and Sanjay Basu, *The Body Economic: Why Austerity Kills: Recessions, Budget Battles, and the Politics of Life and Death* (New York: Basic Books, 2013), 21–3.

84 Ibid., 35; King, Hamm, and Stuckler, "Rapid Large-Scale Privatization and Death Rates in Ex-Communist Countries," 464.

85 On the other hand, although King, Hamm, and Stuckler found an association between mass privatization and reductions in healthcare resources, they did not overall find an association between healthcare resources and life expectancy. Andreev et al., "The Evolving Pattern of Avoidable Mortality in Russia"; King, Hamm, and Stuckler, "Rapid Large-Scale Privatization and Death Rates in Ex-Communist Countries."

86 Julie Margot Feinsilver, *Healing the Masses: Cuban Health Politics at Home and Abroad* (Berkeley: University of California Press, 1993), 39–40.

87 C. W. Keck and G. A. Reed, "The Curious Case of Cuba," *American Journal of Public Health* 102, no. 8 (2012), e15.

88 Feinsilver, *Healing the Masses*, 120.

89 Steve Brouwer, *Revolutionary Doctors: How Venezuela and Cuba Are Changing the World's Conception of Health Care* (New York: Monthly Review Press, 2011), 60–6, quote on 60.

90 Edward W. Campion and Stephen Morrissey, "A Different Model — Medical Care in Cuba," *New England Journal of Medicine* 368, no. 4 (2013), 297–9.

91 Ibid., 297.

92 Keck and Reed, "The Curious Case of Cuba," e15.

93 Ibid.; Felipe Eduardo Sixto, "An Evaluation of Four Decades of Cuban Healthcare," *Association For the Study of the Cuban Economy*, accessed September 10, 2015, http://www.ascecuba.org/c/wp-content/uploads/2014/09/v12-sixto.pdf, 340.

94 Brouwer, *Revolutionary Doctors*, 69.

95 For instance, some have noted that there are charges for some items, like supplies and dental care. Sixto, "An Evaluation of Four Decades of Cuban Healthcare," 328.

96   Feinsilver notes that although many governments speak about the right to healthcare, in Cuba it became a right *and* a responsibility of the government. Feinsilver, *Healing the Masses*, 1.

97   David Blumenthal, "Fidel Castro's Health Care Legacy," *The Commonwealth Fund*, November 28, 106, last accessed January 29, 2017, http://www.commonwealthfund.org/publications/blog/2016/nov/fidel-castros-health-care-legacy.

98   Samuel Moyn, *The Last Utopia: Human Rights in History* (Cambridge, MA: Belknap Press of Harvard University Press, 2010).

99   Ibid., 140–1.

100   Ibid., 222.

101   Tobin makes this point with respect to the human right to health specifically in international law. John Tobin, *The Right to Health in International Law* (Oxford: Oxford University Press, 2012), 32.

102   Colleen M. Flood and Aeyal M. Gross, "Introduction: Marrying Human Rights and Health Care Systems: Contexts for a Power to Improve Access and Equity," in *The Right to Health at the Public/Private Divide: A Global Comparative Study*, 2–4; C. Flood and A. Gross, "Litigating the Right to Health: What Can We Learn from a Comparative Law and Health Care Systems Approach," *Health and Human Rights* 16, no. 2 (2014).

103   Jonathan Wolff, *The Human Right to Health* (New York: W.W. Norton & Company, 2012), 39–91, quote 41.

104   Joe Wright, "Only Your Calamity: The Beginnings of Activism by and for People with AIDS," *American Journal of Public Health* 103, no. 10 (2013), 1788–98.

105   Ibid.

106   Ibid.

107   The document is reproduced in full in ibid., 1794, which is the source for these quotes.

108   Ibid., 1796.

109   Elizabeth Fee and Manon Parry, "Jonathan Mann, HIV/AIDS, and Human Rights," *Journal of Public Health Policy* 29, no. 1 (2008), 54–71.

110   Ibid., 59.

111   Ibid., 63; Jonathan Mann and Daniel Tarantola, "Responding to HIV/AIDS: A Historical Perspective," *Health and Human Rights* (1998).

112   Fee and Parry, "Jonathan Mann, HIV/AIDS, and Human Rights," 61.

113   B. M. Meier and W. Onzivu, "The Evolution of Human Rights in World Health Organization Policy and the Future of Human Rights through Global Health Governance," *Public Health* 128, no. 2, 181.

114   Wolff, *The Human Right to Health*, 59–67.

115   Fee and Parry, "Jonathan Mann, HIV/AIDS, and Human Rights," 62.

116   Michael Kirby, "The Right to Health Fifty Years On: Still Skeptical?" *Health and Human Rights* 4, No. 1 (1999), 17.

117   Fee and Parry, "Jonathan Mann, HIV/AIDS, and Human Rights," 64–5.

118   Ibid., 66.

119   Jonathan M. Mann et al., "Health and Human Rights," *Health and Human Rights* 1, no. 1 (1994): 6–23.

120   Ibid., 13.

121   Ibid., 21.

122   Kari Hannibal and Robert S. Lawrence, "The Health Professional as Human Rights Promoter: Ten Years of Physicians for Human Rights (USA)," *Health and Human Rights* 2, no. 1 (1996): 110–27.

123   Jonathan Mann, "Health and Human Rights: If Not Now, When?" *Health and Human Rights* 2, no. 3 (1997), 115.

124   Alastair T. Iles, "Health and the Environment: A Human Rights Agenda for the Future," *Health and Human Rights* 2, no. 2 (1997), 56.

125   Powel Kazanjian, "The AIDS Pandemic in Historic Perspective," *Journal of the History of Medicine and Allied Sciences* 69, no. 3 (2014), 362.

126 Ibid., 361.

127 Wolff, *The Human Right to Health*, 71; Lisa Forman, "'Rights' and Wrongs: What Utility for the Right to Health in Reforming Trade Rules on Medicines?," *Health and Human Rights* 10, no. 2 (2008), 43.

128 Helena Nygren-Krug, "The Right to Health: From Concept to Practice," in *Advancing the Human Right to Health*, ed. José M. Zuniga, Stephen P. Marks, and Lawrence O. Gostin (Oxford: Oxford University Press, 2013), 40.

129 Brigit C. A. Toebes, *The Right to Health as a Human Right in International Law* (Antwerpen: Instersentia/Hart, 1999), 74.

130 United Nations, *Vienna Declaration and Programme of Action* (1993), last accessed January 12, 2017, http://www.ohchr.org/en/professionalinterest/pages/vienna.aspx.

131 Meier and Onzivu, "The Evolution of Human Rights in World Health Organization Policy and the Future of Human Rights through Global Health Governance," 179–87.

132 Siri Gloppen, "Litigation as a Strategy to Hold Governments Accountable for Implementing the Right to Health," *Health and Human Rights* 10, no. 2 (2008), 23.

133 Many have stressed the significance of General Comment 14, including: Stephen P. Marks, "The Emergence and Scope of the Human Right to Health," in *Advancing the Human Right to Health*, 9–10; Paul O'Connell, "The Human Right to Health in an Age of Market Hegemony," in *Global Health and Human Rights: Legal and Philosophical Perspectives*, ed. John Harrington and Maria Stuttaford (London: Routledge, 2010), 192; Wolff, *The Human Right to Health*, 11–12, 27–35; Gunilla Backman et al., "Health Systems and the Right to Health: An Assessment of 194 Countries," *The Lancet* 372, no. 9655 (2008), 2048–9.

134 United Nations, *General Comment No. 14* (2000), accessed March 28, 2016, http://www.un.org/documents/ecosoc/docs/2001/e2001-22.pdf, 129.

135 Ibid., 130.

136 Ibid., 131–2.

137 United Nations, *International Covenant on Economic, Social and Cultural Rights*, last accessed January 12, 2017, http://www.ohchr.org/en/professionalinterest/pages/cescr.aspx.

138 *General Comment No. 14*, 138–9.

139 Ibid., 139.

140 Ibid., 142–3.

141 Ibid., 144.

142 Forman notes that the "minimum core" originated in General Comment 3, but that General Comment 14 went beyond it by making compliance with the core "non-derogable." Marks, "The Emergence and Scope of the Human Right to Health," 10; Lisa Forman, "What Future for the Minimum Core? Contextualising the Implications of South African Socioeconomic Rights Jurisprudence for the International Human Right to Health," in *Global Health and Human Rights: Legal and Philosophical Perspectives*, ed. John Harrington and Maria Stuttaford (London: Routledge, 2010), 68.

143 Paul Hunt, "The UN Special Rapporteur on the Right to Health: Key Objectives, Themes, and Interventions," *Health and Human Rights* 7, no. 1 (2003), 1–2.

144 Paul Hunt and Sheldon Leader, "Developing and Applying the Right to the Highest Attainable Standard of Health: The Role of the UN Special Rapporteur (2002–2008)," in *Global Health and Human Rights: Legal and Philosophical Perspectives*, ed. John Harrington and Maria Stuttaford (London: Routledge, 2010), 29.

145 Ibid., 29.

146 Gunilla Backman et al., "Health Systems and the Right to Health: An Assessment of 194 Countries," *The Lancet* 372, no. 9655 (2008), 2047–85.

147 Tobin, *The Right to Health in International Law*, 43.

148 Ibid., 71.

149 Flood and Gross, "Introduction: Marrying Human Rights and Health Care Systems: Contexts for a Power to Improve Access and Equity," 9.

150 Ibid.

151   38 percent guaranteed it, for 14 percent it was aspirational (Table I). Jody Heymann et al., "Constitutional Rights to Health, Public Health and Medical Care: The Status of Health Protections in 191 Countries," *Global Public Health* 8, no. 6 (2013), 639–53.

152   See Figure 1, ibid.

153   Nathaniel Bruhn, "Litigating against an Epidemic: HIV/AIDS and the Promise of Socioeconomic Rights in South Africa," *Michigan Journal of Race and Law* 17 (2011), 192–3.

154   Ibid.

155   *Constitution of the Republic of South Africa* (1996), accessed April 2, 2016, http://www.gov. za/documents/constitution-republic-south-africa-1996. This is the source for all quotes from the Constitution in this paragraph.

156   Lisa Forman and Jerome Amir Singh, "The Role of Rights and Litigation in Assuring More Equitable Access to Health Care in South Africa," in *The Right to Health at the Public/Private Divide: A Global Comparative Study*, 302.

157   Charles Ngwena, Rebecca Cook, and Ebenezer Durojaye, "The Right to Health in Post-Apartheid Era in South Africa," in *Advancing the Human Right to Health*, 132.

158   Chris Holden, "Actors and Motives in the Internationalization of Health Businesses," *Business and Politics* 5, no. 3 (2004), 289.

159   Ibid.; Holden, "Privatization and Trade in Health Services: A Review of the Evidence," 685; Richard D. Smith, Rupa Chanda, and Viroj Tangcharoensathien, "Trade in Health-Related Services," *Lancet* 373, no. 9663 (2009), 593–601.

160   Richard D. Smith, Carlos Correa, and Cecilia Oh, "Trade, TRIPS, and Pharmaceuticals," *The Lancet* 373, no. 9664 (2009), 684–91.

161   Ibid., 686.

162   Ibid., 684–91.

163   Ibid.; O'Connell, "The Human Right to Health in an Age of Market Hegemony," 205; Forman, "'Rights' and Wrongs: What Utility for the Right to Health in Reforming Trade Rules on Medicines?" 46.

164   Forman, "'Rights' and Wrongs: What Utility for the Right to Health in Reforming Trade Rules on Medicines?" 43.

165   Ibid.

166   Ibid., 44.

167   Quoted in Julian Borger, "Gore Accused of Working against Cheap AIDS Drugs," *The Guardian*, August 9, 1999, accessed April 1, 2016, http://www.theguardian.com/world/1999/aug/10/uselections2000.usa.

168   Ibid.; Charles Babcock and Ceci Connolly, "AIDS Activists Badger Gore Again," *Washington Post*, June 18, 1999, accessed April 1, 2016, http://www.washingtonpost.com/wp-srv/politics/campaigns/wh2000/stories/gore061899.htm.

169   Forman "'Rights' and Wrongs: What Utility for the Right to Health in Reforming Trade Rules on Medicines?" 44.

170   Samantha Power, "The AIDS Rebel: Letter from South Africa," *The New Yorker*, May 19 2003; Zackie Achmat, "Zackie Achmat – Head of the Treatment Action Campaign. Interview by Pam Das," *Lancet Infectious Disease* 4, no. 7 (2004), 467–70.

171   Mark Heywood, "South Africa's Treatment Action Campaign: Combining Law and Social Mobilization to Realize the Right to Health," *Journal of Human Rights Practice* 1, no. 1 (2009), 17–18.

172   Ibid., 15; Achmat, "Zackie Achmat – Head of the Treatment Action Campaign. Interview by Pam Das."

173   Forman, "'Rights' and Wrongs: What Utility for the Right to Health in Reforming Trade Rules on Medicines?" 44.

174   Ibid.

175   Ibid.

176   A point made by Leslie London, "What Is a Human-Rights Based Approach to Health and Does It Matter?" *Health and Human Rights* 10, no. 1 (2013).

177   Forman, "'Rights' and Wrongs: What Utility for the Right to Health in Reforming Trade Rules on Medicines?" 44.

178   Bruhn, "Litigating against an Epidemic: HIV/AIDS and the Promise of Socioeconomic Rights in South Africa," 195–6.

179   Ibid.

180   Ibid.

181   These points about the Soobramoney case and the quote are from: Forman, "What Future for the Minimum Core? Contextualising the Implications of South African Socioeconomic Rights Jurisprudence for the International Human Right to Health," 70–1. Also see: Aeyal M. Gross, "The Right to Health in an Era of Privatisation and Globalisation: National and International Perspectives," in *Exploring Social Rights: Between Theory and Practice*, ed. Daphne Barak-Erez and Aeyal M. Gross (Oxford: Hart, 2007), 315–17.

182   Bruhn, "Litigating against an Epidemic: HIV/AIDS and the Promise of Socioeconomic Rights in South Africa," 196.

183   Ngwena, Cook, and Durojaye, "The Right to Health in Post-Apartheid Era in South Africa," 133.

184   Gross, "The Right to Health in an Era of Privatisation and Globalisation: National and International Perspectives," 317.

185   Bruhn, "Litigating against an Epidemic: HIV/AIDS and the Promise of Socioeconomic Rights in South Africa," 196–8.

186   Forman, "What Future for the Minimum Core? Contextualising the Implications of South African Socioeconomic Rights Jurisprudence for the International Human Right to Health," 72. See also: Ngwena, Cook, and Durojaye, "The Right to Health in Post-Apartheid Era in South Africa," 134; Bruhn, "Litigating against an Epidemic: HIV/AIDS and the Promise of Socioeconomic Rights in South Africa," 198.

187   Pearlie Joubert, "Grootboom dies homeless and penniless," *Mail & Guardian*, August 8, 2008, last accessed January 12, 2017, http://mg.co.za/article/2008-08-08-grootboom-dies-homeless-and-penniless.

188   Wolff, *The Human Right to Health*, 73.

189   This paragraph relies throughout on Bruhn, "Litigating against an Epidemic: HIV/AIDS and the Promise of Socioeconomic Rights in South Africa," 199–201.

190   This point and the quote from the Supreme Court are from Forman, "What Future for the Minimum Core? Contextualising the Implications of South African Socioeconomic Rights Jurisprudence for the International Human Right to Health," 73.

191   Ibid.

192   Heywood, "South Africa's Treatment Action Campaign: Combining Law and Social Mobilization to Realize the Right to Health," 26.

193   Forman and Singh, "The Role of Rights and Litigation in Assuring More Equitable Access to Health Care in South Africa," 294–300, 318; Shan Naidoo, "The South African National Health Insurance: A Revolution in Health-Care Delivery!," *Journal of Public Health* 34, no. 1 (2012), 149.

194   Shan Naidoo, "The South African National Health Insurance: A Revolution in Health-Care Delivery!" 149.

195   Forman and Singh, "The Role of Rights and Litigation in Assuring More Equitable Access to Health Care in South Africa," 300.

196   Claire Keeton, "Bridging the Gap in South Africa," *Bulletin of the World Health Organization* 88, no. 11 (2010); Naidoo, "The South African National Health Insurance: A Revolution in Health-Care Delivery!" 149–50; Global Health Watch, *South Africa: Building or Destroying Health Systems*, accessed April 14, 2016, http://www.ghwatch.org/sites/www.ghwatch.org/files/B5_1.pdf.

197   Global Health Watch, *South Africa: Building or Destroying Health Systems*.

198   Gavin H. Mooney, *The Health of Nations: Towards a New Political Economy* (London; New York: Zed Books, 2012), 85.

199   In this section, I draw from several chapters of a new edited book, *The Right to Health at the Public/Private Divide*. This work excellently demonstrates the complex interaction between the

right to health and public and private healthcare systems. *The Right to Health at the Public/Private Divide: A Global Comparative Study*, ed. Colleen M. Flood and Aeyal M. Gross (New York: Cambridge University Press, 2014).

200   Jairnilson Paim et al., "The Brazilian Health System: History, Advances, and Challenges," *The Lancet* 377, no. 9779, 1784.

201   Ibid.; Oscar A. Cabrera and Ana S. Ayala, "Advancing the Right to Health through Litigation," in *Advancing the Human Right to Health*, 27.

202   Paim et al., "The Brazilian Health System: History, Advances, and Challenges,", 1784–5; Armando De Negri Filho, "Brazil: A Long Journey Towards a Universal Healthcare System," in *Advancing the Human Right to Health*, 173.

203   *Federative Republic of Brazil Constitution, with 1996 Reforms in English*, accessed April 4, 2016, http://pdba.georgetown.edu/Constitutions/Brazil/english96.html.

204   Cabrera and Ayala, "Advancing the Right to Health through Litigation," 32.

205   James Macinko and Matthew J. Harris, "Brazil's Family Health Strategy — Delivering Community-Based Primary Care in a Universal Health System," *New England Journal of Medicine* 372, no. 23 (2015): 2177–81.

206   Mariana Mota Prado, "Provision of Health Care Services and the Right to Health in Brazil," in *The Right to Health at the Public/Private Divide : A Global Comparative Study*, 319–20; Filho, "Brazil: A Long Journey Towards a Universal Healthcare System," 177; Paim et al., "The Brazilian Health System: History, Advances, and Challenges," 1787.

207   Prado, "Provision of Health Care Services and the Right to Health in Brazil," 319.

208   Ibid.

209   Filho, "Brazil: A Long Journey Towards a Universal Healthcare System," 178.

210   Prado, "Provision of Health Care Services and the Right to Health in Brazil," 331.

211   Filho, "Brazil: A Long Journey Towards a Universal Healthcare System," 178; Paim et al., "The Brazilian Health System: History, Advances, and Challenges," 1785.

212   Octavio Luiz Motta Ferraz, "The Right to Health in the Courts of Brazil: Worsening Health Inequities?" *Health and Human Rights* 11, no. 2 (2009): 33–45.

213   Ibid., 35.

214   Ibid., 33–45.

215   João Biehl et al., "Between the Court and the Clinic: Lawsuits for Medicines and the Right to Health in Brazil," *Health and Human Rights* 14, no. 1 (2012), 36–52.

216   Ibid., 49.

217   Everaldo Lamprea, "Colombia's Right-to-Health Litigation in a Context of Health Care Reform," in *The Right to Health at the Public/Private Divide: A Global Comparative Study*, 139.

218   Ibid., 139; Cabrera and Ayala, "Advancing the Right to Health through Litigation," 32.

219   Lamprea, "Colombia's Right-to-Health Litigation in a Context of Health Care Reform," 144–5.

220   Ibid., 149–51.

221   Cabrera and Ayala, "Advancing the Right to Health through Litigation," 29–30; Alicia Ely Yamin and Oscar Parra-Vera, "How Do Courts Set Health Policy? The Case of the Colombian Constitutional Court," *PLoS Medicine* 6, no. 2 (2009): 0147–50.

222   Lamprea, "Colombia's Right-to-Health Litigation in a Context of Health Care Reform," 133.

223   Homedes and Ugalde, "Why Neoliberal Health Reforms Have Failed in Latin America," 84.

224   Howard Waitzkin, "The Strange Career of Managed Competition: From Military Failure to Medical Success?" *American Journal of Public Health* 84, no. 3 (1994), 482–9. Enthoven laid out his ideas in the late 1970s in two papers in the *New England Journal of Medicine*. Alain C. Enthoven, "Consumer-Choice Health Plan – Inflation and Inequity in Health Care Today: Alternatives for Cost Control and an Analysis of Proposals for National Health Insurance," *New England Journal of Medicine* 298, no. 12 (1978), 650–8; Alain C. Enthoven, "Consumer-Choice Health Plan—a National Health Insurance Proposal Based on Regulated Competition in the Private Sector," *New England Journal of Medicine* 298, no. 13 (1978), 709–20.

225   Adam Gaffney, "What Obamacare Can't Do," *Jacobin*, February 2, 2016, accessed April 5, 2016, https://www.jacobinmag.com/2016/02/gaffney-single-payer-sanders-healthcare-obamacare-aca-clinton.

226   Homedes and Ugalde, "Why Neoliberal Health Reforms Have Failed in Latin America," 91.

227   Sunil Amrith, "Political Culture of Health in India: A Historical Perspective," *Economic and Political Weekly* 42, no. 2 (2007), 114–21.

228   Amrith notes that the success of its early malaria control program "must not be underestimated," even though it would soon "falter." Ibid., 118.

229   Vikram Patel et al., "Assuring Health Coverage for All in India," *The Lancet* 386, no. 10011 (2015), 2423.

230   Y. Balarajan, S. Selvaraj, and S. V. Subramanian, "Health Care and Equity in India," *Lancet* 377, no. 9764 (2011), 505–15.

231   K. Srinath Reddy et al., "Towards Achievement of Universal Health Care in India by 2020: A Call to Action," *Lancet* 377, no. 9767 (2011), 760; Anand Grover, Maitreyi Misra, and Lubhywathi Rangarajan, "Right to Health: Addressing Inequities through Litigation in India," in *The Right to Health at the Public/Private Divide: A Global Comparative Study*, 427.

232   Reddy et al., "Towards Achievement of Universal Health Care in India by 2020: A Call to Action," 760–8.

233   Ravi Duggal, "Health and Development in India: Moving Towards the Right to Health," in *Advancing the Human Right to Health*, 119.

234   Grover, Misra, and Rangarajan, "Right to Health: Addressing Inequities through Litigation in India," 431–2.

235   The facts about this case in this paragraph are drawn from: ibid., 437; Cabrera and Ayala, "Advancing the Right to Health through Litigation," 31; Hunt and Leader, "Developing and Applying the Right to the Highest Attainable Standard of Health: The Role of the UN Special Rapporteur (2002–2008)," 40.

236   Grover, Misra, and Rangarajan, "Right to Health: Addressing Inequities through Litigation in India," 431–2, 441; Cabrera and Ayala, "Advancing the Right to Health through Litigation," 31.

237   Grover, Misra, and Rangarajan, "Right to Health: Addressing Inequities through Litigation in India," 449.

238   Duggal, "Health and Development in India: Moving Towards the Right to Health," 118.

239   Patel et al., "Assuring Health Coverage for All in India," 2425; K. Srinath Reddy, "India's Aspirations for Universal Health Coverage," *New England Journal of Medicine* 373, no. 1 (2015), 3; Reddy et al., "Towards Achievement of Universal Health Care in India by 2020: A Call to Action," 763.

240   Duggal, "Health and Development in India: Moving Towards the Right to Health," 116.

241   Aditya Kalra, "India's Universal Healthcare Rollout to Cost $26 Billion," *Reuters*, October 30, 2014, accessed April 8, 2016, http://in.reuters.com/article/uk-india-health-idINKBN0IJ0VN20141030.

242   Dinesh C. Sharma, "India's BJP Government and Health: 1 Year On," *The Lancet* 385, no. 9982, 2031–2.

243   Gregory P. Marchildon, "Canada: Health System Review," *Health Systems in Transition* 15, no. 1 (2013), 28.

244   Colleen M. Flood, "Litigating Health Rights in Canada: A White Knight for Equity?" in *The Right to Health at the Public/Private Divide: A Global Comparative Study*, 84.

245   Steven Lewis, "A System in Name Only — Access, Variation, and Reform in Canada's Provinces," *New England Journal of Medicine* 372, no. 6 (2015), 498–9; Flood, "Litigating Health Rights in Canada: A White Knight for Equity?" 79–80.

246   Flood, "Litigating Health Rights in Canada: A White Knight for Equity?" 85.

247   The two key sources here are: Flood, "Litigating Health Rights in Canada: A White Knight for Equity?" 94–8; Aeyal Gross, "Is There a Human Right to Private Health Care?" *Journal of Law, Medicine, and Ethics* 41, no. 1 (2013), 138–46.

248   Gross, "Is There a Human Right to Private Health Care?" 139; Flood, "Litigating Health Rights in Canada: A White Knight for Equity?" 94–8.

249   Gross, "Is There a Human Right to Private Health Care?" 140.

250   Ibid.

251 Wendy Glauser, "Private Clinics Continue Explosive Growth," *Canadian Medical Association Journal* 183, no. 8 (2011), e437–8; Alex Peden, "Backgrounder: Court Challenges to One-Tier Medicare," *EvidenceNetwork.ca*, October 15, 2015, accessed April 5, 2016, http://umanitoba.ca/outreach/evidencenetwork/archives/20743.

252 This paragraph thus far is based on: Alex Peden, "Backgrounder: Court Challenges to One-Tier Medicare"; Karen S. Palmer, "Backgrounder: A Primer on the Legal Challenge between Dr. Brian Day and British Columbia – and How It May Affect Our Healthcare System," *EvidenceNetwork.ca*, accessed April 5, 2016, http://umanitoba.ca/outreach/evidencenetwork/archives/25738#sthash.j8PZLeEX.jvsK2ql2.dpuf.

253 A point made by: Flood and Gross, "Conclusion: Contexts for the Promise and Peril of the Right to Health," in *The Right to Health at the Public/Private Divide: A Global Comparative Study*, 458.

254 Gloppen, "Litigation as a Strategy to Hold Governments Accountable for Implementing the Right to Health," 24.

255 Flood and Gross, "Conclusion: Contexts for the Promise and Peril of the Right to Health," in *The Right to Health at the Public/Private Divide: A Global Comparative Study*, 456–80. Quotes on pp. 469, 473.

256 Flood and Gross, "Litigating the Right to Health: What Can We Learn from a Comparative Law and Health Care Systems Approach," 69–70. Also see: Gross, "The Right to Health in an Era of Privatisation and Globalisation: National and International Perspectives," 330–1. Specifically, some have worried about health rights litigation being used for the benefit of the pharmaceutical industry: Alicia Ely Yamin, "Editorial: Promoting Equity in Health: What Role for Courts?" *Health and Human Rights* 16, no. 2 (2014), 7.

257 Alicia Ely Yamin, "Will We Take Suffering Seriously? Reflections on What Applying a Human Rights Framework to Health Means and Why We Should Care," *Health and Human Rights* 10, no. 1 (2008), 51. Also: Alicia Ely Yamin, "Beyond Compassion: The Central Role of Accountability in Applying a Human Rights Framework to Health," *Health and Human Rights* 10, no. 2 (2008), 1–20.

258 Benjamin M. Meier and Alicia E. Yamin, "Right to Health Litigation and HIV/AIDS Policy," *The Journal of Law, Medicine and Ethics* 39 Suppl 1 (2011), 83.

259 Cabrera and Ayala, "Advancing the Right to Health through Litigation," 35.

260 Stein, *Pivotal Decade: How the United States Traded Factories for Finance in the Seventies.*

261 Adam Gaffney, "The Neoliberal Turn in American Health Care," *International Journal of Health Services* 45, no. 1 (2015), 33–52.

262 Here I draw on a framework used in a forthcoming book chapter. Adam Gaffney, David Himmelstein, and Steffie Woolhandler, "The Failure of Obamacare and a Revision of the Single-Payer Proposal After a Quarter Century of Struggle," ed. Howard Waitzkin, *Under the Knife: Beyond Capital in Health* (New York: Monthly Review Press, 2017).

263 There is a large literature on this topic. Good introductions include: John P. Geyman, "Moral Hazard and Consumer-Driven Health Care: A Fundamentally Flawed Concept," *International Journal of the Health Services* 37, no. 2 (2007), 333–51; Malcolm Gladwell, "The Moral-Hazard Myth," *New Yorker*, August 29, 2005. I discuss some of this history as well: Gaffney, "The Neoliberal Turn in American Health Care."

264 Martin S. Feldstein, "The Welfare Loss of Excess Health Insurance," *The Journal of Political Economy* 81 no. 2 (1973), 251, 277. I briefly discuss these points by Feldstein and Hayek in Gaffney, "The Neoliberal Turn in American Health Care."

265 F. A. Hayek, *The Constitution of Liberty: The Definitive Edition* (Chicago: University of Chicago Press, 2011), 421–2.

266 Paul M. Ellwood, Jr. et al., "Health Maintenance Strategy," *Medical Care* 9, no. 3 (1971), 291–8; Bradford H. Gray, "The Rise and Decline of the HMO: A Chapter in U.S. Health-Policy History," in *History and Health Policy in the United States: Putting the Past Back In*, ed. Rosemary Stevens, Charles E. Rosenberg, and Lawton R. Burns (New Brunswick, NJ: Rutgers University Press, 2006), 318; Adam Gaffney and Howard Waitzkin, "The Affordable Care Act and the Transformation of US Health Care," *Cuadernos de Relaciones Laborales* 34 no. 2 (2016), 244–61.

267   Ellwood et al., "Health Maintenance Strategy," 298.

268   Gray, "The Rise and Decline of the HMO: A Chapter in U.S. Health-Policy History," 323–4. On the international spread, see: Karen Stocker, Howard Waitzkin, and Celia Iriart, "The Exportation of Managed Care to Latin America," *New England Journal of Medicine* 340, no. 14 (1999), 1131–6.

269   Howard Waitzkin and Ida Hellander, "The Neoliberal Model Comes Home to Roost in the United States—If We Let It," *Monthly Review* 68, no. 01 (2016).

270   Gaffney, "What Obamacare Can't Do"; Waitzkin and Hellander, "The Neoliberal Model Comes Home to Roost in the United States—If We Let It."

271   "The Medical Industrial Complex," *Health-PAC Bulletin*, November (1969), accessed December 21, 2016, http://www.healthpacbulletin.org/wp-content/uploads/2012/10/1969-Nov.pdf: 1–2. Relman later elaborated on the concept: Arnold S. Relman, "The New Medical-Industrial Complex," *New England Journal of Medicine* 303, no. 17 (1980), 963–70.

272   Charles Webster, *The National Health Service: A Political History*, new ed. (Oxford: Oxford University Press, 2002), 145.

273   Ibid.

274   Ibid., 141.

275   Allyson Pollock, *NHS Plc: The Privatisation of Our Health Care* (London: Verso, 2004), especially: 1–17, 34–124, 157–90. The privatization of long-term care is also described by: Hans Maarse, "The Privatization of Health Care in Europe: An Eight-Country Analysis," *Journal of Health Politics, Policy, and Law* 31, no. 5 (2006), 998–9.

276   Webster, *The National Health Service*, 157.

277   Pollock, *NHS Plc*, 33.

278   Maarse, "The Privatization of Health Care in Europe: An Eight-Country Analysis."

279   Ibid.

280   On the Netherlands experience, see: Pauline V. Rosenau and Christiaan J. Lako, "An Experiment with Regulated Competition and Individual Mandates for Universal Health Care: The New Dutch Health Insurance System," *Journal of Health Politics, Policy, and Law* 33, no. 6 (2008), 1031–55; André den Exter, "Health Care Access in the Netherlands: A True Story," in *The Right to Health at the Public/Private Divide: A Global Comparative Study*, 188–207; Brigit Toebes, "The Right to Health and the Privatization of National Health Systems: A Case Study of the Netherlands," *Health and Human Rights* 9, no. 1 (2006), 102–7; Kieke G. H. Okma, Theodore R. Marmor, and Jonathan Oberlander, "Managed Competition for Medicare? Sobering Lessons from the Netherlands," *New England Journal of Medicine* 365, no. 4 (2011), 287–9; Gaffney, "What Obamacare Can't Do."

281   Anders Anell, "The Public–Private Pendulum—Patient Choice and Equity in Sweden," *New England Journal of Medicine* 372, no. 1 (2015), 1–4; Anna-Sara Lind, "The Right to Health in Sweden," in *The Right to Health at the Public/Private Divide: A Global Comparative Study*, 51–2.

282   Rudolf Klein, "England's National Health Service—Broke but Not Broken," *Milbank Quarterly* 93, no. 3 (2015), 455–8.

283   John Appleby, "NHS Spending: Squeezed as Never Before," *The Kings Fund blog*, October 20 2015, accessed November 24, 2015, http://www.kingsfund.org.uk/blog/2015/10/nhs-spending-squeezed-never.

284   John Lister, "Bleeding Funds," April 4 2016, last accessed January 13, 2017, https://www.morningstaronline.co.uk/a-029a-Bleeding-funds#.VwVLb5MrLwd.

285   Adam Gaffney, "Saving the NHS," *Jacobin*, April 26, 2016, accessed June 1 2016, https://www.jacobinmag.com/2016/04/nhs-junior-doctors-strike-health-privatization.

286   *NHS SOS: How the NHS Was Betrayed—and How We Can Save It*, ed. Raymond Tallis, Jacky Davis, and Jacqueline de Romilly (Oneworld, 2013).

287   Allyson M. Pollock and David B. Price, "From Cradle to Grave," in *NHS SOS: How the NHS Was Betrayed—and How We Can Save It*, ed. Raymond Tallis and Jacky Davis (Oneworld, 2013), 188.

288   On austerity and neoliberalism, see: Labonte and Stuckler, "The Rise of Neoliberalism: How Bad Economics Imperils Health and What to Do About It"; Martin McKee et al., "Austerity:

A Failed Experiment on the People of Europe," *Clinical Medicine* 12, no. 4 (2012), 346–50. On Greece, see: Alexander Kentikelenis et al., "Greece's Health Crisis: From Austerity to Denialism," *Lancet* 383, no. 9918 (2014), 748–53; Charalampos Economou et al., "The Impact of the Crisis on the Health System and Health in Greece," *Economic Crisis, Health Systems, and Health in Europe: Country Experience* (European Observatory on Health Systems and Policies, World Health Organization, 2015), accessed multiple times available as of January 13, 2017, 103–42. On Spain, see: Helena Legido-Quigley et al., "Will Austerity Cuts Dismantle the Spanish Healthcare System?" *British Medical Journal* 346 (2013). On Ireland, see: Sara Ann Burke et al., "From Universal Health Insurance to Universal Healthcare? The Shifting Health Policy Landscape in Ireland since the Economic Crisis," *Health Policy* 120 no. 3 (2015), 235–40. On Portugal, Pedro Barros, "Health Policy Reform in Tough Times: The Case of Portugal," *Health Policy* 106, no. 1 (2012), 17–22.

289   These "four axes" are used as a framework for a discussion of healthcare austerity in a chapter in a forthcoming book (title tentative): Adam Gaffney and Carles Muntaner, "Impact of Austerity Policies on Health Services and Health," *Under the Knife: Beyond Capital in Health*, ed. Howard Waitzkin ed. (New York: Monthly Review Press, 2017). In addition to the articles cited in the notes above, on this topic also see: Martin McKee and David Stuckler, "The Assault on Universalism: How to Destroy the Welfare State," *British Medical Journal* 343 (2011); McKee et al., "Austerity: A Failed Experiment on the People of Europe"; Martin McKee et al., "Universal Health Coverage: A Quest for All Countries but under Threat in Some," *Value Health* 16, no. 1 Suppl (2013): S39–45; Aaron Reeves, Martin McKee, and David Stuckler, "The Attack on Universal Health Coverage in Europe: Recession, Austerity and Unmet Needs," *European Journal of Public Health* 25, no. 3 (2015), 364–5.

290   All quotes from this debate taken from: "Transcript of Second McCain, Obama Debate," accessed April 10, 2016, http://www.cnn.com/2008/POLITICS/10/07/presidential.debate.transcript.

291   Steven Brill, *America's Bitter Pill: Money, Politics, Backroom Deals, and the Fight to Fix Our Broken Healthcare System* (New York: Random House, 2015), 75.

292   Ibid. For a detailed accounting of the legislative process, see: John E. McDonough, *Inside National Health Reform* (Berkeley: University of California Press, 2011), 1–99.

293   Jill Quadagno, "Right-Wing Conspiracy? Socialist Plot? The Origins of the Patient Protection and Affordable Care Act," *Journal of Health Politics, Policy, and Law* 39, no. 1 (2014), 35–56; Adam Gaffney, "How Liberals Tried to Kill the Dream of Single-Payer," *The New Republic*, March 8, 2016, accessed March 8, 2016, https://newrepublic.com/article/131251/liberals-tried-kill-dream-single-payer.

294   Henry J. Kaiser Family Foundation, "Summary of the Affordable Care Act," accessed December 2, 105, http://kff.org/health-reform/fact-sheet/summary-of-the-affordable-care-act/.

295   Michael E. Martinez, Robin A. Cohen, and Emily Zammitti, "Health Insurance Coverage: Early Release of Estimates from the National Health Interview Survey, January–September 2015" (Hyattsville, MD: National Center for Health Statistics, 2016), http://www.cdc.gov/nchs/data/nhis/earlyrelease/insur201602.pdf, Accessed February 15, 2016.

296   Gary Claxton, Cynthia Cox, and Matthew Rae, "The Costs of Care with Marketplace Coverage," *Henry J. Kaiser Family Foundation*, February 11, 2015, accessed February 22, 2015, http://kff.org/health-costs/issue-brief/the-cost-of-care-with-marketplace-coverage/; Henry J. Kaiser Family Foundation, "The 2015 Employer Health Benefits Survey" (2015), accessed September 29, 2015, http://kff.org/health-costs/report/2015-employer-health-benefits-survey/.

297   The source for the 31 million figure is Sara R. Collins et al., "The Problem of Underinsurance and How Rising Deductibles Will Make It Worse—Findings from the Commonwealth Fund Biennial Health Insurance Survey," *The Commonwealth Fund*, May 2015, http://www.commonwealthfund.org/publications/issue-briefs/2015/may/problem-of-underinsurance.

298   Adam Gaffney and Danny McCormick, "The Affordable Care Act: Implications for Health-Care Equity," *The Lancet* 389, no. 10077: 1442–52.

299   Alicia Ely Yamin and Jean Connolly Carmalt, "The United States: Right to Health Obligations in the Context of Disparity and Reform," in *Advancing the Human Right to Health*, 233.

300 Thomas Piketty, *Capital in the Twenty-First Century* (Cambridge, MA: Harvard University Press, 2014).

301 Adam Gaffney, "The Politics of Health," review of *Beyond Obamacare: Life, Death, and Social Policy*, by James. S. House, *Los Angeles Review of Books*, October 26, 2015, accessed October 26, 2016, https://lareviewofbooks.org/review/the-politics-of-health. Raj Chetty et al., "The Association between Income and Life Expectancy in the United States, 2001–2014," *Journal of the American Medical Association* 315 no. 16 (2016), 1750–66.

302 Adam Gaffney, "Is the Path to Racial Health Equity Paved with 'Reparations'? The Politics of Health, Part II: Review of Black Man in a White Coat: A Doctor's Reflections on Race and Medicine by Damon Tweedy and Just Medicine: A Cure for Racial Inequality in American Health Care by Dayna Bowen Matthew," *Los Angeles Review of Books*, March 7, 2016, accessed March 7, 2016, https://lareviewofbooks.org/review/is-the-path-to-racial-health-equity-paved-with-reparations-the-politics-of-health-part-ii.

303 Gaffney, "The Politics of Health"; James S. House and Russell Sage Foundation, *Beyond Obamacare: Life, Death, and Social Policy* (New York: Russell Sage Foundation, 2014); Anne Case and Angus Deaton, "Rising Morbidity and Mortality in Midlife among White Non-Hispanic Americans in the 21st Century," *Proceedings of the National Academy of Sciences* 112, no. 49 (2015), 15078–83.

304 Sabrina Tavernise, "First Rise in U.S. Death Rate in Years Surprises Experts," *New York Times*, June 1, 2016, accessed June 1, 2016, http://mobile.nytimes.com/2016/06/01/health/american-death-rate-rises-for-first-time-in-a-decade.html?_r=0&referer=.

305 "Jeremy Corbyn Launches 'Standing to Deliver'," http://www.jeremyforlabour.com/jeremy_corbyn_launches_standing_to_deliver; Gaffney, "Saving the NHS."

306 Aser Garcia Rada, "Privatisation in Spain Provokes Protests among Doctors," *British Medical Journal* 345 (2012), e7655; Aser Garcia Rada, "Spain's Largest Healthcare Privatisation Plan Is Halted," *British Medical Journal* 348 (2014), g1240; Aser Garcia Rada, "Spanish Doctors Protest against Law That Excludes Immigrants from Public Healthcare," *British Medical Journal* 345 (2012), e5716.

307 Gaffney, "How Liberals Tried to Kill the Dream of Single-Payer."

308 Adam Gaffney et al., "Moving Forward from the Affordable Care Act to a Single-Payer System," *American Journal of Public Health* 106, no. 6 (2016), 987–8.

309 Frank Newport, "Majority in U.S. Support Idea of Fed-Funded Healthcare System," *Gallup* (2016), accessed June 1, 2016, http://www.gallup.com/poll/191504/majority-support-idea-fed-funded-healthcare-system.aspx.

310 "Healthcare Reform to Make America Great Again," accessed December 22, 2016, https://www.donaldjtrump.com/positions/healthcare-reform.

311 Quoted in Robert Costa and Amy Goldstein, "Trump vows 'insurance for everybody' in Obamacare replacement plan," Washington Post, January 15, 2017.]

312 "Report from the Health Care Reform Task Force," published electronically June 22, 2016, accessed July 1, 2016, http://abetterway.speaker.gov/_assets/pdf/ABetterWay-HealthCare-PolicyPaper.pdf.

313 *Congressional Budget Office Cost Estimate: American Health Care Act* (Washington, DC: Congressional Budget Office, 2017), accessed March 13, 2017, https://www.cbo.gov/publication/52486.

314 Adam Gaffney, "If 22 million lose insurance, how many die?" *Theprogressivephysician.net*, published electronically November 11, 2016, accessed November 11, 2106, https://theprogressivephysician.net/2016/11/11/if-22-million-lose-insurance-how-many-die/; David Himmelstein and Steffie Woolhandler, "Repealing the Affordable Care Act will kill more than 43,000 people annually," *The Washington Post*, January 23, 2016, accessed January 23, 2016, https://www.washingtonpost.com/posteverything/wp/2017/01/23/repealing-the-affordable-care-act-will-kill-more-than-43000-people-annually/?utm_term=.bf0142ca36cd.

Conclusion

"Medical care," the surgeon Robert M. Sade approvingly noted in the pages of the *New England Journal of Medicine* in 1971, "is neither a right nor a privilege: it is a service that is provided by doctors and others to people who wish to purchase it."[1] As a description of the status quo, the sentence was partially correct: despite progress—for instance, the broad expansion of healthcare access achieved by the creation of Medicare—there was no universal right to healthcare in the United States in that era (or indeed, today). And at that point, hospitals and doctors could even more or less turn dying people away from their doors, charitably shuttling them to public institutions with the expectation (one hopes) that they wouldn't die *en route*. Such so-called "patient dumping" apparently become more prevalent during the 1980s.[2] Consider this example from that decade, as described in the *Journal of the American Medical Association*:

> [A] patient transferred to Cook County Hospital in Chicago was a 41-year-old man with gunshot wounds to his head, chest, and abdomen. He was in a coma and on a respirator. The reason for the transfer was that he had no insurance.[3]

Gunshot wounds in three body cavities and respiratory failure did not confer a free pass from the healthcare cash nexus. After all, healthcare was not a right, and the 41-year old man seemingly did not—to use Sade's words—"wish to purchase it."

Sade's article was entitled "Medical Care as a Right: A Refutation," and one senses that Sade thought he was on the losing side. Indeed, in the United States in the early 1970s, many were indeed optimistic that the federal government could pass national health insurance, and a legal right to healthcare brought into existence. However, although later reforms would alleviate some of the more outrageous abuses—and although President Barack Obama's ACA expanded healthcare access in more recent years—this did not come to pass. As described in the last chapter, the transformative change of the neoliberal era—undergirded in part by the ideas of economists like one cited by Sade—was rapidly approaching, and the dream of universal healthcare soon began to wilt.

Like many others, Sade counterpoised the notion of the healthcare right and the healthcare commodity. This rights-commodity construct has been followed in this book as well: one of the book's primary aims, in fact, has been to trace the tension between these two configurations of healthcare—what has been termed a healthcare right-commodity dialectic—through history and in different places. To be fair, however, this "dialectic" suggests something of a false dichotomy, as healthcare is provided in a myriad of ways, many of which resist such a binary categorization. For instance, care provided by a traditional healer, between family members or friends, as a form of charity, or in a variety of other ways might not neatly fit into one or the other category. Moreover, although health care has long been both (1) bought and sold, and (2) made available in various forms "outside the cash nexus," it is only after the advent of industrial capitalism, and especially over the course of the twentieth century, that healthcare "rights" and "commodities" emerged in the manner we now think of them. This was the result of three developments traced in this book, which can be briefly recapitulated.

The first development began in the late nineteenth century: governments took steps to create health systems that—incrementally and for a wide variety of often non-egalitarian reasons—created social rights to healthcare. These were not entirely new conceptually, as explored in the first few chapters of this book. As described in Chapter 1, for instance, explicit proposals for universal healthcare-type systems emerged as early as the English Civil War. And as explored in Chapter 2, the articulation of a doctrine of social rights—to some extent extending to healthcare—occurred contemporaneously with the political and civil rights typically associated with the Enlightenment and the French Revolution. Subsequently, Chapter 3 explored what early industrial capitalism meant for the right to health—and healthcare—in an age when "the rights of man" were no longer a prominent aspect of the political discourse. But it was not until the developments described in Chapter 4—when European nations created public health insurance systems—that social rights to healthcare (however limited) moved from concept to policy. And subsequently, as explored in Chapter 6, during the post-Second World War period, nations erected systems of truly universal healthcare, sometimes—as in the United Kingdom and Canada—with most care provided free at point of service, without the class-based tiers common to earlier "compulsory health insurance" systems. Thus did the first true social rights to healthcare emerge.

The second development was the corporatization and consolidation of the healthcare sector, which followed larger developments in capitalism itself. For instance, although Sade champions the "healthcare as commodity" concept, he envisions healthcare sold by the individual physician to the individual patient. In reality, however, over the course of the twentieth century, this "seller" was increasingly not the traditional black-bag-toting solo family practitioner of yore, but a large business enterprise. The "Coming of the Corporation," as Paul Starr called it in his 1982 history of US healthcare, *The Social Transformation of American Medicine*, has admittedly been uneven and partial, but it is nonetheless a crucial fact of the political economy of contemporary healthcare.[4] This corporate transformation is truly global in reach, with implications for both high and low-income nations.[5] Although specifics differ from nation to nation, the twentieth century saw the emergence and/or growth of a wide range of powerful healthcare enterprises: the global for-profit "managed care" insurance industry, a pharmaceutical industry of enormous wealth and influence, for-profit hospitals and (frequently) profit-oriented not-for-profit hospitals, and varied commercial providers ranging from corporate dialysis chains and cancer centers to nursing homes and hospices.[6] More recently, there has also been a trend towards greater consolidation within each of the three major pillars of what can be termed "healthcare capital"—hospital systems, insurance companies, and pharmaceutical companies—amounting to a transition towards larger business enterprises, which again reflects broader dynamics in capitalism.[7]

The third development—the birth and growth of the human right to health *movement*—emerged contemporaneously with this growing corporatization. These two developments were, in fact, interconnected. For instance, as explored in Chapter 7, in the context of the AIDS epidemic, pharmaceutical companies' essential denial of HIV medications to poor nations—often with the support of rich nation governments—provoked grassroots political resistance that employed "human right to health" language and concepts. Similarly, market-style healthcare reforms and "managed care"-style care denials contributed, to some extent, to the formation of the human right to health movement in high-income nations.[8] Thus, although the human right to health *concept* had its ideological underpinnings in the rights documents and declarations of the post-Second World War era, it was only during the 1980s and especially the 1990s that it emerged as a powerful language and movement. Universal healthcare and human rights thus became discursively and politically intertwined in a novel and sometimes powerful way.

This third development, it's worth noting, has not yet run its course: the human right to healthcare remains a battle cry among activists looking to establish, defend, or expand systems of universal healthcare. Where it will lead, however, is not clear: there is no certainty in such struggles, and the expanding power—and relentless greed—of healthcare capital constitutes an imposing bulwark to progressive change.

This leads to the second aim of this book, as set forth in the introduction: *why* was a right to healthcare created in some places, at some times, and not in others? There is—it is important to note—a literature concerning this sort of question from the broader perspective of the welfare state. This book in no way amounts to a comparative analysis of the predictors of universal healthcare, a task others have pursued.[9] However, it seems reasonable to conclude from the developments surveyed in this book that Esping-Andersen's assertions about the role of left power in bringing about a more decommodified form of a welfare state seem to have some general parallels in the realm of healthcare. In Germany, for instance, even though compulsory health insurance was the work of a highly conservative government (and even though it created only a limited and stratified right to healthcare), it was at least in part a response to the political threat posed by the Social Democratic Party (SPD). In Britain, the creation of the NHS emerged from the ideology and ultimately the electoral victory of a working-class political organization, the Labour Party. In Canada, as noted, the first provincial experiment with a universal healthcare system was the work of the leftist Cooperative Commonwealth Federation. And, as described in Chapter 6, a number of novel efforts towards universal healthcare systems in Latin America were undertaken by leftist parties or movements. Again, the approach here has not been systematic, but it nonetheless seems fair to assert the following: that some of the more uniquely decommodified universal healthcare systems—i.e. those that provide (often free) care to all without tiers or stratification—emerged in part as a result of Left and working-class political power and/or ideological pressure.[10]

This is, of course, very far from an original conclusion. Indeed, it was made by Vicente Navarro—a key figure in progressive healthcare thought in recent decades—some time ago: "In all countries," he wrote, "the major force behind the establishment of an NHP [national health program] has been the labor movement (and its political instruments—the socialist parties) in its pursuit of the welfare state."[11] It is also true that no one single factor will fully explain the emergence or characteristics of a nation's healthcare system. For instance, in the US context, historian Colin Gordon has emphasized that a purely class-based viewpoint disregards the role of racial and gender dynamics.[12] For instance, he notes that the prospect of national health insurance "posed a more direct threat to the southern racial order," a dynamic which led to resistance and which provides at "least a partial explanation for the failure of national health insurance in the United States."[13] That racism has been wielded to undercut support for universal welfare programs seems difficult to deny. Similarly, a structuring of the welfare state around the (usually) male breadwinner meant that early systems of compulsory health insurance often effectively denied benefits to many or most women.[14] Gender dynamics thus played a role in limiting the scope of "universal" healthcare systems in some places. Yet none of this reduces the essential fact that in most places we look, the ideological taproots of universal, decommodified healthcare systems run sharply leftward, from the nineteenth century Erfurt program to today.

Although historical analyses about the right to healthcare can no doubt be revealing and useful, they nonetheless leave unanswered the most important questions. Should a human right to healthcare, for instance, remain a goal in the twenty-first century, in our age of rapid technological advancement, rising inequality, and political reaction? Can, and should, such a right ever be achieved not only within national borders, but across them? And are there practical pitfalls in an employing rights-based rhetoric to advance the cause of healthcare universalism?

The intensive care unit—where I mostly work—provides a strange vantage point for thinking about healthcare rights, and especially the question of trans-national healthcare equality. In the ICU, lives can sometimes be saved through the intensive application of medical science and advanced technology; at the same time, it's a setting where the provision of highly expensive (and sometimes inappropriate) care to those who are beyond all aid is far from rare. Under-standably, the expansion of critical care services might thus be seen as a low priority, especially for low- or middle-income nations, from the perspective of healthcare rights. Yet this misses the point. The fact that people continue to unnecessarily die in some nations because of lack of access to critical care—or for that matter to cancer care, surgical care, or whatever high-technology life-saving or life-improving care is available to the rich and not the poor—is a violation of the equal right to healthcare. This is, admittedly, an atypical way to look at the question of healthcare rights: the focus, at least when the discussion is on low-income nations, is often on basic care and "essential" medications. And no doubt, health systems and governments must work with the resources currently at their disposal, and of course they must prioritize. But an *awareness* of the reality of transnational inequality need not lead to an *acceptance* of it, lest the notion of equality and healthcare rights lose all currency.

Thus, though it is no doubt a distant goal, an equal right to healthcare—whether for PTSD or pancreatic cancer, a gunshot wound or a gangrenous gall bladder—should be the goal both within nations but also among nations. An equal global human right to healthcare, when so phrased, is no doubt radical, and perhaps even utopian-sounding. However, it is as defensible as any other universal global human right. Indeed, as Upendra Baxi argues, health is actually a *precondition* for the protection of other rights: "Health . . . is a sine qua non for accessibility, exercise and enjoyment of all other human rights . . . one may not have all the human rights without first being *alright*."[15]

Creating new rights to healthcare thus remains a difficult, yet critical task. At the same time, it is worth acknowledging that there are potential pitfalls in a rights-based approach. There is a real danger, for instance, that the "right to healthcare" could become an increasingly aspirational but decreasingly meaningful rhetorical gesture, devoid of a clear connection to an explicit political program. It's cheap to talk about the right to healthcare, and indeed, politicians increasingly endorse it. The risk is that this "right" becomes severed from the essential tool necessary for its realization: the creation of a universal health system in which individuals can obtain equitable care on the basis of their medical needs, not economic status. On a similar level, "universal healthcare" can also become emptied of meaning. Indeed, it may already be being slowly modified into what some now call "universal health coverage," an increasingly invoked paradigm that is sometimes used to describe quasi-universal systems that provide tiered, unequal benefits—like that of the US or Colombia.[16] Despite the "universal" moniker, such systems often provide healthcare benefits based on one's economic status, an arrangement conducive to the prerogatives of corporate healthcare entities like insurers (in contradistinction to fully public, equitable systems). Indeed, following Trump's election in late 2016, Congressional Republicans took this downgraded version of universalism a step further, calling for a system of "universal access" to health insurance products for those who want (and presumably, can afford) to buy them.[17] Universal "access" to *buy* healthcare should be seen as the commoditization of universal healthcare itself.

Still, whatever the potential pitfalls of the "human right to health" discourse may be, the justice of the underlying cause seems clear: increasingly prosaic as rhetoric, this right remains no less radical as praxis. The real danger, then, is not that we will be outmaneuvered in the rhetorical field, but that will be bested—by the powerful few—in the arena of political struggle.

"Very brief," Bertrand Russell once wrote about our fellow members of the human race, "is the time in which we can help them, in which their happiness or misery is decided. Be it ours to shed sunshine on their path, to lighten their sorrows by the balm of sympathy, to give them the pure joy of a never-tiring affection, to strengthen failing courage, to instill faith in hours of despair."[18] Be it ours too, then, to help our fellows escape suffering and to live—to the greatest extent possible—in better health of body and of mind, for the very longest that nature permits them.

Healthcare, of course, is not health, and despite much progress, its benefits remain limited and its delivery very far from perfect. Still, when provided with the highest standards of humanity and science, healthcare can do a great deal to ease human suffering, improving both the number and the happiness of our brief years. Yet the commoditization of healthcare—there should be little doubt—violently cuts short its salubrious potential, constraining its benefits to some, and subordinating the medical mission to the motives and dynamics of capital. In contrast, if healthcare were made an essential right of humankind, its benefits would be universalized, its purpose made more noble, and its capacity to aid multiplied beyond measure. This will not come easily, but it is also well within the realm of what we can achieve together.

Notes

1   Robert M. Sade, "Medical Care as a Right: A Refutation," *New England Journal of Medicine* 285, no. 23 (1971), 1289.
2   David A. Ansell and Robert L. Schiff, "Patient Dumping: Status, Implications, and Policy Recommendations," *Journal of the American Medical Association* 257, no. 11 (1987), 1500–2.
3   Ibid., 1501.
4   Paul Starr, *The Social Transformation of American Medicine* (New York: Basic Books, 1982), 420–9.
5   For the low-income nation scene especially, see: John Lister, *Health Policy Reform: Global Health Versus Private Profit* (Faringdon: Libri Publishing, 2013).
6   A prominent description of this transformation was that of Arnold S. Relman, "The New Medical-Industrial Complex," *New England Journal of Medicine* 303, no. 17 (1980), 963–70.
7   These developments around "healthcare capital" are discussed in a chapter of a book forthcoming at the time of writing: Adam Gaffney, David Himmelstein, and Steffie Woolhandler, "The Failure of Obamacare and a Revision of the Single- Payer Proposal After a Quarter Century of Struggle," in Howard Waitzkin (ed.), *Under the Knife: Beyond Capital in Health* (New York: Monthly Review Press, 2017).
8   As earlier noted, Flood and Gross count these two dynamics among many others as leading to the right to health movement. Colleen M. Flood and Aeyal M. Gross, "Introduction: Marrying Human Rights and Health Care Systems: Contexts for a Power to Improve Access and Equity," in *The Right to Health at the Public/Private Divide: A Global Comparative Study* (New York: Cambridge University Press, 2014), 2–4; Colleen M. Flood and Aeyal M. Gross, "Litigating the Right to Health: What Can We Learn from a Comparative Law and Health Care Systems Approach," *Health and Human Rights* 16, no. 2 (2014), 63–4.
9   Others have approached this question from a variety of perspectives. From a comparative perspective, see: Jacob S. Hacker, "The Historical Logic of National Health Insurance: Structure

and Sequence in the Development of British, Canadian, and U.S. Medical Policy," *Studies in American Political Development* 12, no. 01 (1998), 57–130. For good and brief discussions of the major categories of explanations from the US perspective see: Colin Gordon, *Dead on Arrival: The Politics of Health Care in Twentieth-Century America* (Princeton, NJ: Princeton University Press, 2005), especially pp. 1–8, and Jill S. Quadagno, *One Nation, Uninsured: Why the U.S. Has No National Health Insurance* (New York: Oxford University Press, 2005), 202–7.

10   It is also worth pointing to a study by Bambra that sought, along the lines of Esping-Andersen, to quantify the degree of decommodification of health systems, and which found that among 18 OECD nations, the United Kingdom, Canada, three Nordic nations, as well as New Zealand belonged to the most decommodified cluster. This study quantified decommodification using three metrics: the percentage of private health spending to GDP, the percentage of private hospitals beds to total beds, and the percentage of the nation covered by the public system. See: Clare Bambra, "Worlds of Welfare and the Health Care Discrepancy," *Social Policy and Society* 4, no. 01 (2005), 31–41. An important omission here seems to be the lack of a metric to describe out-of-pocket spending burden. Additionally, the degree to which hospital beds are private and public may be of less importance from the perspective of healthcare rights than other factors. For instance, in Canada, hospitals may be private, but universal health insurance entitles all individuals to free access to them. Bambra computes an index of health system decommodification in another study as well: Clare Bambra, "Cash Versus Services: 'Worlds of Welfare' and the Decommodification of Cash Benefits and Health Care Services," *Journal of Social Policy* 34, no. 02 (2005), 195–213.

11   Vicente Navarro, *The Politics of Health Policy: The US Reforms, 1980–1994* (Cambridge, MA: Blackwell, 1994), xii–xiii. See also: Vicente Navarro, "Why Some Countries Have National Health Insurance, Others Have National Health Services, and the United States Has Neither," *International Journal of Health Services* 19, no. 3 (1989), 383–404.

12   Gordon, *Dead on Arrival*, 8.

13   Ibid., 209.

14   Ibid., 92.

15   Upendra Baxi, "The Place of the Human Right to Health and Contemporary Approaches to Global Justice: Some Impertinent Interrogations," in *Global Health and Human Rights: Legal and Philosophical Perspectives*, ed. John Harrington and Maria Stuttaford (London: Routledge, 2010), 13.

16   I draw here on the argument of Howard Waitzkin, "Universal Health Coverage: The Strange Romance of the Lancet, MEDICC, and Cuba," *Social Medicine* 9, no. 2 (2015), 93–7.

17   Robert Pear and Thomas Kaplan, "G.O.P Plans to Replace Health Care Law with 'Universal Access'," *The New York Times*, December 15, 2016, accessed December 27, 2016, http://www.nytimes.com/2016/12/15/us/politics/paul-ryan-affordable-care-act-repeal.html?_r=0.

18   Bertrand Russell, *A Free Man's Worship* (Portland, ME: Thomas Bird Mosher, 1923), 26.

Index

228 · Index

neoliberalism 4, 132, 149, 152, 164–6, 168, 173–4, 185–6, 189, 193–5, 197, 199–200; and healthcare 170–5; and the right to health in law 178–81; and the right to health movement 175–8
Netherlands 189, 195–6
nevirapine 184–5
New Deal era 4, 95–9, 105, 124–5, 128, 149, 165; rights and healthcare in 99–104
New Liberalism 78–81
Newell, Kenneth 142–3
Nicaragua 118, 141, 144, 149–52, 165, 170–2
Nigeria 169
Nixon, Richard 140–1, 148–9, 151, 194–5, 198
nursing 121–2

Obama, Barack 195, 197–8, 215
Obamacare 200
Occupy movement 199
O'Connor, Feargus 58
Old Age Pensions Act (1909) 79–80
Origen 17

paganism 11
Paine, Thomas 42–3, 46–7, 106
patent protections 181–2. *See also* intellectual property
patient dumping 215
Patient Protection 195
payment for healthcare 25, 27, 62; in antiquity 10–13
Pennington, Kenneth 22
pensions 43, 74–5, 80, 83, 101
People's Budget (1909) 80
Perkins, Frances 101, 124
Petty, William 25
pharmaceutical industry 85, 177–8, 181–6, 188–9, 191–2, 217
philanthropy: and Christianity 17; *philanthropia* 9, 12, 16–18; *philoptôchos* 17
Physicians for Human Rights 177
Physicians Forum 128
Piketty, Thomas 199
Pinochet, Augusto 141, 170–1
Plague of Cyprian 17
plagues. *See* Black Death; epidemics; *individual plagues*
Plato 6–7
Plautus 9
Pliny the Elder 11
Poen, Monte M. 127
polio 151

political rights 24, 47, 134
Pollock, Allyson 196–7
poor, the: in antiquity 9–13; deserving 22, 39; in the French Revolution 39, 42–4, 46, 48; and health insurance 78, 87; in the Middle Ages 16–25, 27, 100; natural rights of 19–23; in the nineteenth century 53–5, 57–60, 64–6, 68; in the twentieth century 99–100, 106; undeserving 22
Poor Law Act (1601) 61
Poor Law Amendment Act (1834) 61
Poor Law Commission 57–8, 62
poor laws 22–3, 26, 53, 55–61, 74, 77–80, 82–3, 106, 119, 122, 146, 169
population growth 55
Portugal 197
post-colonialism 4
poverty. *See* poor, the; and health insurance 80
pre-existing conditions 198, 200
Price, David 197
primary healthcare 117
privatization of health systems 3, 164, 167, 171–2, 174, 186, 191–3, 196, 199–200
Progressive Party (US) 83
Prometheus 9
property 8, 19–21, 42, 47, 100–1. *See also* housing
protectionism 74
Provision of Meals Act (1906) 79
public health 54–9, 67, 96, 103, 152, 172, 186, 189
Public Health Act (1848) 61, 63, 68
public physicians 12–13

quality of healthcare 40–1. *See also* hospitals (conditions in)
quality of life 58

racial inequality 37, 88, 145–6, 148, 199, 218. *See also* Civil Rights movement; universal suffrage
Raynal, Abbé 38
Reagan, Ronald 149, 151, 166–7, 194
Red Scare 86–7, 126–8. *See also* McCarthyism
reforms. *See* health system reform
Reign of Terror 45–7
religion 41. *See also individual religions*
Renaissance 22
retirement 121. *See also* pensions
revolutions 48, 59, 63–4, 66; American Revolution 41–3, 48; French Revolution